Pediatric Rehabilitation

Editors

MARY MCMAHON
AMY HOUTROW

PEDIATRIC CLINICS OF NORTH AMERICA

www.pediatric.theclinics.com

Consulting Editor
TINA L. CHENG

June 2023 • Volume 70 • Number 3

ELSEVIER

1600 John F. Kennedy Boulevard • Suite 1800 • Philadelphia, Pennsylvania, 19103-2899

http://www.theclinics.com

THE PEDIATRIC CLINICS OF NORTH AMERICA Volume 70, Number 3
June 2023 ISSN 0031-3955, ISBN-13: 978-0-323-93905-8

Editor: Kerry Holland
Developmental Editor: Axell Ivan Jade M. Purificacion

The Pediatric Clinics of North America (ISSN 0031-3955) is published bimonthly by Elsevier Inc., 360 Park Avenue South, New York, NY 10010-1710. Months of issue are February, April, June, August, October, and December. Periodicals postage paid at New York, NY and additional mailing offices. Subscription prices are $279.00 per year (US individuals), $827.00 per year (US institutions), $351.00 per year (Canadian individuals), $1100.00 per year (Canadian institutions), $419.00 per year (international individuals), $1100.00 per year (international institutions), $100.00 per year (US students and residents), $100.00 per year (Canadian students and residents), and $165.00 per year (international residents and students). To receive students/resident rare, orders must be accompanied by name of affiliated institution, date of term, and the signature of program/residency coordinator on institution letterhead. Orders will be billed at individual rate until proof of status is received. Foreign air speed delivery is included in all *Clinics* subscription prices. All prices are subject to change without notice. **POSTMASTER:** Send address changes to *The Pediatric Clinics of North America*, Elsevier Health Sciences Division, Subscription Customer Service, 3251 Riverport Lane, Maryland Heights, MO 63043. **Customer Service: 1-800-654-2452 (US and Canada). From outside of the US and Canada: 1-314-447-8871. Fax: 1-314-447-8029. For print support, E-mail: JournalsCustomerService-usa@elsevier. com. For online support, E-mail: JournalsOnlineSupport-usa@elsevier.com.**

Reprints. For copies of 100 or more, of articles in this publication, please contact the Commercial Reprints Department, Elsevier Inc., 360 Park Avenue South, New York, NY 10010-1710. Tel.: 212-633-3874; Fax: 212-633-3820; E-mail: reprints@elsevier.com.

The Pediatric Clinics of North America is also published in Spanish by McGraw-Hill Inter-americana Editores S.A., Mexico City, Mexico; in Portuguese by Riechmann and Affonso Editores, Rua Comandante Coelho 1085, CEP 21250, Rio de Janeiro, Brazil; and in Greek by Althayia SA, Athens, Greece.

The Pediatric Clinics of North America is covered in *MEDLINE/PubMed (Index Medicus)*, *Excerpta Medica*, *Current Contents*, *Current Contents/Clinical Medicine*, *Science Citation Index*, *ASCA*, *ISI/BIOMED*, and *BIOSIS*.

PROGRAM OBJECTIVE
The goal of the *Pediatric Clinics of North America* is to keep practicing physicians and residents up to date with current clinical practice in pediatrics by providing timely articles reviewing the state-of-the-art in patient care.

TARGET AUDIENCE
All practicing pediatricians, physicians, and healthcare professionals who provide patient care to pediatric patients.

LEARNING OBJECTIVES
Upon completion of this activity, participants will be able to:
1. Review congenital and acquired spinal cord injury and dysfunction in children.
2. Discuss successful strategies for youth returning to educational settings post traumatic brain injury.
3. Recognize chronic pain in children and management.

ACCREDITATIONS
Physician Credit

The Elsevier Office of Continuing Medical Education (EOCME) is accredited by the Accreditation Council for Continuing Medical Education (ACCME) to provide continuing medical education for physicians.

The EOCME designates this journal-based activity for a maximum of 16 *AMA PRA Category 1 Credit*(s)™.-Physicians should claim only the credit commensurate with the extent of their participation in the activity.

All other healthcare professionals requesting continuing education credit for this journal-based activity will be issued a certificate of participation.

ABP Maintenance of Certification Credit

Successful completion of this CME activity, which includes participation in the activity and individual assessment of and feedback to the learner, enables the learner to earn up to 16 MOC points in the American Board of Pediatrics' (ABP) Maintenance of Certification (MOC) program. It is the CME activity provider's responsibility to submit learner completion information to ACCME for the purpose of granting ABP MOC credit.

DISCLOSURE OF CONFLICTS OF INTEREST
The EOCME assesses conflict of interest with its instructors, faculty, planners, and other individuals who are in a position to control the content of CME activities. All relevant conflicts of interest that are identified are thoroughly vetted by EOCME for fair balance, scientific objectivity, and patient care recommendations. EOCME is committed to providing its learners with CME activities that promote improvements or quality in healthcare and not a specific proprietary business or a commercial interest.

The planning committee, staff, authors, and editors listed below have identified no financial relationships or relationships to products or devices they or their spouse/life partner have with commercial interest related to the content of this CME activity:
David Baker, PsyD, ABPP-CN; Priya D. Bolikal, MD; Glendaliz Bosques, MD; Joline E. Brandenburg, MD; Caitlin Lee Chicoine, MD; Andrew B. Collins, MD; Loren T. Davidson, MD; Michael Dichiaro, MD; Sherilyn W. Driscoll, MD; Mary E. Dubon, MD; Maya C. Evans, MD; Angela Garcia, MD; Matthew T. Haas, MD; Kimberly C. Hartman, MD, MHPE; Lainie K. Holman, MD, MFA; Amy J. Houtrow, MD, PhD, MPH; Robyn A. Howarth, PhD; Jessica M. Jarvis, PhD; Lynette Jones, MSN, RN-BC; Sarah Lewis, DPT; Christopher D. Lunsford, MD; Rajkumar Mayakrishnan, BSc, MBA; Matthew J. McLaughlin, MD, MS; Mary P. McMahon, MD; Paola Mendoza-Sengco, MD; Kevin P. Murphy, MD; Marisa Osorio, DO; David W. Pruitt, MD; Marion Quirici, PhD; Amy E. Rabatin, MD; Sarah Rubin, MD, MsCl; Cristina Sanders, DO; Amit Sinha, MD, MBA; Sarah J. Tlustos, PhD, ABPP-CN; Stephanie Tow, MD; Raymond W. Tse, MD; Sathya Vadivelu, DO; Jilda Vargus-Adams, MD, MSc; Joshua A. Vova, MD

The planning committee, staff, authors, and editors listed below have identified financial relationships or relationships to products or devices they or their spouse/life partner have with commercial interest related to the content of this CME activity:
Phoebe Scott-Wyard, DO, FAAP, FAAPMR: Consultant: Hanger Clinic

UNAPPROVED/OFF-LABEL USE DISCLOSURE
The EOCME requires CME faculty to disclose to the participants:

1. When products or procedures being discussed are off-label, unlabelled, experimental, and/or investigational (not US Food and Drug Administration [FDA] approved); and
2. Any limitations on the information presented, such as data that are preliminary or that represent ongoing research, interim analyses, and/or unsupported opinions. Faculty may discuss information about pharmaceutical agents that is outside of FDA-approved labelling. This information is intended solely for CME and is not intended to promote off-label use of these medications. If you have any questions, contact the medical affairs department of the manufacturer for the most recent prescribing information.

TO ENROLL

To enroll in the *Pediatric Clinics of North America* Continuing Medical Education program, call customer service at 1-800-654-2452 or sign up online at http://www.theclinics.com/home/cme. The CME program is available to subscribers for an additional annual fee of USD 324.00.

METHOD OF PARTICIPATION

In order to claim credit, participants must complete the following:
1. Complete enrolment as indicated above.
2. Read the activity.
3. Complete the CME Test and Evaluation. Participants must achieve a score of 70% on the test. All CME Tests and Evaluations must be completed online.

In order to claim MOC points, participants must complete the following:
1. Complete steps listed above for claiming CME credit
2. Provide your specialty board ID#, birth date (MM/DD), and attestation.
3. Online MOC submission is only available for the American Board of pediatrics' (ABP) Maintenance of Certification (MOC) program

CME INQUIRIES/SPECIAL NEEDS

For all CME inquiries or special needs, please contact elsevierCME@elsevier.com

Contributors

CONSULTING EDITOR

TINA L. CHENG, MD, MPH
BK Rachford Professor and Chair of Pediatrics, University of Cincinnati, Director, Cincinnati Children's Research Foundation, Chief Medical Officer, Cincinnati Children's Hospital Medical Center, Cincinnati, Ohio

EDITORS

MARY McMAHON, MD
Professor of Physical Medicine and Rehabilitation and Pediatrics, Aaron W. Perlman Division Chief, Pediatric Rehabilitation Medicine, Department of Pediatrics, University of Cincinnati College of Medicine, Cincinnati, Ohio

AMY J. HOUTROW, MD, PhD, MPH
Endowed Professor of Physical Medicine and Rehabilitation and Pediatrics, Division of Pediatric Rehabilitation Medicine, Department of Physical Medicine and Rehabilitation, University of Pittsburgh, University of Pittsburgh School of Medicine, UPMC Children's Hospital of Pittsburgh, Pittsburgh, Pennsylvania

AUTHORS

DAVID BAKER, PsyD, ABPP-CN
Assistant Professor, Department of Rehabilitation, University of Colorado School of Medicine, Children's Hospital Colorado, Aurora, Colorado

PRIYA D. BOLIKAL, MD
Assistant Professor, Clinical Pediatrics and Clinical Neurology and Rehabilitation Medicine, University of Cincinnati College of Medicine, Cincinnati Children's Hospital Medical Center, Cincinnati, Ohio

GLENDALIZ BOSQUES, MD
Associate Professor, Department of Neurology, Chief of Pediatric Rehabilitation Medicine, Pediatric Neurosciences Program, Dell Medical School, The University of Texas at Austin, Dell Children's Medical Center, Austin, Texas

JOLINE E. BRANDENBURG, MD
Assistant Professor, Physical Medicine and Rehabilitation, Assistant Professor, Pediatrics, Chair, Division of Pediatric Rehabilitation Medicine, Departments of Physical Medicine and Rehabilitation, and Pediatric and Adolescent Medicine, Mayo Clinic, Rochester, Minnesota

ANDREW B. COLLINS, MD
Assistant Professor, Departments of Pediatrics, and Neurology and Rehabilitation Medicine, University of Cincinnati College of Medicine, Attending Physician, Divisions of

Pediatric Rehabilitation Medicine and Pediatric Pain Medicine, Cincinnati Children's Hospital Medical Center, Cincinnati, Ohio

LOREN T. DAVIDSON, MD
Clinical Professor, Physical Medicine and Rehabilitation, UC Davis Department of Physical Medicine and Rehabilitation, University of California, Davis, Shriners Children's Northern California, Sacramento, California

MICHAEL DICHIARO, MD
Associate Professor, Department of Rehabilitation, University of Colorado School of Medicine, Children's Hospital Colorado, Aurora, Colorado

SHERILYN W. DRISCOLL, MD
Associate Professor, Physical Medicine and Rehabilitation, Division of Pediatric Rehabilitation Medicine, Departments of Physical Medicine and Rehabilitation, and Pediatric and Adolescent Medicine, Mayo Clinic, Rochester, Minnesota

MARY E. DUBON, MD
Division of Pediatric Rehabilitation Medicine, Department of Physical Medicine and Rehabilitation, Spaulding Rehabilitation Hospital, Harvard Medical School, Department of Physical Medicine and Rehabilitation, Kelley Adaptive Sports Research Institute, Department of Sports Medicine, Boston Children's Hospital, Boston, Massachusetts

MAYA C. EVANS, MD
Associate Professor, Physical Medicine and Rehabilitation, UC Davis Department of Physical Medicine and Rehabilitation, University of California, Davis, Shriners Children's Northern California, Sacramento, California

ANGELA GARCIA, MD
Assistant Professor, Department of Physical Medicine and Rehabilitation, University of Pittsburgh, Attending Physician, UPMC Children's Hospital of Pittsburgh, Pittsburgh, Pennsylvania

MATTHEW T. HAAS, MD
Assistant Professor, Physical Medicine and Rehabilitation, Northwestern University Feinberg School of Medicine, Shirley Ryan AbilityLab, Chicago, Illinois

KIMBERLY C. HARTMAN, MD, MHPE
Children's Mercy Kansas City, University of Missouri-Kansas City School of Medicine, Department of Physical Medicine and Rehabilitation, University of Kansas School of Medicine, Kansas City, Missouri

LAINIE K. HOLMAN, MD, MFA
Associate Clinical Professor, Cleveland Clinic Lerner College of Medicine, Chair, Pediatric Rehabilitation, Cleveland Clinic Children's Hospital for Rehabilitation, Cleveland, Ohio

AMY J. HOUTROW, MD, PhD, MPH
Endowed Professor of Physical Medicine and Rehabilitation and Pediatrics, Division of Pediatric Rehabilitation Medicine, Department of Physical Medicine and Rehabilitation, University of Pittsburgh, University of Pittsburgh School of Medicine, UPMC Children's Hospital of Pittsburgh, Pittsburgh, Pennsylvania

ROBYN A. HOWARTH, PhD
Department of Physical Medicine and Rehabilitation, Children's Healthcare of Atlanta, Atlanta, Georgia

JESSICA M. JARVIS, PhD
Department of Physical Medicine and Rehabilitation, University of Pittsburgh, Pittsburgh, Pennsylvania

CAITLIN LEE CHICOINE, MD
Assistant Professor of Clinical Pediatrics, Division of Pediatric Rehabilitation Medicine, Cincinnati Children's Hospital Medical Center, University of Cincinnati College of Medicine, Cincinnati, Ohio

SARAH LEWIS, DPT
Rehabilitation Medicine, Seattle Children's Hospital, Seattle, Washington

CHRISTOPHER D. LUNSFORD, MD
Assistant Professor, Departments of Orthopaedics and Pediatrics, Duke University Health System, Durham, North Carolina

MATTHEW J. McLAUGHLIN, MD, MS
Children's Mercy Kansas City, University of Missouri- Kansas City School of Medicine, Department of Physical Medicine and Rehabilitation, University of Kansas School of Medicine, Kansas City, Missouri

PAOLA MENDOZA-SENGCO, MD
Assistant Professor of Clinical Pediatrics and Clinical Neurology and Rehabilitation Medicine, Division of Pediatric Rehabilitation Medicine, Cincinnati Children's Hospital Medical Center, University of Cincinnati College of Medicine, Cincinnati, Ohio

KEVIN P. MURPHY, MD
Pediatric Physiatrist, Medical Director, Pediatric Rehabilitation Services, Department of Physical Medicine and Rehabilitation, Sanford Health Systems, Bismarck North Dakota and Northern Minnesota, CEO and Medical Director, Northland Pediatric Rehabilitation Medicine LLC, Duluth, Minnesota

MARISA OSORIO, DO
Associate Professor, Department of Rehabilitation Medicine, University of Washington, Seattle Children's Hospital, Rehabilitation Medicine, Seattle, Washington

DAVID W. PRUITT, MD
Professor, Clinical Pediatrics and Clinical Neurology and Rehabilitation Medicine, University of Cincinnati College of Medicine, Cincinnati Children's Hospital Medical Center, Cincinnati, Ohio

MARION QUIRICI, PhD
Assistant Professor, Disability Studies and Global Anglophone Literature, Department of English, Kennesaw State University, Kennesaw, Georgia

AMY E. RABATIN, MD
Assistant Professor, Physical Medicine and Rehabilitation, Assistant Professor, Pediatrics, Pediatric Physiatrist, Division of Pediatric Rehabilitation Medicine, Departments of Physical Medicine and Rehabilitation, and Pediatric and Adolescent Medicine, Mayo Clinic, Rochester, Minnesota

SARAH RUBIN, MD, MSCI
Department of Critical Care Medicine, University of Pittsburgh, Pittsburgh, Pennsylvania

CRISTINA SANDERS, DO
Pediatric Physiatrist, Pediatric Rehabilitation Medicine, Monument Health Department of Neurology and Rehabilitation, Monument Health System, Rapid City, South Dakota

PHOEBE SCOTT-WYARD, DO, FAAP, FAAPMR
Associate Clinical Professor, Division of Pediatric Rehabilitation, Department of Orthopedics, Rady Children's Hospital, University of California, San Diego, San Diego, California

AMIT SINHA, MD, MBA
Department of Physical Medicine and Rehabilitation, University of Pittsburgh, Pittsburgh, Pennsylvania

SARAH J. TLUSTOS, PhD, ABPP-CN
Assistant Professor, Department of Rehabilitation, University of Colorado School of Medicine, Children's Hospital Colorado, Aurora, Colorado

STEPHANIE TOW, MD
US Paralympics Swimming, University of Colorado, Anschutz Medical Campus, Children's Hospital Colorado, Aurora, Colorado

RAYMOND W. TSE, MD
Associate Professor, Division of Plastic Surgery, Department of Surgery, University of Washington, Division of Craniofacial and Plastic Surgery, Department of Surgery, Seattle Children's Hospital, Seattle, Washington

SATHYA VADIVELU, DO
Children's Mercy Kansas City, University of Missouri- Kansas City School of Medicine, Department of Physical Medicine and Rehabilitation, University of Kansas School of Medicine, Kansas City, Missouri

JILDA VARGUS-ADAMS, MD, MSc
Professor of Clinical Pediatrics and Clinical Neurology and Rehabilitation Medicine, Division of Pediatric Rehabilitation Medicine, Cincinnati Children's Hospital Medical Center, University of Cincinnati College of Medicine, Cincinnati, Ohio

JOSHUA A. VOVA, MD
Department of Physical Medicine and Rehabilitation, Children's Healthcare of Atlanta, Atlanta, Georgia

Contents

Pediatric rehabilitation medicine (PRM) physicians are subspecialists in the field of physical medicine and rehabilitation trained to promote the health and function of children with disabilities (CWD) across their lifespans. Management strategies employed include prescribing medications, therapy, and adaptive equipment (braces and mobility devices) to optimize function and allow participation. PRM physicians collaborate with other providers to mitigate the negative consequences of health conditions and injuries. Their work is interdisciplinary because CWD with either temporary or permanent impairments needs treatments, services, and support that extend beyond the clinical environment. Owing to this, PRM physicians are essential members of the health neighborhood for CWD.

Early identification of cerebral palsy (CP) facilitates optimal care, support, and outcomes for children and their families. Ideally, infants with risk factors or developmental deviations should be evaluated early using standardized assessments of neurodevelopment and brain imaging. If a diagnosis of CP or high risk for CP (HRCP) is established, specialized, evidence-informed therapy and family support should be initiated. With task-specific motor skill training and an enriched environment, infants with CP show greater gross motor and cognitive gains. These enhanced outcomes are only achievable with early diagnosis and subsequent intervention.

Over two-thirds of pediatric critical illness survivors will experience functional impairments that persist after discharge, that is, post–intensive care syndrome in pediatrics (PICS-p). Risk factors include child and family characteristics, invasive procedures, and social determinants of health. Approaches to remediate PICS-p include early rehabilitation, minimizing sedation, psychosocial resources for caregivers, delivery of family-centered care, and longitudinal screening for PICS-p. Challenges include

mechanism of SCI/D has dramatic implications for function and risk of co-morbidities throughout the lifespan. Optimal care of children with SCI/D is multidisciplinary and the pediatrician is a very important member of this team. This review highlights functional prognosis and important health maintenance issues to prevent complications and maximize independence. It is intended to assist the pediatrician in the care of this unique patient population.

Spasticity results from an abnormality of the central nervous system and is characterized by a velocity-dependent increase in muscle tone or stiffness. In children, it can cause functional impairments, delays in achieving developmental or motor milestones, participation restrictions, discomfort, and musculoskeletal differences. Unique to children is the ongoing process of a maturing central nervous system and body, which can create the appearance of worsening or changing spasticity. Treatment options include physical interventions such as stretching, serial casting, and bracing; oral and injectable medications; and neurosurgical procedures such as selective dorsal rhizotomy and intrathecal baclofen pump.

Care for pediatric cancer survivors must include scheduled, thorough evaluations of potential chronic and late effects resulting from multidimensional cancer treatments. Assessment of functional independence with activities and participation is critical in assuring that survivors can optimally access their environments and pursue educational, occupational, and leisure activities appropriate to their interests and capabilities. Owing to their expertise in both rehabilitation and habilitation, pediatric physiatrists are of great benefit in the care of survivors of pediatric cancer.

Neonatal brachial plexus palsies (NBPP) occur in 1.74 per 1000 live births with 20% to 30% having persistent deficits. Dysfunction can range from mild to severe and is correlated with the number of nerves involved and the degree of injury. In addition, there are several comorbidities and musculoskeletal sequelae that directly impact the overall functional development. This review addresses the nonsurgical and surgical management options and provides guidance for pediatricians on monitoring and when to refer for specialty care.

Owing to the lack of trained professionals in amputee care, the pediatrician is often required to assist in the care of children with limb deficiencies. An overview of the causes and epidemiology of limb deficiency is provided, as well as an evaluation and diagnostic workup. Important considerations for surgical interventions are discussed and an introduction to prosthetic prescribing and care of the amputee is described. Common overuse syndromes and mental health issues are also reviewed. Finally, resources for funding of prosthetic devices, as well as support and education for clinicians and families are provided.

Back pain is common, in up to 30% of children, increasing with age. Eighty percent is benign, mechanical type, improving within 2 weeks of conservative care. Required for those not improving is in-depth evaluation, including MRI, laboratory, and peer consultations. Spondylolysis and spondylolisthesis comprise almost 10% of pediatric back pain, often caused by lumbar hyperextension activities and treated conservatively in most cases. Osteoid osteomas and osteoblastomas constitute the most common benign spinal tumors in childhood. Aggressive and malignant tumors of the spine are rare but when present require tertiary care referral and a comprehensive oncology team for optimal life-sustaining outcomes.

Chronic pain in children is a relatively prevalent cause of functional disability. Contributing factors to this pain are best viewed through the biopsychosocial model. Although evidence is lacking for individual aspects of treatment, interdisciplinary care is considered the best treatment approach for children with chronic pain. Interdisciplinary care can include medication management with daily and as-needed medications, physical and occupational therapy focusing on function and movement, and psychological treatment with cognitive-behavioral therapy and acceptance focused treatment. In children with severe pain and disability, intensive interdisciplinary pain treatment may be needed to improve pain and function.

Functional neurologic disorders are common in the pediatric population. Recently, there has been a renewed focus on functional neurologic disorders, leading to improvements in diagnosis and management. This review focuses on updates in clinical presentation, diagnosis, pathophysiology (including neuroimaging), and treatment of functional neurologic disorders in the pediatric population.

Approximately 25% of children in the United States participate in appropriate amounts of physical activity. That percentage is even lower for children with disabilities. Adaptive sports and physical activity opportunities are increasing in the United States. Health care providers are encouraged to discuss physical activity in the clinical setting and to help to promote physical activity for all individuals, including children with disabilities.

Christopher D. Lunsford and Marion Quirici

The negative impact of ableism on healthcare, and the health of people with disabilities, can be mitigated by recognizing and addressing anti-disability bias. However, ableism is not yet being addressed as a threat to health in the same manner as other societal inequities. This article provides a primer on ableism and disability justice, through the lens of critical disability studies, as well as actionable recommendations on anti-ableist language etiquette and clinical best practices. With the knowledge of disability justice and anti-ableism, pediatricians can ensure that every child with a disability has the best chance to thrive.

PEDIATRIC CLINICS OF NORTH AMERICA

SERIES OF RELATED INTEREST

Physical Medicine and Rehabilitation Clinics
www.pmr.theclinics.com

THE CLINICS ARE AVAILABLE ONLINE!
Access your subscription at:
www.theclinics.com

Foreword

Pediatric Rehabilitation Medicine: It's Go Time

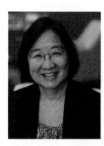

Tina L. Cheng, MD, MPH
Consulting Editor

Physical Medicine and Rehabilitation (PM&R), also called physiatry, has been practiced for centuries. Historically, patients with disabilities were treated with light, thermotherapy, manipulation, massage, instrumentation, movement, and other modalities.[1] In ancient China, movement was thought to promote health. Believing in the afterlife, Egyptians crafted devices for mummies. Canes were discovered in the tomb of Tutankhamun, confirming that the pharaoh suffered from clubfoot.[1]

PM&R's development in the United States was tied to wars. Prosthetics were developed for survivors of amputations in the Civil War in the mid to late 1800s, and later, wars reemphasized the importance of the field. It was not until the early twentieth century that PM&R was recognized by the medical establishment and organized medicine. The American College of Radiology and Physiotherapy, later the American Congress of Rehabilitation Medicine, was founded in 1923 (100-year birthday!). Members included radiologists, physical therapy physicians (the term for physiatrists at that time), and physiotherapists. Physical therapy physicians later promoted physical medicine as a medical specialty, and the American Society of Physical Therapy Physicians, the organization that became the American Academy of Physical Medicine and Rehabilitation, was founded in 1938.

In 1941, the United States entered the Second World War, where PM&R was an essential specialty. The AMA established the Section on PM&R in 1945, and the American Board of Physical Medicine became incorporated in 1947.

Like other areas of medicine, focus on the unique needs of children developed later. The polio epidemic in the mid twentieth century contributed to the recognition of the need for pediatric-focused PM&R.[2] The American Board of Pediatric Rehabilitation Medicine (ABPMR) offers subspecialty certification in Pediatric Rehabilitation Medicine (PRM) in order to enhance the quality of care available to individuals with pediatric rehabilitation needs and their families. Subspecialty certification in PRM by the ABPMR began in 2003. Accreditation of Pediatric Rehabilitation training programs as a subspecialty of PM&R also began in the early 2000s.

PM&R focuses on multidisciplinary interventions and medications with the goal of restoration of a person's function after injury or illness. PRM addresses the prevention, diagnosis, treatment, and management of congenital and childhood-onset physical impairments, including related or secondary medical, physical, functional, psychosocial, cognitive, and vocational limitations or conditions, with an understanding of the life course of disability.

Medical and public health advancements have changed the epidemiology of health conditions among children. There has been a steady rise of chronic health conditions among infants, children, and youth,[3] requiring focus on the care models provided by Pediatric Rehabilitation Medicine. To address the needs of children, adolescents, and families, the field must grow so that every child's abilities are optimized, promoted, valued, and celebrated.

Tina L. Cheng, MD, MPH
University of Cincinnati
Cincinnati Children's Hospital Medical Center
3333 Burnet Avenue MLC 3016
Cincinnati, OH 45229-3026, USA

E-mail address:
Tina.cheng@cchmc.org

REFERENCES

1. Arabi H. Physical medicine and rehabilitation: from the birth of a specialty to its recognition. Cureus 2021;13(9):e17664. https://doi.org/10.7759/cureus.17664. PMID: 34650846; PMCID: PMC8489541.
2. Alexander M, Turk MA, Ayyangar R. Dr Jessie Wright: breaking new ground in pediatric physical medicine and rehabilitation. PM R 2013;5(9):739–46. https://doi.org/10.1016/j.pmrj.2013.07.006.
3. Perrin JM, Anderson LE, Van Cleave J. The rise in chronic conditions among infants, children, and youth can be met with continued health system innovations. Health Aff (Millwood) 2014;33(12):2099–105. https://doi.org/10.1377/hlthaff.2014.0832. PMID: 25489027.

Preface

Focus on Functioning: The Field of Pediatric Rehabilitation Medicine

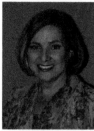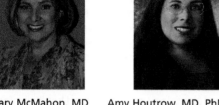

Mary McMahon, MD   Amy Houtrow, MD, PhD, MPH
Editors

We are honored to be invited to edit the first issue of *Pediatric Clinics of North America* dedicated to the field of Pediatric Rehabilitation Medicine (PRM). PRM is one of the youngest pediatric subspecialities, and many pediatricians have not yet had an opportunity to collaborate with members of our field. We hope this historic issue will provide valuable insights as to how PRM can partner with pediatricians to improve the function and lives of children with disabilities and their families in our care.

Rehabilitation Medicine, also known as Physiatry or Physical Medicine and Rehabilitation (PM&R), was founded the 1940s and was well established by the 1970s. The field aims to enhance or restore functional ability and improve the quality of life for individuals living with a disability, whether that disability is likely temporary or permanent. This is often accomplished in the setting of multidisciplinary teams. Early on, the field of PM&R was focused on the care of adult patients, but recognition soon followed that children's lives are also significantly impacted by medical conditions or traumatic events that result in impairments amenable to rehabilitation interventions.

Early pioneers in the field of PRM advocated for formal training and recognition for the specialty of PRM, and the first certification exam was offered in 2003. Although the number of training programs for PRM has increased dramatically in the past decade, the number of certified physicians is still quite small, presently at 376. At the same time, the number of children living with disability is growing, thanks to advances in acute care medicine and survivorship. This is resulting in a lack of access to rehabilitation care and a growing concern for health inequities. The field of PRM is actively considering opportunities to increase the number of certified physicians through increasing medical student's and resident's awareness of the specialty and broadening access to training programs. Increasing pediatricians' understanding

Pediatr Clin N Am 70 (2023) xvii–xix
https://doi.org/10.1016/j.pcl.2023.02.001
0031-3955/23/© 2023 Published by Elsevier Inc.

pediatric.theclinics.com

and knowledge of the impact of impairment and disability on the lives of their patients and the value of rehabilitation medicine is another opportunity to decrease health disparities for this population of children often multiply marginalized in society. Our hope is this first issue of *Pediatric Clinics of North America* dedicated to PRM will serve an important contribution toward this goal.

Another major aim of this issue is for pediatricians to gain insight into the breadth of our field and awareness as to when seeking out consultations and collaborations with PRM physicians would be helpful for their patients. We wish to express that this issue provides a small sampling of the very broad field of PRM. The topics were chosen for their timeliness and application to a large range and number of patients as well as as a means of demonstrating the scope of the field. The specialty of PM&R is often viewed as a field of medicine that is most helpful toward the back end of the continuum of care. We hope this issue highlights the important contributions we can make in the acute setting, including the pediatric intensive care unit. We also hope to feature some of the unique approaches and perspectives that our field brings and how we can serve as strong collaborators with a broad range of medical and surgical specialties, such as Developmental and Behavioral Pediatrics, Neurodevelopmental Disabilities, Orthopedics, Neurosurgery, and Neurology as well as allied health professionals. Each specialty brings a distinctive approach to the evaluation and management of children with disabilities, and only by working together can we provide the best possible outcomes. Our field strives to be a champion for the importance of interdisciplinary care across the spectrum of care, from the hospital to communities. We look forward to the day when PRM has a considerable presence at all children's hospitals, and its importance will be viewed comparably to all other pediatric specialties, because children with disabilities, like all other children, deserve the highest-quality health care to help them thrive and grow.

As we look toward the future, we recognize the increasing value of team-based collaborative care that is focused on outcomes important to children and their families, such as optimizing function in daily life. As medical care advances, the population of children and young adults with disabilities will continue to grow. More people will be living with the sequelae of chronic disease, whether it is from long-COVID, congenital heart disease, or rare genetic conditions. Furthermore, we recognize the importance of addressing health disparities and attending to the underlying causes of health disparities (poverty, discrimination, and their downstream impacts). Because children with disabilities are more likely to be poor and from minoritized backgrounds, and are discriminated based on their disabilities, the field of PRM seeks to advocate for children with disabilities to have a fair and just opportunity to be healthy and live their lives to the fullest.

We are humbled and grateful to serve as the editors for this first issue of *Pediatric Clinics of North America* with a focus on PRM and the opportunity to increase the understanding and awareness of our field in pediatrics. We owe immense gratitude to the early pioneers in PRM, whose compassion and commitment for children living with disabilities led to the creation of this field of medicine. We would like to thank all the contributing authors for their time and expertise in creating this issue. We enjoyed the opportunity to collaborate and interact with some of the leading experts in PRM. These contributors continue to be pioneers of our young field. They are creating and growing PRM clinical and training programs around the country, advancing the science of our field, and they serve as an inspiration to us. We would like to sincerely thank Tina Cheng, Editor for the *Pediatric Clinics of North America*, for inviting the field of PRM for its first issue in this important and historic publication. Last, we express our genuine gratitude to Axell Ivan Jade M. Purificacion and the publishing staff of *Pediatric Clinics of North America* for their patience and help with this issue.

Mary McMahon, MD
Pediatric Rehabilitation Medicine
Cincinnati Children's Hospital Medical Center
University of Cincinnati College of Medicine
Cincinnati, OH, USA

Amy Houtrow, MD, PhD, MPH
University of Pittsburgh School of Medicine
Pittsburgh, PA, USA

E-mail addresses:
mary.mcmahon@cchmc.org (M. McMahon)
houtrow@upmc.edu (A. Houtrow)

Pediatric Rehabilitation Medicine Physicians

Your Essential Medical Home Neighbors for Children with Disabilities

Glendaliz Bosques, MD[a],*, Amy J. Houtrow, MD, PhD, MPH[b],
Lainie K. Holman, MD, MFA[c]

KEYWORDS

- Children • Disability • Rehabilitation • Physiatry • Neighborhood health • Advocacy
- Medical home

KEY POINTS

- Pediatric rehabilitation medicine (PRM) physicians are subspecialists who are trained and dedicated to promoting the health, functioning, and well-being of children with disabilities across their life span.
- The role of the PRM physician is to minimize the impacts of impairments and to optimize a child's ability to do activities and participate in life events regardless of existing health conditions and associated impairments.
- PRM physicians serve as the leaders of an interdisciplinary and interprofessional team to maximize the child's development and function, by managing chronic impairments, ameliorating complications, and optimizing access and participation.

INTRODUCTION

Childhood-onset disabilities have been present since the beginning of time. Survivorship, inclusion, and the management and care for individuals with childhood-onset disabilities have progressed and transformed through time (**Fig. 1**). The modernization of medicine has allowed us to expand our management of medical conditions leading

[a] Department of Neurology, Pediatric Neurosciences Program, Dell Medical School at The University of Texas at Austin, Dell Children's Medical Center, 4910 Mueller Boulevard Suite 300, Austin, TX 78723, USA; [b] Department of Physical Medicine & Rehabilitation, University of Pittsburgh, UPMC Children's Hospital of Pittsburgh, 4401 Penn Avenue, Pittsburgh, PA 15224, USA; [c] Cleveland Clinic Lerner College of Medicine, Pediatric Rehabilitation, Cleveland Clinic Children's Hospital for Rehabilitation, 2801 Martin Luther King Jr Drive, Cleveland, OH 44104, USA
* Corresponding author.
E-mail address: Glendaliz.Bosques@austin.utexas.edu

Pediatr Clin N Am 70 (2023) 371–384
https://doi.org/10.1016/j.pcl.2023.01.001
0031-3955/23/© 2023 Elsevier Inc. All rights reserved.

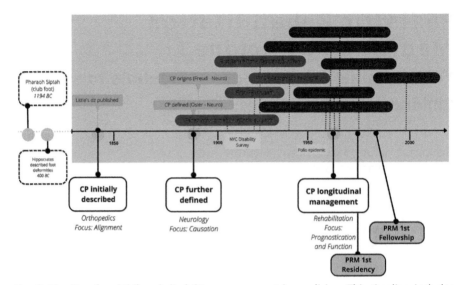

Fig. 1. Timeline for childhood disability management in medicine. This timeline includes how the care of CP, the most common disability in children, transformed in the last century. Interest in the longitudinal management of this and other childhood-onset disabilities resulted in the origins of PRM as a subspecialty.

to a steady increase in childhood-onset disabilities in the past decades. Pediatric rehabilitation medicine (PRM) physicians are important members of the health neighborhood for the care of children with temporary or permanent disabilities. PRM physicians diagnose medical conditions; assess associated impairments, activity limitations, and participation restrictions; devise and implement treatment plans; recommend strategies to optimize functioning such as through the management of disease, prescribing adaptive equipment, and advocating for accommodations; lead rehabilitation teams focused on full participation in society; and collaborate with health and community providers to assure that children with disabilities have the opportunity to thrive.

Rehabilitation: The New Kid on the Pediatrics Block

The pioneers of the PRM field have been advocating since the 1950s, illuminating the importance of understanding and identifying the needs of children with disabilities and the functional impact of health/medical conditions (see **Fig. 1**) Dr Harriett Gillette, one of those pioneers, reported that children with disabilities required (1) means of communication, (2) ability to care for self, (3) education, (4) security, (5) love and recognition, (6) ability to move.[1] These early PRM physicians who cared for children with disabilities, including children with cerebral palsy (CP) and spina bifida; made significant contributions to CP prognostication, orthosis use, and understanding of child development; and paved the pathway for the field of PRM.[1–4] As pediatricians they saw that this population required additional care beyond primary medical management. This interest made them pursue additional training and experience in the budding field of rehabilitation. In the beginning, there were no formal training pathways; the only option was for pediatricians to pursue a second residency in physical medicine and rehabilitation (PM&R). The first combined pediatrics and PM&R residency and PRM department were founded at the University of California in 1982 by Dr Gabriella Molnar.[5] The 5-year combined training program allowed for graduates to obtain board certification in both pediatrics and PM&R. The number of these combined training programs grew relatively quickly and peaked in the 1990s, but the programs struggled to fill their positions and programs began to slowly decline in number. Around this same time, the field successfully advocated for the American Board of Medical Specialties to approve a subspeciality certification in PRM. The Accreditation Council for Graduate Medical Education (ACGME) approved program requirements for accreditation of fellowship training in PRM in 2002 and in 2003 the American Board of Physical Medicine and Rehabilitation (ABPMR) offered the first PRM certification examination. Presently, there are two training pathways that would allow one to sit for the PRM subspeciality examination (**Fig. 2**). There are a growing number of accredited fellowship training programs and a small number of triple board programs (allowing graduates to qualify for pediatric, PM&R, and PRM subspecialty certification).

Pediatric Rehabilitation Medicine Physician Role in Disability Management

The role of the PRM physician is to minimize the impact of impairments and to optimize a child's ability to engage in activities and participate in life events regardless of existing health conditions and associated impairments. The PRM physician integrates the biopsychosocial model in their practice. This framework for approaching and managing children with disabilities follows the International Classification of Functioning, Health and Disabilities (ICF), as proposed by the World Health Organization (WHO). The ICF frames disability as an umbrella term for impairments at the level of the body structure or system, activity restrictions at the level of the person, and

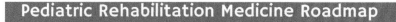

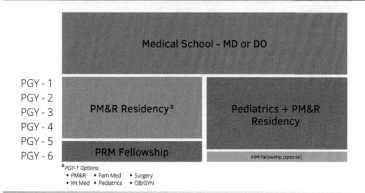

Fig. 2. PRM physician training roadmap. After completing medical or osteopathic school (4 years), additional training is obtained to subspecialize in PRM. Physicians may complete a triple board residency in pediatrics and PM&R (5 years) with an optional additional year for a clinical research fellowship, or they may complete a residency in PM&R (4 years) and a PRM fellowship (2 years; combined training of 6 years). After completing training, specialists are board eligible for PM&R, Pediatrics (if they completed triple board residency program), and the PRM subspeciality certificate. Despite PRM's origin within pediatrics, there is currently not a pathway for physicians who are not trained in PM&R to be trained or certified in PRM. This has sparked debate within the field, given the tremendous need for PRM providers.

participation restrictions at the level of the person in society.[6] (**Fig. 3** *for an example of how this framework is used for a child with CP.*) Disability is understood to be influenced not only by one's medical diagnoses but also by environmental and personal factors that can hinder or facilitate functioning.[6] Rosenbaum and colleagues[7] presents this approach as the "F-words" in childhood disability: (1) function, (2) family, (3) fitness, (4) fun, (5) friends, and (6) future (**Fig. 4**).

PRM physicians bring all these, from fun to function, together. Aside from history taking and a physical examination, PRM physicians are trained to diagnose (using laboratory studies, imaging, and electrodiagnostics), treat, and direct a rehabilitation plan that provides the best possible outcome for patients. In addition, they employ therapeutic exercise to treat disorders that produce pain, impairment, and disability. The focus is to develop a comprehensive program where the patient as a whole—body and environment—are addressed.

According to the latest report from 2021 US Census data, the percentage of children with a disability continues to increase.[9] PRM physicians serve a variety of medical conditions that result in childhood-onset disabilities (**Table 1**). Medical conditions may be congenital or acquired and include disorders of the brain, spinal cord, peripheral nerves, and neuromuscular conditions, among others. Children without chronic disabilities may also have episodic care needs with sports injuries or other issues that affect function temporarily.

Primary care pediatricians, as the nexus of the medical home, are responsible for specialty referrals and care coordination.[10,11] The surrounding community of health care providers that serve individuals whose needs exceed the capacity of the medical home can be considered health neighbors.[12] This includes PRM physicians, who are

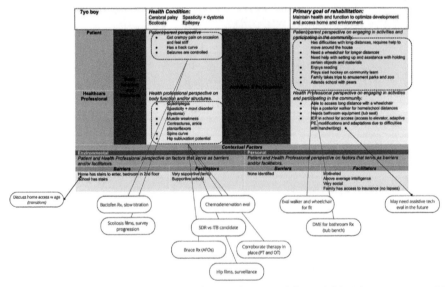

Fig. 3. Example of PRM management within ICF framework for a child with CP. A 7-year-old boy with CP was referred to PRM physician for rehabilitation needs and tone management. After history taking and physical examination, the PRM physician proposes a plan of care, which will include anticipatory guidance, rehabilitation interventions, equipment, devices (including braces, if needed), and medical or pharmacological interventions. Columns indicate ICF framework for assessing the patient. Bubbles a PRM physician's proposed recommendations.

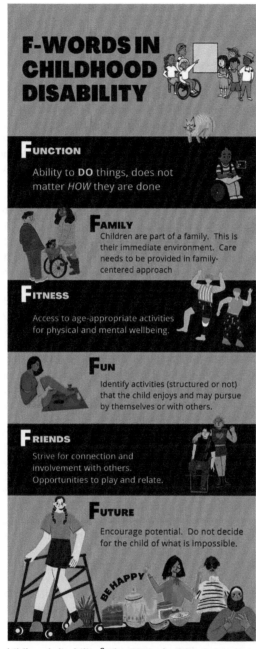

Fig. 4. F-words in childhood disability.[8] The PRM physician integrates the biopsychosocial model into their practice. Rosenbaum and colleagues reconceptualized the ICF framework into the F-words of childhood disability. PRM physicians recommend rehabilitation interventions that assist in developing capacity, performance, and FUNCTION. Care is provided in a FAMILY and patient-centered approach within the context of personal factors (family). By identifying specialized equipment, devices, environmental modifications, and accommodations to improve access to participating in desired activities, PRM physicians tackle FITNESS,

particularly valuable health neighbors for children with disabilities. An important aspect of the health neighborhood is communication between providers, an understanding of each provider's role, and collaboration toward optimal outcomes.[12] In addition to medical providers, the health neighborhood often includes nonmedical community providers as well, such as those from schools and social service organizations.[13]

As a member of the health neighborhood, the PRM physician plays a crucial role in the care of children with congenital and acquired disabilities. The PRM physician focuses on functional goal-setting and attainment through collaborating with therapists and clinicians in neurology, neurosurgery, orthopedic surgery, developmental pediatrics, psychiatry, psychology, and others. This unique attention to the functional abilities of a child connects traditional diagnosis and treatment to real-world access and ability at home, at school, and at avocation.

Settings in Which Pediatric Rehabilitation Medicine Services Are provided

Inpatient services (consults and inpatient rehabilitation programs)

PRM physicians are mainly located within academic centers, with the majority offering services in hospital-based inpatient services or clinics.[14] In the inpatient setting, PRM physicians fulfill multiple roles in the continuum of care (**Fig. 5**). Initial rehabilitation care is ideally in the framework of early consultation and comanagement in acute care settings (**Table 2**). This can take the form of early mobilization, dysautonomia management, skin protection, bowel and bladder management, and initial education regarding traumatic injuries or acute illness.[15] Early consultation in the acute setting facilitates a longitudinal relationship with children and families, making the transition to the post-acute rehabilitation phase more streamlined and informed. Once acute medical problems stabilize, more focused therapies can begin in the hospital setting, ideally with recommendations from the PRM physician and communication with the primary service, with an eye toward disposition to home or to an inpatient rehabilitation program (IPR) for more intensive therapies.

The PRM physician is best suited for conversations around the functional prognosis and the typical trajectory of recovery from various injuries and illnesses. It is vital to help families navigate the unfamiliar landscape they are encountering. For the vast majority of families confronted with acute illness and injury, it is also their first significant encounter with the medical system, and certainly with parenting a child with disabilities. As an expert in the post-acute setting (after the acute care hospitalization), the PRM physician recommends the optimal rehabilitation setting and interventions. Further, the PRM physician can engage with the parents as they embark on the journey of recovery to set realistic goals.

Generally, a patient is appropriate for transfer to a comprehensive IPR program after acute medical problems are stabilized, and if there are functional changes that will benefit from intensive, high-frequency rehabilitative interventions. The PRM physician serves as the leader of this interdisciplinary and interprofessional team to maximize the child's return to a level of function that is compatible with a safe discharge to home and the community (**Fig. 6**). Typically, IPR will require more than one therapy discipline's focus (eg, physical therapy [PT] for mobility, endurance, and/or strengthening;

FUN, and FRIENDS. All interventions and recommendations are provided to maintain health, access experiences, and unlock the potential of each child with a disability to prepare them for the FUTURE.

Table 1
Medical conditions for which pediatric rehabilitation medicine physicians can be good neighbors

	Congenital	Acquired
Brain/cerebellum	Cerebral palsy Genetic disorders (hereditary spastic paraparesis, Frederich's ataxia, etc.) Perinatal infections Perinatal stroke Migration deformities (schizencephaly, septo-optic dysplasia, Dandy–Walker variant, etc.) Developmental disorders	Traumatic brain injuries Strokes (including anoxic brain injuries) Encephalitis (infectious or inflammatory; ie. anti-NMDA, ADEM) Multiple sclerosis (and other autoimmune disorders) Tumors Functional neurological disorders
Spinal cord	Spina bifida and other neural tube defects Spinal muscular atrophy	Traumatic spinal cord injuries Transverse myelitis, acute flaccid myelitis, and other inflammatory or autoimmune myelopathies Strokes Infectious myelitis Tumors
Peripheral nerve	Brachial plexus palsy Hereditary polyneuropathies (Charcot-Marie-Tooth, etc.)	Guillain-Barré syndrome AIDP, CIDP Traumatic nerve injuries
Muscular and skeletal (MSK)	Myopathies Muscular dystrophies Arthrogryposis and other congenital contractures Limb differences	Polytrauma Idiopathic toe walking Limb loss/amputation MSK presentation of genetic conditions (ie, trisomy 21) Rheumatological condition Tumors Sports injuries Chronic pain

occupational therapy [OT] for activities of daily living, visuospatial deficits, or upper limb function; and/or speech-therapy [SLP] for language, communication, cognition, oromotor skills, swallowing, and feeding). Patients requiring an IPR level of care must be able to tolerate at least 3 h of therapies per day, 5 days per week (see **Fig. 5**). Owing to the intensity of this type of rehabilitation, the patients should be recommended for this level of care and then medically cleared before admission by a PRM physician. The comprehensive IPR team consists of the aforementioned disciplines (PT, OT, and SLP) in addition to psychology, social work, recreational therapy, music therapy, child life specialist, nutrition, education, care coordination, and often organized support groups for family members. The IPR team can also help families access various resources for financial support and advocacy.

School reentry coordination and communication are an integral part of this transition, given that a patient's function—even after some recovery—may still require accommodations and modifications to optimize academic success.[16] Both educators and peers should be included in understanding the individual's new level of function to ensure a supportive and engaged reentry. In some settings, a school liaison is available to facilitate communication with the school and ensure appropriate goal-setting and support in the academic setting.

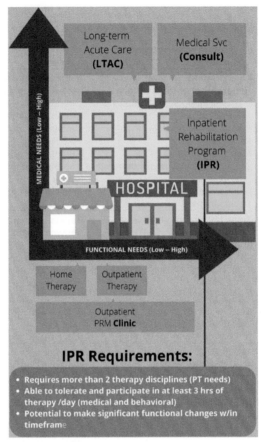

Fig. 5. PRM physicians and post-acute levels of care. PRM physicians are leaders in the interdisciplinary and interprofessional rehabilitation team of patients. They are experts in identifying the optimal level of care and setting for rehabilitation interventions.

Outpatient clinics and programs

In the outpatient setting, most PRM physicians will have a continuity rehabilitation clinic to longitudinally follow patients with childhood-onset conditions. Given that many conditions benefit greatly from collaborative, multidisciplinary same-point care, pediatric physiatrists (PRM physicians) often direct or participate in interdisciplinary clinics. Examples of patient populations that are often cared for in this setting include: spina bifida, CP, neuromuscular disorders (ie, muscular dystrophy), acquired brain injury, childhood cancer, limb difference/amputee, arthrogryposis, among many others.

In these outpatient settings, the PRM physician is the expert in evaluating and prescribing equipment to improve access and function in the community, overseeing therapeutic goals, ensuring interventions progress and effectiveness, and in making sure that the school is providing the least restrictive environment for learning. PRM physicians are skilled in tone and spasticity management and can also recommend pharmacological management, including chemodenervation (botulinum toxin injections), neurolysis (alcohol injections), evaluation and management of intrathecal baclofen pumps, and candidacy for surgical interventions.

Table 2		
Early consultation considerations		
PRM Early Consultation		
Trauma	• Initial GCS < 13	Reasons:
	• Closed head injury requiring OR management	• Impaired cognition
	• Open head injuries (including penetrating trauma)	• Changes in swallowing function/ feeding
	• Spinal cord injury	• New weakness or paralysis
	• Obvious paralysis	• Mobility changes
	• Limb loss (aka amputation) ± compartment syndrome	• Changes in tone, spasticity
	• Extensive burns	• Autonomic dysfunction or dysregulation
	• Polytrauma (>2 limb fractures; >7dd in PICU)	• Decline in function or skills (even if chronic disability)
Neuro	• Functional neurological disorder	
	• Stroke, AVM/hemorrhages	
	• ADEM, anti-NMDA encephalitis and others	
	• Transverse myelitis, AFM	
	• Guillain–Barré syndrome	
	• Tumors (brain or spine)	

Children's custom equipment must be frequently evaluated for growth and functional change. It is subject to the specific documentation for medical necessity, coverage, and reimbursement that does not generally apply to adults. For example, a prescribed custom wheelchair frame should last a child five years, during periods of rapid growth, and intellectual and psycho-social development.[17] Wheelchairs and other equipment require ongoing evaluation and maintenance, and the PRM physician is best situated to assist with technology updates and changes. Although personal durable medical equipment (DME) is often covered by insurance, the infrastructure supporting it (ramps, vehicles, home modifications) are not, and are generally expensive, therefore best coordinated with knowledgeable guidance.

Telemedicine (virtual)
In an era of emerging technology, PRM physicians are also able to provide increased access via telehealth for patients with mobility challenges. There remains work to be done in this area to facilitate video/remote access for patients who have limitations in hearing, verbal communication, and vision, but telehealth holds promise for patients who have difficulty accessing care.[18]

Transitions (beyond pediatric settings)
As children with congenital or genetic conditions are living longer and often with better quality of life, another crucial role for the PRM physician is managing the transition of adolescents with disabilities to not only adult clinicians but to a greater level of independence -something their peers without disabilities are able to access with relative ease. Indeed, there are potential safety risks if this transition is not managed with care. A young adult with a disability, especially with communication or cognitive challenges, can easily find themselves in an acute situation where their set of medical issues is poorly understood. As for all young people transitioning, youth with disabilities should be encouraged to develop self-direction and autonomy. Supported decision-making may be needed for some youth with disabilities

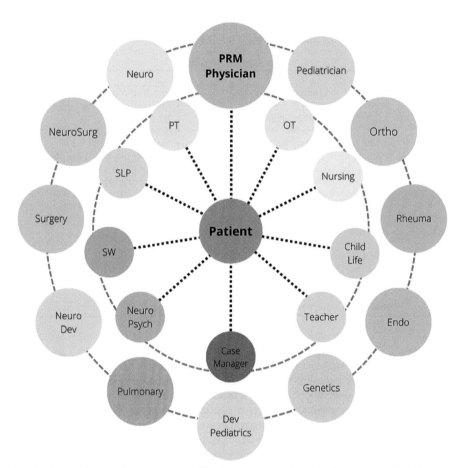

Fig. 6. Comprehensive inpatient rehabilitation team members. Each patient's rehabilitation team composition may look different. The PRM physician provides management through an interdisciplinary and interprofessional framework, centered on the patient's and the family's goals.

and occasionally guardianship is necessary. PRM physicians can help the family navigate the legal options so that youth with disabilities are supported in the least restrictive fashion.

In addition, the transition to adulthood requires the consultation of new subspecialties (women's health, cancer screenings, immunizations, etc.). Here again, the rehabilitation team is best positioned to aid in the transition to adulthood. Unique considerations include college choice and access, vocational skills assessment and placement, needs surrounding guardianship and financial security, health insurance stability, housing, transportation, safety, and reproductive health and sexuality education. In many regions, this transition to adult clinicians is not readily available, and the former children must be cared for by pediatric clinicians who then must consider the unique needs of adults. In addition, many physicians may not feel comfortable treating patients with disabilities or may be unaware of how to provide accessible care.[19] PRM physicians can help ease the transition by providing a warm hand-off or may stay involved as the individual's physiatrist well into adulthood. Further PRM physicians serve as strong advocates for advancing the system of care to assure people with disabilities do not face health care discrimination.

Educational transitions are often stressful for youth with disabilities and their families, so special attention to this transition is often a key focus of PRM physician's activities when youth age out of public education system. As good health neighbors, the PRM physician can work with the school on the transition plan and engage vocational rehabilitation supports as appropriate. Although economic self-sufficiency might not be feasible or even a goal, supporting youth with disabilities to engage in activities that are meaningful for them can help foster fulfillment. Similarly, during the transition years, the PRM physician can help develop strategies for an independent living if desired by the youth with disabilities.

Pediatric Rehabilitation Medicine Role in the Community (Advocacy)

Children's health is the extent to which children are "able or enabled to (a) develop and realize their potential; (b) satisfy their needs; and (c) develop the capacities that allow them to interact successfully with their biological, physical, and social environments."[20,21] PRM physicians understand childhood disability as an environmentally contextualized health-related limitation in a child's existing or emergent capacity to perform developmentally appropriate activities and participate, as desired in society.[22]

It is well recognized that children with disabilities face a multitude of barriers to fully participate in life events and realize their full health potential. PRM physicians work to help address these barriers by taking an anti-ableist approach that emphasizes that all children are worthy of the opportunity to be as healthy and functional as possible and engage in lives that bring them fulfillment and joy. Advocacy is often a less visible but important role of the PRM physician. Advocacy can be conducted on behalf of one particular child, such as advocating for inclusive educational services, or for a group of children, such as advocating for policies that help ensure children with disabilities can access the supports and services they need. As a good neighbor to the medical home, the PRM physician can offer their expertise in optimizing medical management and community resources to support functioning. For example, advocacy conducted during the coronavirus disease-2019 pandemic by PRM physicians included ensuring that individualized educational plans (IEPs) were carried out appropriately, promoting guidelines to lower the risk of severe acute respiratory syndrome coronavirus 2 infection, pivoting to telehealth, and working with vendors to ensure that children with disabilities received needed equipment and supplies.[20,22–25]

Pediatric Rehabilitation Medicine Role in Medical Education and Research

Because PRM physicians mostly practice in academic medical centers, they are often heavily involved in teaching medical students, residents, and fellows, as well as health professionals from other disciplines, such as speech and language pathology, PT, and OT. Providing medical education regarding disabilities to clinicians-in-training is one mechanism to reduce health care discrimination. From an innovation perspective, the research PRM physicians conduct spans preclinical to the health care system. PRM physicians often participate in multidisciplinary research as coinvestigators or principal investigators for studies that focus on functional outcomes.

SUMMARY

As the population of children with disability grows, the need for PRM physicians is growing.[26] As of the last report in 2021, there are 348 certified PRM physicians in the nation leaving many children with lack of access to rehabilitation medicine.[27–29] To ensure health equity (ie, a fair and just opportunity to be as healthy as possible),[30] children with disabilities need access to high-quality care that helps them thrive. PRM physicians, as members of the health neighborhood, provide important health services focused on optimizing function and helping children with disabilities participate in their homes and communities as desired.

CLINICS CARE POINTS

- The pediatric rehabilitation medicine (PRM) physician integrates the biopsychosocial model in their practice. This framework for approaching and managing children with disabilities follows the International Classification of Functioning, Health and Disabilities, as proposed by the World Health Organization in the care of chronic medical problems and conditions.

- Initial rehabilitation care is ideally in the framework of early consultation and comanagement in acute care settings. This can take the form of early mobilization, dysautonomia management, skin protection, bowel and bladder management, and initial education regarding traumatic injuries or acute illness.

- PRM physicians are well versed in evaluating and prescribing medical devices, durable medical equipment, orthoses, and prostheses. Children without chronic disabilities may also have episodic care needs with sports injuries or complications that may affect function.

- To ensure health equity, children with disabilities need access to high-quality care that helps them thrive, which should include PRM physicians as an essential part of their health neighborhood.

REFERENCES

1. Gillette HE. Rehabilitation of the crippled child. J Med Assoc Ga 1950;39(8): 332–5.
2. Molnar GE, Gordon SU. Cerebral palsy: predictive value of selected clinical signs for early prognostication of motor function. Arch Phys Med Rehabil 1976;57(4): 153–8.
3. Gillette HE. Systems of therapy in cerebral palsy. Springfield, IL: Charles C. Thomas Ltd; 1969.
4. Badell-Ribera A, Swinyard CA, Greenspan L, et al. Spina bifida with myelomeningocele: evaluation of rehabilitation potential. Arch Phys Med Rehabil 1964;45: 343–4.
5. Murphy KP, Gabriella E. Molnar MD: grandmother of pediatric rehabilitation medicine. J Pediatr Rehabil Med 2022;15(1):249–51. https://doi.org/10.3233/prm-220009.
6. World Health Organization (WHO). International classification of functioning, disability and health: ICF. 2001. Available at: http://apps.who.int/iris/bitstream/handle/10665/42407/9241545429.pdf;jsessionid=FC469AEA887C64AF68F30E4 7574AA9F2?sequence=1. Accessed July 14, 2019.
7. Rosenbaum P, Gorter JW. The 'F-words' in childhood disability: I swear this is how we should think! Child Care Health Dev 2012;38(4):457–63.
8. Camden C, Kay D, Rosenbaum P, et al. The F-Words in childhood disability: a values statement for children, families and service providers. Ann Phys Rehabil Med 2014;57:e345.

9. US Census Bureau. Childhood Disability in the United States: 2019. Available at: https://www.census.gov/library/publications/2021/acs/acsbr-006.html. Accessed June 4, 2022.

10. Cooley WC. Redefining primary pediatric care for children with special health care needs: the primary care medical home. Curr Opin Pediatr 2004;16(6): 689–92.

11. Cooley WC, McAllister JW. Building medical homes: improvement strategies in primary care for children with special health care needs. Pediatrics 2004;113(5 Suppl):1499–506.

12. Greenberg JO, Barnett ML, Spinks MA, et al. The "medical neighborhood": integrating primary and specialty care for ambulatory patients. JAMA Intern Med 2014;174(3):454–7.

13. Garg A, Sandel M, Dworkin PH, et al. From medical home to health neighborhood: transforming the medical home into a community-based health neighborhood. J Pediatr 2012;160(4):535–6.e1.

14. Houtrow AJ, Pruitt DW, Zigler CK. Gender-based salary inequities among pediatric rehabilitation medicine physicians in the United States. Arch Phys Med Rehabil 2020;101(5):741–9.

15. Foster K, Branco RG. Bringing pediatric rehabilitation to the intensive care*. Pediatr Crit Care Med 2019;20(6):586–7.

16. Carney J, Porter P. School reentry for children with acquired central nervous systems injuries. Dev Disabil Res Rev. 2009;15(2):152–8.

17. RESNA Position on the Application of Power Wheelchairs for Pediatric Users. 2008. Available at: http://www.rstce.pitt.edu/RSTCE_Resources/Resna_position_on_Peds_wheelchair_Users.pdf. Accessed August 24, 2022.

18. Hsu N, Monasterio E, Rolin O. Telehealth in pediatric rehabilitation. Phys Med Rehabil Clin N Am 2021;32(2):307–17.

19. Lagu T, Haywood C, Reimold K, et al. "I Am Not The Doctor For You": Physicians' Attitudes About Caring For People With Disabilities. Health Aff 2022;41(10): 1387–95.

20. Sholas MG, Apkon SD, Houtrow AJ. Children with disabilities must be more than an afterthought in school reopening. JAMA Pediatr 2021;175(4):423–4.

21. Stein REK. Children's health, the nation's wealth: assessing and improving child health. Ambul Pediatr 2005;5(3):131–3.

22. Beardsley J, Houtrow A, Verduzco-Gutierrez M. Letter to the Editor on "Disrupted access to therapies and impact on well-being during the COVID-19 pandemic for children with motor impairment and their caregivers.". Am J Phys Med Rehabil 2021;100(11):1033.

23. Levin-Decanini T, Henderson C, Mistry S, et al. Decreased access to therapeutic services for children with disabilities during COVID-19 stay-at-home orders in Western Pennsylvania. J Pediatr Rehabil Med 2022. https://doi.org/10.3233/PRM-200799.

24. Brandenburg JE, Holman LK, Apkon SD, et al. School reopening during COVID-19 pandemic: considering students with disabilities. J Pediatr Rehabil Med 2020; 13(3):425–31.

25. Houtrow A, Harris D, Molinero A, et al. Children with disabilities in the United States and the COVID-19 pandemic. J Pediatr Rehabil Med 2020;13(3):415–24.

26. Houtrow AJ, Pruitt DW. Meeting the growing need for pediatric rehabilitation medicine physicians. Arch Phys Med Rehabil 2016;97(4):501–6.

27. ABPMR - 2019 Pediatric Rehabilitation Medicine Examination Results. Available at: https://www.abpmr.org/NewsCenter/Detail/examination-results-certification-prm-2019. Accessed June 4, 2022.
28. ABPMR - 2020 Pediatric Rehabilitation Medicine Examination Results. Available at: https://www.abpmr.org/NewsCenter/Detail/2020-prm-exam-results. Accessed June 4, 2022.
29. ABPMR - 2021 pediatric rehabilitation examination results. Available at: https://www.abpmr.org/NewsCenter/Detail/prm-exam-2021. Accessed June 4, 2022.
30. Houtrow A, Martin AJ, Harris D, et al. Health equity for children and youth with special health care needs: a vision for the future. Pediatrics 2022;149(Suppl 7). https://doi.org/10.1542/peds.2021-056150F.

Early Cerebral Palsy Detection and Intervention

Paola Mendoza-Sengco, MD*, Caitlin Lee Chicoine, MD,
Jilda Vargus-Adams, MD, MSc

KEYWORDS

- CP • Cerebral palsy • Early detection • Early intervention • High risk for CP

KEY POINTS

- Cerebral palsy (CP) is the most common physical disability of childhood.
- Using standardized guidelines, CP can be accurately diagnosed in infants younger than 6 months of age.
- If a diagnosis of CP or high risk for CP is established, specialized, evidence-informed therapy and family support should be initiated.

INTRODUCTION AND BACKGROUND

Cerebral palsy (CP) is defined as a nonprogressive motor disorder with impaired movement or posture that is the result of an injury or anomaly of the developing brain (generally occurring before the age of 3 years). Although CP must result in activity limitation, it is an umbrella diagnosis and includes a wide range of impairments, severities, and comorbidities. Affecting 1 in 312 school-aged children in the United States, CP is the most common physical disability of childhood.[1]

CP can result from any situation that can affect the fetal or infant brain including malformations, infection, trauma, or hypoxia/ischemia from any cause. Prematurity is the most common risk factor for CP due to the increased likelihood of impaired cerebral perfusion accompanying hemodynamic instability, bleeding, or other insults.[2,3] Multiple gestation, small for gestational age, maternal illness, birth asphyxia, and neonatal seizures are other risk factors.[2,3]

The motor disabilities of CP can range from movement disorders (particularly spasticity and dystonia) to weakness to impaired motor control and balance. Frequently, children with CP experience all of these challenges, albeit to varying degrees.

Division of Pediatric Rehabilitation Medicine, Cincinnati Children's Hospital Medical Center, University of Cincinnati College of Medicine, 3333 Burnet Avenue, MLC 4009, Cincinnati, OH 45229-3026, USA
* Corresponding author. Cincinnati Children's Pediatric Rehabilitation Medicine, 3333 Burnet Avenue, MLC 4009, Cincinnati, Ohio 45229.
E-mail address: PaolaMaria.Mendoza-Sengco@cchmc.org

Pediatr Clin N Am 70 (2023) 385–398
https://doi.org/10.1016/j.pcl.2023.01.014
0031-3955/23/© 2023 Elsevier Inc. All rights reserved.
pediatric.theclinics.com

Because CP can result from any number of underlying brain insults, genetic conditions, or other etiologies, the range of associated comorbidities and complications is large. Among the more common issues for children with CP are epilepsy, intellectual disability, pain, and limited mobility. Hip and spine issues, behavior disorders, incontinence, and sleep problems also impact a significant minority of children with CP. Children with more significant gross motor impairments (especially those who rely upon wheelchairs for mobility) are more likely to also have significant impairments with fine motor skills, self-care, communication, and feeding.

This article discusses risk factors and early presentation of CP in young infants along with the recommended algorithm that can aid early and accurate diagnosis and in turn help initiate timely CP-specific treatment and surveillance for complications.

DISCUSSION
Importance of Early Detection of Cerebral Palsy

Early identification of children with CP is key to maximizing outcomes for children and families. Primarily, early detection facilitates early intervention and support for children with CP and their caregivers, which is believed to improve outcomes and reduce stressors and complications.[3] Although the evidence is still developing on this front, it is reasonable to argue that the benefits must outweigh the risks because the risks of early intervention are very small.

The process of diagnosis and information sharing for parents should occur as early as possible because it helps families to learn about their child's condition as soon as they can. When parents are not provided with an early diagnosis, their mental health suffers with more reported stress and depression.[4,5] Parents of children with CP prefer to learn early about their child's CP and to take advantage of opportunities to seek skilled intervention.[4–6] With early diagnosis, families benefit from the knowledge they gain, the capacity to take action to help their child, and early, ongoing support from care team members and other parents.[6]

Once a diagnosis is established, early intervention with evidence-informed therapy is indicated. It is important to intervene early because the neonatal and infant nervous system is highly sensitive to inputs and stimulation.[7] To maximize neurodevelopment and particularly to address plasticity in nerves and other tissues, infants with CP should be engaged in activities that stimulate their motor cortex. Without the appropriate inputs of active movement generation and interaction with the environment around them, infant brain development is likely to be circumscribed.[8] Early diagnosis means that therapy and home programming can commence at a younger age and be more effective in facilitating brain refinement and the development of motor skills.[3] These activities may also foster cognitive development and the growth of musculoskeletal tissues.[8]

An additional goal of early diagnosis is an early entry into surveillance and comprehensive care. When an infant is diagnosed with CP, they should begin to receive services from an integrated, interdisciplinary, CP-specific care team. This means that their medical management will include timely assessments and evaluations for comorbidities such as hip displacement, decreased bone mineral density, and learning problems, among others. Comprehensive care results in lower rates of orthopedic complications.[9] Engagement with such a care team also affords children and families the opportunity to learn about and access the most effective treatment options. When children with CP are not diagnosed early, their engagement with a CP-specific care team can be delayed by years, resulting in missed opportunities for interventions and support leading to worse outcomes.[3,10]

Table 1			
Historical risk factors for cerebral palsy[2]			
Preconception	**Prenatal**	**Perinatal**	**Postnatal**
• History of stillbirth or miscarriage	• Genetic abnormality	• Prematurity	• Stroke
• Chromosomal abnormality	• Multiple gestation	• Intrapartum hypoxicischemic event	• Accidental or nonaccidental brain injury before age 2 years
• Assisted reproduction technology	• Male sex	• Neonatal encephalopathy or seizures	• Surgical complications
• Low socioeconomic income status	• Congenital anomalies	• Infection, such as meningitis	• Infection, such as meningitis
• Maternal chronic illness	• Intrauterine growth restriction	• Jaundice	
	• Infection, such as chorioamnionitis	• hypoglycemia	
	• Maternal substance abuse		

Elements of early diagnosis of cerebral palsy

CP is a clinical diagnosis made based on a combination of historical risk factors, examination, and imaging findings.

Risk Factors

History is the first key component in evaluating an infant for CP. This should include a discussion about any movement or tone abnormalities observed by the family, a review of the infant's developmental milestones, and an assessment of known risk factors for CP. Several risk factors have been identified in the preconception, prenatal, perinatal, and postnatal periods (**Table 1**). Although prematurity is the greatest risk factor for the development of CP[2] most children with CP were not born prematurely.

Infants with CP may show delays and deviations in motor development even in the neonatal period. Red flags for CP include any abnormalities in the neurologic examination, including persistent head lag or hand fisting past 4 months of age or stiffness/spasticity, as well as asymmetries, including early hand preferences before 18 months, or delays in achieving motor milestones like sitting by 9 months of age or inability to weight bear through the plantar surface of feet.[3] Parents may report early standing postures (worrisome for lower extremity spasticity), early handedness (worrisome for contralateral impairment), or unusual floor mobility (such as bunny-hopping rather than creeping) without recognizing these findings as concerns. Any and all such findings should prompt careful evaluation.

Clinical Neurologic Examination

A diagnosis of CP requires the identification of motor dysfunction on neurologic examination. The Hammersmith Infant Neurological Examination (HINE) is a standardized examination for children between 3 and 24 months of age that has predictive value in the early detection of CP.[11] The global score can range from 0 to 78, and cutoff scores for age have been identified that indicate risk for abnormal neuromotor development. Asymmetries between the right and left sides are also noted.

Neuroimaging

Neuroimaging is a standard component of the evaluation for CP. MRI of the brain is preferred to identify parenchymal abnormalities that affect motor function.[12] Such abnormalities can support, but are not themselves sufficient for, a diagnosis of CP.

Normal imaging also does not preclude the diagnosis of CP, provided that clinical criteria are met.[3]

The most predictive patterns of injury are[1] as follows:

- White matter injury, such as periventricular leukomalacia
- Cortical and deep gray matter lesions, such as basal ganglia lesions, multicystic encephalomalacia, or stroke
- Brain malformation, such as lissencephaly, polymicrogyria, or schizencephaly

Subtle white matter lesions may not be apparent during infancy due to incomplete myelination and plasticity. In these cases, repeat MRI at age two may be beneficial to further characterize the underlying etiology of a clinical presentation consistent with CP. Examples of abnormal brain MRI findings in children with CP are shown in **Fig. 1**.

Standardized Motor Assessments

In addition to the standardized infant neurologic examination provided by the HINE, several other standardized assessments can be used in the early diagnosis of CP, including:

- Prechtl's General Movement Assessment (GMA)[13]
- Test of Infant Motor Performance (TIMP)[14]
- Developmental Assessment of Young Children (DAYC)[15]
- Alberta Infant Motor Scale (AIMS)[14,16]
- Motor Assessment of Infants (MAI)[17]
- Neuro Sensory Motor Development Assessment (NSMDA)[16]

Scores on the HINE and the above motor assessments should not be interpreted in isolation. Diagnostic accuracy is increased when findings from imaging, infant neurologic examination, and motor assessment are interpreted collectively.[12]

Algorithm for early diagnosis of cerebral palsy

Evidence-based algorithms for early diagnosis of CP have been established, using different standardized assessments in combination with neurologic examination and brain imaging. Visit the QR code in **Fig. 2** for a summary of this approach to diagnosis. When the diagnosis of CP is suspected but uncertain, an interim diagnosis of "high risk for cerebral palsy" (HRCP) can be used.[3] It is valuable to make note of the specific concern for CP to ensure the infant receives appropriate, CP-specific therapy interventions as well as surveillance for potential comorbidities..

Before 5 months of corrected age, the most useful tools for early diagnosis of CP are the GMA, HINE, and brain MRI.[3] A retrospective study showed that the sensitivity and specificity for a diagnosis of CP were 95% and 97% for absent fidgety movements on GMA, 88% and 62% for HINE global score less than 57 at 3 months, and 79% and 99% for abnormal neuroimaging.[12] When these three assessments were viewed together, their combined sensitivity and specificity for a diagnosis of CP improved to 97.86% and 99.22%.[12,18]

After 5 months of corrected age, the most predictive elements for CP diagnosis are the HINE, DAYC, and brain MRI.[3,12,18] Abnormal HINE and DAYC have been reported as 90% and 89% predictive, respectively, of a diagnosis of CP.[3,12,18]

Early assessments can provide prognostic information for families regarding the severity of their child's condition. HINE global scores below 50 suggest likely bilateral CP, whereas higher global scores (50 to 73) or significant asymmetries (more than 5) indicate likely unilateral CP.[3,12,19] Global scores under 40 indicated a low likelihood of independent ambulation without an assistive device.[3,12] In addition, some MRI

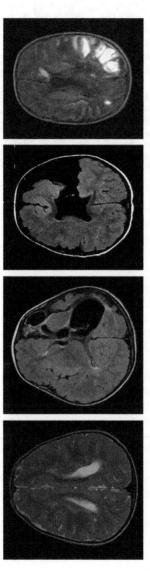

Fig. 1. Brain MRI findings in CP. From left to right: (1) periventricular leukomalacia in a child with spastic diplegia; (2) left cystic encephalomalacia resulting from early ischemic insult in a child with right spastic hemiplegia; (3) left open lip schizencephaly causing right spastic hemiplegia; and (4) severe hypoxic ischemic injury with cortical laminar necrosis in a child with spastic quadriplegic CP.

Fig. 2. QR code for algorithm for early diagnosis of CP or high risk for CP.

findings (such as grade IV intraventricular hemorrhage with parenchymal involvement, significant brain malformation, global hypoxic-ischemic injury, or basal ganglia injury) may portend a diagnosis of nonambulatory CP.[3]

Differential diagnosis of cerebral palsy

CP is a broad umbrella diagnosis that is made clinically and encompasses a wide range of static injuries or anomalies to the developing brain resulting in motor dysfunction. However, it is appropriate to maintain a differential diagnosis when performing an early assessment for CP, as not all disorders causing motor concerns in infancy and early childhood will fall underneath this umbrella. Although children with CP commonly present with developmental delays, not all children with delayed development (such as those with early autism or intellectual disability) meet the criteria for a diagnosis of CP. Progressive neurologic conditions, such as leukodystrophies or mutations in methyl CpG-binding protein 2 (MECP2)-related disorders like Rett syndrome, can mimic the CP phenotype in early childhood before significant regression is observed. Unilateral weakness related to brachial plexus palsy may be mistaken for hemiparetic CP. Neuromuscular conditions, such as spinal muscular atrophy or congenital muscular dystrophies, can cause motor dysfunction in young children but arise from pathology in the muscle or peripheral nervous system rather than the brain and therefore do not qualify as CP; this group of disorders should especially be considered when motor dysfunction is accompanied by hypotonia.

Cerebral palsy-specific early intervention

Targeted interventions for infants with CP or HRCP fall under three general themes: (1) skills development, (2) complications prevention, and (3) parental support.

Skills Development
Motor. Once a diagnosis of CP or HRCP has been established, immediate referral to home-based and/or ambulatory-based therapies to start a diagnosis-specific motor intervention is recommended. Commencing motor interventions during this critical period of neural development optimizes motor and cognitive outcomes in these infants and avoids maladaptive brain plasticity.[8] CP-specific motor interventions differ from

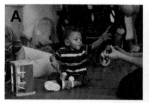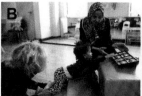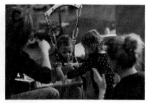

Fig. 3. (A–C) Examples of CP-specific early intervention activities. (*From* Cincinnati Children's Hospital Medical Center Perlman Center Specialty Program, with permission.)

generic early intervention with basic principles of (1) facilitating infant self-initiated active movements rather than just passive stretching or massage, (2) setting up the play environment to create an enriched experience, and (3) scaffolding developmental skills to promote progress.[8] Although the distribution of limb involvement may evolve in the early years due to neuroplasticity and development, it is important to delineate unilateral versus bilateral involvement in these infants at the time of diagnosis as treatment interventions, long-term outcomes, and complications differ.[3]

Goals, Activity, and Motor Enrichment (GAME) is a home-based intensive therapy approach that has been found to be beneficial for infants with unilateral or bilateral involvement.[20] This intensive intervention utilizes motor learning principles that are goal-oriented and activity-based with an emphasis on coaching parents on creating an enriched play environment that would facilitate practicing motor tasks and progression of skills. Randomized controlled trials showed that this intervention resulted in advanced motor and cognitive outcomes in participants at 12 months when compared with standard care[20] Examples of CP-specific activity-based early intervention therapy with social engagement are depicted in **Fig. 3**.

For children with unilateral CP, traditional upper extremity intensive therapy adopts a bimanual (BIM) approach to improve the use of the impaired hand as an assist in play or functional activities. On the contrary, constraint-induced movement therapy (CIMT) uses a unimanual approach wherein the uninvolved arm is constrained in a glove, cast, or mitt to encourage forced use and improved function of the weak arm. There are various protocols incorporating different duration and frequency of this intervention as well as the type of constraint used. It has been shown to be effective in improving hand function in infants with unilateral CP or HRCP compared with massage.[21] Trials (ie, REACH and APPLES) are ongoing to investigate its superiority over BIM.[22,23] An infant with CP undergoing CIMT is pictured in **Fig. 4**.

The task of reciprocal stepping is theorized to be controlled by primitive central pattern generators in the spinal cord activated by the brainstem and basal ganglia.[24] Repetitive activation of this automatic reciprocal mechanism eventually leads to the interplay of higher brain centers which in turn translates to an improvement of voluntary control of walking skills following neurologic injury.[24] Partial body-weight-supported treadmill training (BWSTT), as depicted in **Fig. 5**, is one method used in neurologic rehabilitation in adults with stroke and children with CP that facilitates motor learning of reciprocal walking through multiple repetitions and active participation with the effect of gravity reduced or minimized.[25] Commercial BWSTT systems are available in different sizes and can be placed over any treadmill. Although BWSTT appears to be a feasible and safe intervention for infants and toddlers with CP, additional research is needed to determine its efficacy in this age group.[25]

Cognition. Strong evidence supports the efficacy of incorporating environmental enrichment, multiple sensory modalities, family engagement, and adaptive technology

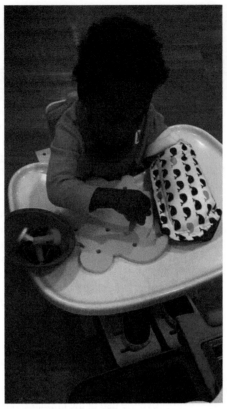

Fig. 4. Infant with right hemiplegic CP undergoing constraint-induced movement therapy. (*From* Cincinnati Children's Hospital Medical Center Perlman Center Specialty Program, with permission.)

in task-specific activities wherein an infant's self-generated movements produce a desired consequence.[26] This strategy facilitates active learning which, in turn, correlates with long-term positive cognitive outcomes.[26] Conditional evidence argues against the use of generic developmental education that focuses on passive movement, patterning, and/or reflex integration.[26]

Communication. Fifty percent of children with CP may experience difficulties with reciprocal verbal expression and up to 32% are nonverbal.[27] Lack of verbal skills at 2 years old correlates with poor communication outcomes at 4 years old for children with CP.[27] Although young infants with CP or HRCP are nonverbal, their capacity for socialization and communication can be fostered with face-to-face talk, singing, using emotions when communicating, using baby talk, and teaching parents to read their babies' micro-expressions. In children who are nonverbal but show emerging verbal skills, parent-child transaction therapy such as the Hanen method ("It Takes Two to Talk") promotes reciprocal communication and expressive language skills.[28]

Feeding. Infants with CP or HRCP are at risk for malnutrition and adverse outcomes when they experience impaired oromotor skills impacting diet progression, safety in swallowing, and efficacy in feeding.[29,30] Some preliminary evidence supports use of

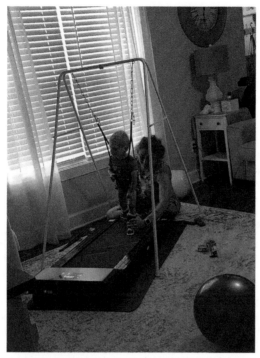

Fig. 5. Infant with bilateral CP undergoing home bodyweight-supported treadmill training. With permission from Aissia Hughes.

softer food consistencies and proper upright positioning.[29,30] There is insufficient evidence for neuromuscular stimulation and oral sensorimotor training. In infants and children with aspiration, use of gastrostomy tube may be the only viable means to support adequate nutrition.[30,31] One in 15 children with CP will require gastrostomy tube feeding.[32]

COMMON COMORBIDITIES
Epilepsy

One in four children with CP will have epilepsy[32] for which standard antiepileptic pharmacologic management is recommended.

Visual Impairment

One in 10 children with CP will have a visual impairment[32] that could negatively impact their mobility, and the way they access their environment and learn. There is conditional evidence to support early surgical correction of strabismus[33] and visual training with use of color contrast cues for cortical visual impairment.[34]

Sleep Disorders

Twenty percent of children with CP will suffer from sleep disorders[32] that not only negatively impact their quality of life but the well-being of their families as well. Evidence supports the early implementation of positive sleep hygiene practices, controlled crying and comforting, gradual extinction, and consideration of melatonin for sleep initiation difficulties.[35–37] Sleep positioning systems and acupuncture are not recommended.[36] A referral to sleep clinic for sleep apnea management may be indicated. If sleep is interrupted by pain from muscle spasms, enteral antispasmodics, and botulinum toxin injections can be considered.[38]

Hypertonia

There is limited evidence on pharmacologic management of hypertonia for children with CP under 2 years old.[39] However, when hypertonia threatens comfort, positioning, caregiving, skin and joint integrity, or progression of motor skills, medication management with enteral antispasmodics and botulinum toxin injections may be beneficial and is considered standard of care for infants and children with CP in high income countries.[39] Documentation of a standardized assessment for tone as well as a discussion of risks and benefits helps inform decisions and monitor treatment response. Ideally, hypertonia treatment would be coupled with stretching and/or motor intervention to maximize benefits.

Musculoskeletal Sequelae

Children with hypertonic CP, especially if non-ambulatory, are at increased risk for preventable joint malalignment and hip dislocation. Use of ankle braces or orthotics can help mitigate development of contractures and promote early weightbearing and walking skills.[40] The timing of orthosis introduction to achieve a balance of joint support and promoting mobility remains variable and controversial. One in three children with CP will experience hip displacement.[32] Anteroposterior pelvic radiographs every 6 to 12 months beginning at 12 months of age is recommended in accordance with surveillance guidelines.[9,41] Establishing a standing program by using a stander or walker when developmentally appropriate can also help prevent hip subluxation in infants with limited weightbearing abilities.[42]

Comprehensive Interdisciplinary Care Model

Because CP is a lifelong condition with varying severity and co-morbidities, infants with this condition deserve individualized yet comprehensive care.[10] Infants with known prenatal or newborn risk factors could benefit from early referrals to pediatric neurologists or pediatric rehabilitation physicians even while still admitted in neonatal intensive care units (NICU). These specialists can reinforce early diagnosis, manage tone abnormalities, optimize development, prescribe appropriate orthotics and equipment. Some infants without prenatal or newborn detectible risk factors may later be diagnosed in early detection clinics staffed by pediatric neurologists, developmental pediatricians and/or pediatric rehabilitation physicians.[43–45] Long-term needs are ideally followed by an interdisciplinary CP team. Although various care models exist, a common theme is the placement of families at the center of goal-setting and shared decision-making surrounding prevention, treatment and care coordination that impact the child's function and participation.[10,46]

Caregiver Support

Parents and caregivers of infants with CP or HRCP may experience inadvertent trauma, anxiety, and even depression brought on by a new diagnosis and or perceived burden of care.[4,5,47,48] Parental coaching on infant bonding, facilitating their child's developmental progress by carryover of therapy activities and exercises in an enriched home environment, and emotional support can lead to healthy adjustment and engagement and long-term favorable functional outcomes in their child and family unit.[4,49] Support from a skilled care coordinator can help families more readily access community and financial resources.

SUMMARY

CP is a disorder of movement and posture resulting from nonprogressive disturbances in a fetal or infant brain. Although it is characterized by primarily motor deficits, CP is heterogenous in severity and can be associated with disturbances in communication and/or cognition, as well as behavior, seizure, and/or musculoskeletal disorders and may result in a considerable lifetime burden of care. Through a combination of historical risk factors, validated infant neurologic examination, standardized motor assessment, and neuroimaging, CP can be reliably diagnosed in infants less than 6 months of age. When infants present with motor abnormalities but lack some of the essential criteria for diagnosing CP with certainty, an interim designation of HRCP is recommended to ensure early access to parent education and to diagnosis-specific interventions during a critical period of neuroplasticity.[3]

CLINICS CARE POINTS

- Affecting 1 in 312 school-aged children in the United States, cerebral palsy (CP) is the most common physical disability in childhood.[1]
- CP is associated with multiple comorbidities: 1 in 2 have intellectual disability, 1 in 4 are nonverbal, 1 in 15 require tube feeding, 1 in 4 have epilepsy, 1 in 3 have hip displacement, and 3 in 4 live in chronic pain.[32]
- CP can be accurately diagnosed in infants less than 6 months of age using a combination of risk factors, Hammersmith Infant Neurological Examination, standardized motor assessment tools, and neuroimaging. Normal neuroimaging does not rule out CP.[3]
- When a diagnosis of CP cannot yet be established with certainty, the interim diagnosis of high risk for CP (HRCP) should be assigned.[3,50]
- Infants with CP and HRCP benefit from an early diagnosis because motor and cognitive outcomes are better with the initiation of diagnosis-specific early intervention and parent support.[3,26]

DISCLOSURE

The authors have nothing to disclose.

REFERENCES

1. McGuire DO, Tian LH, Yeargin-Allsopp M, et al. Prevalence of cerebral palsy, intellectual disability, hearing loss, and blindness, National Health Interview survey, 2009-2016. Disability and Health Journal 2019;12(3):443–51.
2. Nelson KB. Causative factors in cerebral palsy. Clin Obstet Gynecol 2008;51(4): 749–62.
3. Novak I, Morgan C, Adde L, et al. Early, accurate diagnosis and early intervention in cerebral palsy: advances in diagnosis and treatment. JAMA Pediatr 2017; 171(9):897–907.
4. Spittle AJ, Anderson PJ, Lee KJ, et al. Preventive care at home for very preterm infants improves infant and caregiver outcomes at 2 years. Pediatrics 2010;126: e171–8.
5. Cheshire A, Barlow JH, Powell LA. The psychosocial well-being of parents of children with cerebral palsy: a comparison study. Disabil Rehabil 2010;32:1673–7.

6. Baird G, McConachie H, Scrutton D. Parents' perceptions of disclosure of the diagnosis of cerebral palsy. Arch Dis Child 2000;83:475–80.

7. Johnston MV. Plasticity in the developing brain: implications for rehabilitation. Dev Disabil Res Rev 2009;15:94–101.

8. Martin JH, Chakrabarty S, Friel KM. Harnessing activity-dependent plasticity to repair the damaged corticospinal tract in an animal model of cerebral palsy. Dev Med Child Neurol 2011;53(suppl 4):9–13.

9. Shrader MW, Wimberly L, Thompson R. Hip Surveillance in Children with Cerebral Palsy. J Am Acad Orthop Surg 2019;27(20):760–8.

10. Schwabe A. Comprehensive Care in Cerebral Palsy. Phys Med Rehabil Clin 2020; 31(1):1–13.

11. Romeo DM, Ricci D, Brogna C, et al. Use of the Hammersmith Infant Neurological Examination in infants with cerebral palsy: a critical review of the literature. Dev Med Child Neurol 2015;58(3):240–5.

12. Bosanquet M, Copeland L, Ware R, et al. A systematic review of tests to predict cerebral palsy in young children. Dev Med Child Neurol 2013;55(5):418–26.

13. Einspieler C, Marschik PB, Bos AF, et al. Early markers for cerebral palsy: insights from the assessment of general movements. Future Neurol 2012;7:709–17.

14. Barbosa VM, Campbell SK, Sheftel D, et al. Longitudinal performance of infants with cerebral palsy on the Test of Infant Motor Performance and on the Alberta Infant Motor Scale. Phys Occup Ther Pediatr 2003;23(3):7–29.

15. Maitre NL, Slaughter JC, Aschner JL. Early prediction of cerebral palsy after neonatal intensive care using motor development trajectories in infancy. Early Hum Dev 2013;89(10):781–6.

16. Spittle AJ, Lee KJ, Spencer-Smith M, et al. Accuracy of Two Motor Assessments during the First Year of Life in Preterm Infants for Predicting Motor Outcome at Preschool Age. PLoS One 2015;10(5):e0125854.

17. Rose-Jacobs R, Cabral H, Beeghly H, et al. The Movement Assessment of Infants (MAI) as a Predictor of Two-Year Neurodevelopmental Outcome for Infants Born at Term Who Are at Social Risk. Pediatr Phys Ther: Winter 2004;16 - Issue 4: 212–21.

18. Morgan C, Romeo D, Chorna O, et al. The pooled diagnostic accuracy of three tests for diagnosing cerebral palsy early in high risk infants: a case control study. J Clin Med 2019;8:1879.

19. Hay K, Nelin M, Carey H, et al. Hammersmith Infant Neurological Examination Asymmetry Score Distinguishes Hemiplegic Cerebral Palsy From Typical Development. Pediatr Neurol 2018;87:70–4.

20. Morgan C, Novak I, Dale R. Single blind randomised controlled trial of GAME (Goals - Activity - Motor Enrichment) in infants at high risk of cerebral palsy. Res Dev Disabil 2016;55:256–67.

21. Eliasson AC, Holmefur M. The influence of early modified constraint-induced movement therapy training on the longitudinal development of hand function in children with unilateral cerebral palsy. Dev Med Child Neurol 2015;57:89–94.

22. Boyd RN, Ziviani J, Sakzewski L, et al. REACH: study protocol of a randomised trial of rehabilitation very early in congenital hemiplegia. BMJ Open 2017;7(9): e017204.

23. Chorna O, Heathcock J, Key A, et al. Early childhood constraint therapy for sensory/motor impairment in cerebral palsy: a randomised clinical trial protocol. BMJ Open 2015;5(12):e010212. https://doi.org/10.1136/bmjopen-2015-010212.

24. MacKay-Lyons M. Central pattern generation of locomotion: a review of the evidence. Phys Ther 2002;82:69–83.

25. Mattern-Baxter K, Louper J, Zou C, et al. Low-Intensity vs High-Intensity Home-Based Treadmill Training and Walking Attainment in Young Children With Spastic Diplegic Cerebral Palsy. Arch Phys Med Rehabil 2020;101(2):204–12.

26. Morgan C, Fetters L, Adde L, et al. Early Intervention for Children Aged 0 to 2 Years With or at High Risk of Cerebral Palsy International Clinical Practice Guideline Based on Systematic Reviews. JAMA Pediatr 2021;175(8):846–58.

27. Coleman A, Weir K, Ware RS, et al. Predicting functional communication ability in children with cerebral palsy at school entry. Dev Med Child Neurol 2015;57(3):279–85.

28. Pennington L, Akor WA, Laws K, et al. Parent-mediated communication interventions for improving the communication skills of preschool children with non-progressive motor disorders. Cochrane Database Syst Rev 2018;7(7):CD012507.

29. Khamis A, Novak I, Morgan C, et al. Motor learning feeding interventions for infants at risk of cerebral palsy: a systematic review. Dysphagia 2020;35(1):1–17.

30. Weir K, McMahon S, Barry L, et al. Oropharyngeal aspiration and pneumonia in children. Pediatr Pulmonol 2007;42(11):1024–31.

31. Ferluga ED, Sathe NA, Krishnaswami S, et al. Surgical intervention for feeding and nutrition difficulties in cerebral palsy: a systematic review. Dev Med Child Neurol 2014;56(1):31–43.

32. Novak I, Hines M, Goldsmith S, et al. Clinical prognostic messages from a systematic review on cerebral palsy. Pediatrics 2012;130(5):e1285–312.

33. Ghasia F, Brunstrom-Hernandez J, Tychsen L. Repair of strabismus and binocular fusion in children with cerebral palsy: gross motor function classification scale. Invest Ophthalmol Vis Sci 2011;52(10):7664–71.

34. Malkowicz DE, Myers G, Leisman G. Rehabilitation of cortical visual impairment in children. Int J Neurosci 2006;116(9):1015–33.

35. Simard-Tremblay E, Constantin E, Gruber R, et al. Sleep in children with cerebral palsy: a review. J Child Neurol 2011;26(10):1303–10.

36. Halal CSE, Nunes ML. Education in children's sleep hygiene: which approaches are effective? a systematic review. J Pediatr 2014;90(5):449–56.

37. Angriman M, Caravale B, Novelli L, et al. Sleep in children with neurodevelopmental disabilities. Neuropediatrics 2015;46(3):199–210.

38. Binay Safer V, Ozbudak Demir S, Ozkan E, et al. Effects of botulinum toxin serotype A on sleep problems in children with cerebral palsy and on mothers sleep quality and depression. Neurosciences 2016;21(4):331–7.

39. Ayala L, Winter S, Byrne R, et al. Assessments and Interventions for Spasticity in Infants With or at High Risk for Cerebral Palsy: A Systematic Review. Pediatr Neurol 2021;118:72–90.

40. Zhao X, Xiao N, Li H, et al. Day vs. day-night use of ankle-foot orthoses in young children with spastic diplegia: a randomized controlled study. Am J Phys Med Rehabil 2013;92(10):905–11.

41. Wynter M, Gibson N, Willoughby KL, et al. Australian hip surveillance guidelines for children with cerebral palsy: 5 - year review. Dev Med Child Neurol 2015;57:808–20. https://doi.org/10.1111/dmcn.12754.

42. Macias-Merlo L, Bagur-Calafat C, Girabent-Farres M, et al. Effects of the standing program with hip abduction on hip acetabular development in children with spastic diplegia cerebral palsy. Disabil Rehabil 2016;38(11):1075–81.

43. te Velde A, Tantsis E, Novak I, et al. Age of Diagnosis, Fidelity and Acceptability of an Early Diagnosis Clinic for Cerebral Palsy: A Single Site Implementation Study. Brain Sci 2021;11(8):1074.

44. Maitre NL, Burton VJ, Duncan AF, et al. Network Implementation of Guideline for Early Detection Decreases Age at Cerebral Palsy Diagnosis. Pediatrics 2020; 145(5):e20192126.
45. Hubermann L, Boychuck Z, Shevell M, et al. Age at Referral of Children for Initial Diagnosis of Cerebral Palsy and Rehabilitation: Current Practices. J Child Neurol 2016;31(3):364–9.
46. Vargus-Adams J, Paulson A. Functional Assessment and Goals of Management. In: Glader L, Stevenson R, editors. Children and Youth with Complex cerebral palsy: care and management. London: McKeith Press; 2019. p. pp15–29.
47. te Velde A, Morgan C, Novak I, et al. Early Diagnosis and Classification of Cerebral Palsy: An Historical Perspective and Barriers to an Early Diagnosis. J Clin Med 2019;8(10):1599.
48. Pousada M, Guillamón N, Hernández-Encuentra E, et al. Impact of caring for a child with cerebral palsy on the quality of life of parents: a systematic review of the literature. J Dev Phys Disabil 2013;25:545–77.
49. Rentinck ICM, Ketelaar M, Jongmans MJ, et al. Parents of children with cerebral palsy: a review of factors related to the process of adaptation. Child Care Health Dev 2007;33:161–9.
50. Maitre N, Byrne R, Duncan A. High Risk for cerebral palsy" designation: A clinical consensus statement. J Pediatr Rehabil Med: An Interdisciplinary Approach Throughout the Lifespan 2022;15:165–74.

Promoting Functional Recovery in Critically Ill Children

Amit Sinha, MD, MBA[a], Sarah Rubin, MD, MSCI[b],
Jessica M. Jarvis, PhD[a],*

KEYWORDS

- Post–intensive care syndrome in pediatrics (PICS-p)
- Pediatric intensive care unit (PICU) • Post-ICU morbidity • Recovery • Rehabilitation

KEY POINTS

- Post–intensive care syndrome in pediatrics (PICS-p) is composed of new or worsening impairments in physical, cognitive, social, and mental health for the child and their family.
- Addressing PICS-p requires a multilevel and longitudinal approach.
- An interdisciplinary team, including intensivists, rehabilitation specialists, and social workers, is essential for the prevention and management of PICS-p.
- Monitoring outcomes via validated measures of core outcomes and starting with focused patient populations can facilitate the implementation and evaluation of approaches to address PICS-p.

INTRODUCTION

The landscape of pediatric critical care has changed since the establishment of pediatric intensive care units (PICUs) in the 1950s. The number of children who become critically ill each year in the United States has been steadily increasing by approximately 3% each year.[1] More than two-thirds of children admitted to the PICU have a previously diagnosed condition, and half have impaired or abnormal functioning at their baseline.[2,3] Although PICU mortalities have decreased drastically to 2% to 3% in high-resource countries, rates of new morbidity and readmission have increased.[2,3] This evolution has driven a paradigm shift in pediatric critical care from a focus on surviving pediatric critical illness to examining trajectories of recovery and promoting child and family functioning in the longer term.[4]

[a] Department of Physical Medicine and Rehabilitation, University of Pittsburgh, 3471 Fifth Avenue, Suite 910, Pittsburgh, PA 15213, USA; [b] Department of Critical Care Medicine, University of Pittsburgh, 4401 Penn Avenue, Faculty Pavilion, 2nd Floor, Pittsburgh, PA 15224, USA
* Corresponding author.
E-mail address: Jmjarvis@pitt.edu

Pediatr Clin N Am 70 (2023) 399–413
https://doi.org/10.1016/j.pcl.2023.01.008
0031-3955/23/© 2023 Elsevier Inc. All rights reserved.

POST–INTENSIVE CARE SYNDROME IN PEDIATRICS

The persistence of PICU-acquired impairments across physical, cognitive, or mental health domains experienced by survivors of pediatric critical illness has been termed *post-intensive care syndrome in pediatrics* (PICS-p).[5,6] Manning and colleagues[7] created a conceptual model of PICS-p to depict this phenomenon and describe the impact on components unique to pediatrics, such as the impact on their continued development and family. PICS-p impairments are reported across domains of physical health (health status, mobility, activities of daily living, fatigue, and pain), cognition (attention, memory, executive functioning), emotional/mental health (anxiety, depression, acute- and posttraumatic stress, behavior), and social and family functioning (reintegration in the home, community, and school/work, family communication and cohesion).[8–10]

Fig. 1 is a version of the PICS-p framework, depicting the impact of critical illness on the child and their family, the types of impairments experienced, and modified with author consent to highlight the association between post-PICU impairments and hospital readmission, and how all these components are impacted by their social and political context.

Physical Functioning

The World Health Organization developed the International Classification of Functioning, Disability, and Health to provide a common framework to conceptualize functional health and disabilities.[11] This framework considers functioning in 3 different ways: functional status and physical structures (eg, muscle strength); activities (eg, ability to complete tasks such as brushing teeth or transferring from bed to chair); and participation (eg, engagement in sets and sequences of meaningful life events, such as school field trips or family celebrations). Rates of impaired physical

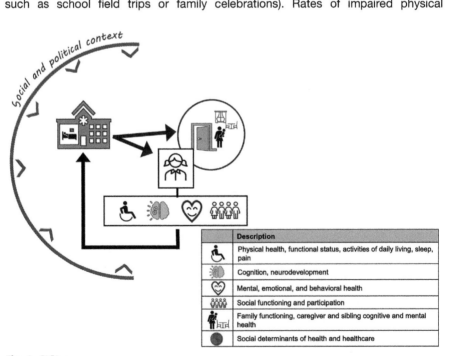

	Description
♿	Physical health, functional status, activities of daily living, sleep, pain
🧠	Cognition, neurodevelopment
💟	Mental, emotional, and behavioral health
👨‍👩‍👧‍👦	Social functioning and participation
👫	Family functioning, caregiver and sibling cognitive and mental health
⬤	Social determinants of health and healthcare

Fig. 1. PICS-p.

functioning range from 10% to 82% at PICU discharge, depending on how functioning was conceptualized and measured.[12–17] When using the Pediatric Evaluation of Disability Inventory, a proxy/patient-reported outcome measure of children's ability to perform activities across physical, social, and cognitive domains, to compare level of functioning pre-PICU, impairments were reported in 82% and 28% of children at PICU discharge and 6 months after, respectively. Using the Functional Status Scale, trajectories of recovery differ between survivors; for example, although approximately two-thirds of survivors report impairments persist for several months to years after discharge,[16,18] in a prospective cohort study by Pinto and colleagues,[6] morbidities and mortalities increased in the initial 3 years after discharge.

Cognitive Health

Cognitive dysfunction following critical illness in children includes difficulties with attention, memory, and executive function, increased cognitive fatigue, delayed neurodevelopment, and worsened academic performance.[19,20] Reported prevalence of new cognitive dysfunction in children following critical illness ranges from 3% to 73%, depending on the specificity of the measure, timing of assessment, and cohort characteristics.[21] Among children with sepsis and meningitis requiring critical care, up to 42% report cognitive impairment or neurodevelopmental delays following illness.[22] After cardiac arrest, 47% of children requiring extracorporeal membrane oxygenation report persistent learning difficulties.[23] Furthermore, there is emerging evidence cognitive impairments may persist or worsen over the first year.[24]

Emotional Health

Children receive a median of 11 stressful and painful procedures in a single PICU day.[25] Unsurprisingly, 64% of children demonstrate the symptoms for acute stress disorder during their PICU admission.[26] Emotional dysfunction after PICU admission can manifest as anxiety, depression, behavior difficulties, and posttraumatic stress disorder (PTSD).[19,27–30] PTSD is the most common psychiatric diagnosis after PICU. Prevalence of PTSD among critically ill children varies from 13% to 32% within 12 months of discharge.[31,32] Other post-PICU psychiatric comorbidities include hyperactivity, depression, sleep disturbance, cognitive fatigue, and conduct disorders.[33–35]

Social/Familial Health

Pediatric critical illness is a highly stressful experience for caregivers and siblings of the patient and can negatively impact their mental health and family cohesion.[36–38] A third of caregivers report moderate to severe anxiety or moderate to severe depression after PICU.[30] One study reported 10% of caregivers receive a new mental health diagnosis within 6 months of their child's critical illness, 110% higher than projected.[39] Critical illness also impacts child and family social networks, relationship functioning, and work or school attendance. One prospective cohort study reported 43% of children had missed 7 or more days of school and 14% had missed 30 or more days of school 3 months after PICU.[40]

Risk Factors and Social Determinants of Health

Individual risk factors for PICS-p are outlined in **Table 1**. Although an in-depth review of the PICU care equity and related health disparities is out of the scope of this review, it is necessary to briefly discuss the impact of the social and political factors that influence health and health care when discussing trajectories of functional recovery.[41–43] Access to care is the opportunity to have health needs fulfilled through

Table 1
Risk factors for post–intensive care syndrome in pediatrics

Risk Factor	Description	Reference
Caregiver language and ethnicity	Non-English speaking is associated with worse outcomes, for example, increased mortality	59,98
Socioeconomic status	Lower income, education, and geographic location increase risk for PICU admission and poor PICU outcome	41
Child's baseline status	Prior chronic condition	23,47
Admitting diagnosis	Neurologic conditions, sepsis, multiorgan dysfunction	48
Invasive procedures	Invasive mechanical ventilation, receipt of extracorporeal membrane oxygenation	49
Sedation requirements	Length of deep sedation	27,58

timely and appropriate care.[44] Access to care opportunities results from the interaction between an individual's abilities/resources (eg, mobility, transportation) and the health care system characteristics (eg, geographic location, physical layout), both of which are influenced by social and political policies and norms. Unfortunately, there is an abundance of literature demonstrating access to care is inequitable, that is, access differences that are unjust, for children with disabilities, children of color, and children with lower-socioeconomic status in both the hospital and the community.[45–47] The *Conceptual Model of Disability and Disparities* demonstrates the impact of disability on access to care and how access to care experiences influence the abling/disabling process.[48] Thus, given the complexity and vulnerability of the PICU population, the authors posit that it is crucial to include examination of and support for access to care for all services developed and implemented to assure equitable care and recovery for all children.

MANAGEMENT OF POST–INTENSIVE CARE SYNDROME IN PEDIATRICS

Given the breadth of the impact of PICS-p, there are several approaches emerging to optimize the functioning of PICU survivors. These approaches include prevention, identification, and intervention during and after the PICU and may be targeted at the level of the individual/family or health care system. **Fig. 2** illustrates the existing approaches across the care continuum, and components are summarized in later discussion.

Prognostication and Screening

Identifying those at risk for PICS-p presents several challenges. First, functional impairments can be difficult to detect in very young children until they are older or after resuming home and family life, emphasizing the need for repeated screening, including after hospital discharge.[14] Second, there is currently no validated measure to assess PICS-p. Existing measures of functional outcomes tend to be validated only for a specific diagnosis or narrow age group and may not detect all of the deficiencies associated with PICS-p.[27,49] Given the importance of early identification to guide resource distribution and care coordination, multimodal approaches to screening and prognostication may be necessary, such as sing both caregiver/patient-reported outcome measures and clinical data, including serum, physiologic,

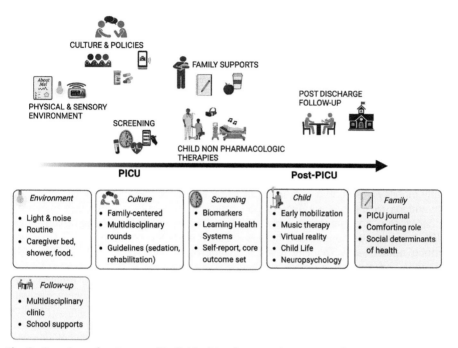

Fig. 2. Overview of system- and individual-level approaches to remediate PICS-p.

and imaging biomarker data. For example, serum-derived vascular endothelial growth factor 1 day after PICU admission was associated with decreased functional status at hospital discharge for 44 children with acquired brain injury; heart rate variability metrics within the first 24 hours of admission predicted organ dysfunction and mortality in a cohort of more than 7000 critically ill children, and decreased connectivity strength in paralimbic tracks identified via resting state functional MRI and diffusion tensor imaging was associated with neurocognitive impairment among 12 children with cardiac arrest.[50–52]

Pediatric Intensive Care Unit–Based Care

System level
Environmental modifications, such as limiting noise from alarms and shift change, keeping the child on a familiar routine, and decorating the room with familiar items, are suggested to prevent some of the psychological sequalae of critical care.[53–57] Interventions to optimize PICU culture include approaches to care delivery, such as providing family-centered care, the equity in care allocation and care quality, availability of translators, and educational materials and resources in non-English languages.[57–63] Policies and training to promote family-centered care include protocols to improve communication (**Table 2**), incorporating caregivers in goal setting and care planning, provision of resources that support caregiver presence, for example, a place to sleep and nutritious food, and remote/telehealth options to engage caregivers in care planning when they cannot be at the PICU bedside.[58,64–66] Implementation of multidisciplinary rounds within the PICU facilitates referral of necessary services and care coordination (**Fig. 3**). Last, adherence to pediatric critical care guidelines for pain and sedation management, mechanical ventilation, and delirium prevention may prevent development of PICS-p.[63,67–70]

Table 2
Improving communication during pediatric critical care through the acronym HICCC

Component	Description
Honest	Straightforward, upfront, and candid
Inclusive	Listening to and implementing caregiver feedback and concerns
Compassionate	Caring about the patient and family
Comprehensive & Clear	Concise descriptions and rationales
Coordinated	Care team roles are defined and expectations listed

Individual level

Early mobility has been a primary focus of rehabilitation therapies of PICU-based interventions to prevent impairment and promote recovery.[71,72] Although feasibility, acceptability, and safety of early mobilization and rehabilitation therapies in the PICU has been demonstrated, there is a lack of evidence on efficacy.[73–77] However, among adults, early mobility resulted in improved outcomes, such as increased strength and shorter durations of mechanical ventilation and lengths of intensive care unit (ICU) stay.[78] Furthermore, caregivers report less stress 6 months after discharge if their child received PICU-based rehabilitation therapies, compared with those who did not.[79] Thus, the 2022 Society of Critical Care Medicine Clinical Practice Guidelines for critically ill pediatric patients recommend incorporation of a standardized early mobility protocol outlining criteria to participate in early mobility, the contraindications, and mobility activities and goals.[70]

Nonpharmacologic approaches to supporting children's comfort and mental health, such as providing music or music therapy, virtual reality, and comfort-care holding, are emerging as potentially effective alternatives to decreasing stress and pain without

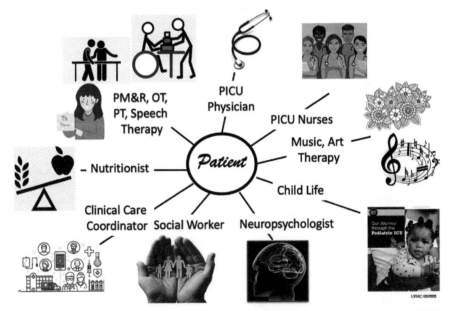

Fig. 3. Disciplines involved in multidisciplinary PICU care. OT, occupational therapy; PM&R, physical medicine and rehabilitation; PT, physical therapy.

the potentially deleterious effects associated with analgesics and sedatives.[80–86] These studies primarily demonstrate feasibility, acceptability, and safety. However, there is promising results among critically ill adults to encourage continued exploration of these approaches. For example, listening to music during mechanical ventilation resulted in decreased self-reported anxiety and less medication use, compared with usual care in a randomized control trial of 373 patients across 12 different ICUs.[87] Additional interventions to support both child and caregiver include caregivers reading to their child and PICU diaries.[88,89] The latter involves working with families to create a written record detailing daily events about their child's condition and care during the PICU hospitalization in their own words. These diaries may address gaps in a child's memory regarding their critical illness hospitalization and provide clarity and context about their experience. Among adults, ICU diaries have been associated with a reduction in the incidence of PTSD, anxiety, and depression, as well as improve health-related quality of life.[90] Last, but possibly most importantly for addressing PICS-p, are approaches of bundled care. The *ABCDEF Bundle* (**Fig. 4**), also known as "A2F Care" and "PICU Liberation," aims to minimize pain and sedation, decrease unnecessarily prolonged mechanical ventilation, prevent immobility, and facilitate family engagement.[91]

Post–Pediatric Intensive Care Unit Follow-Up

The creation of post-PICU follow-up clinics is a postacute approach to optimize recovery through recognition of PICs-p, provision of referrals for health care and school accommodations requests, care coordination, and connection with psychosocial support. There is significant variability in the design of post-ICU clinics; however, families report high satisfaction and value from attending.[92–94] Common components of these clinics are multidisciplinary engagement (eg, therapists, social workers, intensivists, physiatrists, neuropsychologists) and screening for child and family functional outcomes.[8,27] Developing such clinics can be complicated and time consuming, given the heterogeneity of the PICU population diagnoses, conditions, and ages coupled with the resources necessary to support multidisciplinary care.

To guide the successful development of post-PICU follow-up clinics, Butcher and colleagues[95] provide the following "5 S's" to consider when implementing a post-ICU clinic:

- Space: Affordability; availability; accessibility; maximum occupancy
- Staff: Disciplines; scheduling; compensation
- Stuff: Funding; technology; equipment
- Screening: Eligibility criteria; outcomes to assess; process to identify; timing of follow-up
- Selling it: Awareness; advocacy; assuring attendance

A. Assessing, preventing, and managing pain

B. Both spontaneous breathing and awakening trials

C. Choice of analgesia and sedation

D. Delirium assessment, prevention, and management

E. Early mobility and exercise

F. Family engagement and empowerment

Fig. 4. Components of the *ABCDEF Bundle* for addressing PICS-p.

Addressing these considerations inevitably depends on the resources and expertise available at individual institutions. Partnering *between* PICU physicians and established follow-up clinics provides a potentially universal solution to space and equipment. Particularly multidisciplinary, specialty clinics, such as Complex Care or Pediatric Rehabilitation Medicine clinics, can provide access to many of the support services patients require after ICU admission. Determining which patients will be offered follow-up visits may also depend on the number of staff available to participate in post-ICU clinics. Who should be involved and mode of follow-up (eg, in-person, virtual, asynchronous) require careful consideration. Beginning with a focused patient population and expanding gradually as additional funding and resources are identified may facilitate the feasibility of starting and sustaining this care. Incorporating a diverse set of stakeholders, both end users and providers, in clinic design and optimizations can optimize care, facilitate efforts to promote awareness of PICS-p, advocate for clinic attendance, and promote retention across longitudinal care.[92,96,97]

THE ROLE OF PEDIATRIC REHABILITATION MEDICINE

Pediatric physiatrists are well poised to champion this space of optimizing recovery for survivors of pediatric critical illness, given their unique focus on child functioning versus a specific organ system. Pediatric rehabilitation medicine spans the health care continuum from the PICU to postacute and ambulatory care, while consistently focusing on optimizing function through effective collaboration and communication with other health care professionals. Pediatric physiatrists are ideally equipped to identify and manage weakness and functional limitations in the PICU and can also help educate families about PICS-p and assist in coordination of care for patients who are able to transition home. For those pediatric patients who have more significant functional deficits, they can identify those who would benefit from transfer to a pediatric acute inpatient rehabilitation unit before discharge home.

FUTURE DIRECTIONS

There has been a rapid evolution of research aimed at characterizing and facilitating functional recovery for children and families after pediatric critical illness; however, significant hurdles still lay ahead. Resources and tools for PICS-p education and identification will be necessary to maintain momentum for improving functional recovery of survivors of pediatric critical illness.[96] In addition, evidence on PICS-p intervention efficacy and guidelines for equitable implementation are necessary to drive development of health policies for clinical implementation. Last, children and families admitted into the PICU reported a higher prevalence of adverse social determinants of health and prior adverse childhood experiences compared with the general population.[94,95,97] Taken together with the high proportion of children from historically marginalized communities within the PICU population, additional research on best practices to screen for and intervene on adverse social determinants of health and assure equitable opportunity to access care is crucial to assure every child has the opportunity to achieve their optimal health.

SUMMARY

Pediatric critical illness can have a long-lasting, negative impact on children and families across a variety of different functional domains. Preventing, identifying, and treating PICS-p requires coordinated care among a multidisciplinary team of health care professions and intentional development of guidelines and policies that assure equitable implementation of evidence-based care during and after the PICU admission. Clinicians and researchers should evaluate their local needs, barriers, and facilitators for addressing PICS-p and collaborate with lived experience experts to design the longitudinal support necessary for recovery in the longer term.

CLINICS CARE POINTS

- Children, their caregivers, and their siblings may experience new or worsening impairments after pediatric intensive care unit discharge, known as post–intensive care syndrome in pediatrics. Post–intensive care syndrome in pediatrics education and awareness for families, health care providers (eg, primary care physicians), and educators are necessary to improve identification and treatment.

- Within the pediatric intensive care unit, there are several promising interventions addressing post–intensive care syndrome in pediatrics at an individual and a system level. Protocolizing a bundled approach may be best, given the wide range of potential impairments.

- Follow-up assessment and care are necessary, but resource intensive. There is need for careful consideration of who should be a part of follow-up care, mode of delivery, and the level of specificity desired for outcome data (eg, general vs specific) to drive measure selection, although outcomes should always align with family priorities.

- Efforts to promote survivorship should incorporate addressing social determinants of health and equitable access.

DISCLOSURE

This work was supported in part by the Eunice Kennedy Shriver National Institute of Child Health & Human Development of the National Institutes of Health under Award Number K23HD106011 (J.M. Jarvis). The content is solely the responsibility of the authors and does not necessarily represent the official views of the National Institutes of Health. The authors have nothing else to disclose.

ACKNOWLEDGMENTS

The authors acknowledge Ericka Fink, MD, MS and Katie Hayden, MSN for their expertise, time, and guidance during this review.

REFERENCES

1. Heneghan JA, Rogerson C, Goodman DM, et al. Epidemiology of Pediatric Critical Care Admissions in 43 United States Children's Hospitals, 2014–2019. Pediatr Crit Care Med 2022;23(7):484–92.
2. Namachivayam P, Shann F, Shekerdemian L, et al. Three decades of pediatric intensive care: Who was admitted, what happened in intensive care, and what happened afterward. Pediatr Crit Care Med 2010;11(5):549–55.
3. Pollack MM, Holubkov R, Funai T, et al. Pediatric Intensive Care Outcomes: Development of New Morbidities During Pediatric Critical Care. Pediatr Crit Care Med 2014;15(9):821–7.
4. Heneghan J, Pollack MM. Morbidity: Changing the outcome paradigm for pediatric critical care. Pediatr Clin North Am 2017;64(5):1147–65. Morbidity.
5. Herrup EA, Wieczorek B, Kudchadkar SR. Characteristics of postintensive care syndrome in survivors of pediatric critical illness: A systematic review. World J Crit Care Med 2017;6(2):124.

6. Pinto NP, Rhinesmith EW, Kim TY, et al. Long-term function after pediatric critical illness: Results from the Survivor Outcomes study. Pediatr Crit Care Med 2017; 18(3):122–30.

7. Manning JC, Pinto NP, Rennick JE, et al. Conceptualizing Post Intensive Care Syndrome in Children—The PICS-p Framework. Pediatr Crit Care Med 2018; 19(4):298–300.

8. Fink EL, Maddux AB, Pinto N, et al. A Core Outcome Set for Pediatric Critical Care. Crit Care Med 2020;48(12):1819–28.

9. Choong K. PICU-acquired complications: the new marker of the quality of care. ICU Manag 2019;19(2):84–8.

10. Fayed BN, Cameron S, Fraser D, et al. Priority outcomes in critically ill children. A patient and parent perspective 2020;29(5):94–103.

11. The World Health Organization. International classification of functioning, disability, and health: children & youth version. ICF-CY; 2007. https://doi.org/10.1017/CBO9781107415324.004. Published online.

12. Choong K, Fraser D, Al-Harbi S, et al. Functional Recovery in Critically Ill Children, the "WeeCover" Multicenter Study. Pediatr Crit Care Med 2018;19(2): 145–54.

13. Ong C, Lee JH, Leow MKS, et al. Functional outcomes and physical impairments in pediatric critical care survivors: A scoping review. Pediatr Crit Care Med 2016; 17(5):e247–59.

14. Khetani MA, Albrecht E, Jarvis JM, et al. Determinants of change in home participation among critically ill children. Dev Med Child Neurol 2018;60(8):793–800.

15. Jarvis JM, Fayed N, Fink EL, et al. Caregiver dissatisfaction with their child's participation in home activities after pediatric critical illness. BMC Pediatr 2020; 20(1):415.

16. Jarvis J, Houtrow A, Treble-Barna A, et al. #442: Post pediatric neurocritical care recovery: A whole child and family perspective. Pediatr Crit Care Med 2021; 22(Supplement 1 3S):13.

17. Bossen D, de Boer RM, Knoester H, et al. Physical Functioning After Admission to the PICU: A Scoping Review. Crit Care Explor 2021;3(6):e0462.

18. Carlton EF, Pinto N, Smith M, et al. Overall health following pediatric critical illness: A scoping review of instruments and methodology. Pediatr Crit Care Med 2021;22(12):1061–71.

19. Als LC, Tennant A, Nadel S, et al. Persistence of neuropsychological deficits following pediatric critical illness. Crit Care Med 2015;43(8 PG-312–315):e312–5.

20. Als LC, Nadel S, Cooper M, et al. Neuropsychologic Function Three to Six Months Following Admission to the PICU With Meningoencephalitis, Sepsis, and Other Disorders. Crit Care Med 2013;41(4):1094–103.

21. Chaiyakulsil C. ROC and, 2021 undefined. Pediatric postintensive care syndrome: high burden and a gap in evaluation tools for limited-resource settings. ncbi.nlm.nih.gov. Available at: https://www.ncbi.nlm.nih.gov/pmc/articles/PMC8426094/. Accessed November 20, 2022.

22. Kachmar AG, Irving SY, Connolly CA, et al. A systematic review of risk factors associated with cognitive impairment after pediatric critical illness. Pediatr Crit Care Med 2018;19(3):e164–71.

23. Elias MD, Achuff BJ, Ittenbach RF, et al. Long-term outcomes of pediatric cardiac patients supported by extracorporeal membrane oxygenation. Pediatr Crit Care Med 2017;18(8):787–94.

24. Hall TA, Greene RK, Lee JB, et al. Post-Intensive Care Syndrome in a Cohort of School-Aged Children and Adolescent ICU Survivors: The Importance of

Follow-up in the Acute Recovery Phase. J Pediatr Intensive Care 2022. https://doi.org/10.1055/s-0042-1747935.

25. Baarslag MA, Jhingoer S, Ista E, et al. How often do we perform painful and stressful procedures in the paediatric intensive care unit? A prospective observational study. Aust Crit Care 2019;32(1):4–10.

26. Nelson LP, Lachman SE, Goodman K, et al. Admission Psychosocial Characteristics of Critically Ill Children and Acute Stress. Pediatr Crit Care Med 2020;22(2):194–203.

27. Pinto NP, Maddux AB, Dervan LA, et al. A Core Outcome Measurement Set for Pediatric Critical Care. Pediatr Crit Care Med 2022;23(11):893–907.

28. Manning JC, Hemingway P, Redsell SA. Long-term psychosocial impact reported by childhood critical illness survivors: A systematic review. Nurs Crit Care 2014;19(3):145–56.

29. Colville G, Kerry S, Pierce C. Children's factual and delusional memories of intensive care. Am J Respir Crit Care Med 2008;177(9):976–82.

30. Rodríguez-Rey R, Alonso-Tapia J, Colville G. Prediction of parental posttraumatic stress, anxiety and depression after a child's critical hospitalization. J Crit Care 2018;45:149–55.

31. Nelson LP, Gold JI. Posttraumatic stress disorder in children and their parents following admission to the pediatric intensive care unit: A review. Pediatr Crit Care Med 2012;13(3):338–47.

32. Nelson LP, Lachman SE, Li SW, et al. The effects of family functioning on the development of posttraumatic stress in children and their parents following admission to the PICU. Pediatr Crit Care Med 2019;20(4):e208–15.

33. Kudchadkar SR, Aljohani OA, Punjabi NM. Sleep of critically ill children in the pediatric intensive care unit: A systematic review. Sleep Med Rev 2014;18(2):103–10.

34. Colville GA, Pierce CM, Peters MJ. Self-Reported Fatigue in Children Following Intensive Care Treatment. Pediatr Crit Care Med 2019;20(2):e98–101.

35. Rennick JE, Dougherty G, Chambers C, et al. Children's psychological and behavioral responses following pediatric intensive care unit hospitalization: the caring intensively study. BMC Pediatr 2014;14(1):276.

36. Abela KM, Wardell D, Rozmus C, et al. Impact of paediatric critical illness and injury on families: An updated systematic review. J Pediatr Nurs 2020;51:21–31.

37. Shudy M, de Almeida ML, Ly S, et al. Impact of pediatric critical illness and injury on families: A systematic literature review. Pediatrics 2006;118(Supplement_3):S203–18.

38. Colville G, Darkins J, Hesketh J, et al. The impact on parents of a child's admission to intensive care: Integration of qualitative findings from a cross-sectional study. Intensive Crit Care Nurs 2009;25(2):72–9.

39. Logan GE, Sahrmann JM, Gu H, et al. Parental mental health care after their child's pediatric intensive care hospitalization. Pediatr Crit Care Med 2020;21(11):941–8.

40. Kastner K, Pinto N, Msall ME, et al. PICU follow-up: The impact of missed school in a cohort of children following PICU admission. Crit Care Explor 2019;1(8):1–4.

41. Modification of social determinants of health by critical illness and consequences of that modification for recovery: an international qualitative study. BMJ Open 2022;12(9):e060454. Available at: https://bmjopen.bmj.com/content/12/9/e060454.abstract. Accessed November 20, 2022.

42. Zambrano LD, Ly KN, Link-Gelles R, et al. Investigating Health Disparities Associated With Multisystem Inflammatory Syndrome in Children After SARS-CoV-2 Infection. Pediatr Infect Dis J 2022;41(11):891–8.

43. Zurca AD, Suttle ML, October TW. An Antiracism Approach to Conducting, Reporting, and Evaluating Pediatric Critical Care Research. Pediatr Crit Care Med 2022;23(2):129–32.

44. Levesque J, Harris M, Russell G. Patient-centred access to health care: conceptualising access at the interface of health systems and populations. Int J Equity Health 2013;12(18):1–9.

45. Mitchell H, Reddy A, Perry M, et al. Racial, ethnic, and socioeconomic disparities in paediatric critical care in the USA. Lancet Child Adolesc Health 2021;5: 739–50. Available at: https://pubmed.ncbi.nlm.nih.gov/34370979/.

46. Kuo DZ, Goudie A, Cohen E, et al. Inequities in health care needs for children with medical complexity. Health Aff 2014;33(12):2190–8.

47. McGowan SK, Sarigiannis KA, Fox SC, et al. Racial Disparities in ICU Outcomes: A Systematic Review. Crit Care Med 2022;50(1):1–20.

48. Meade MA, Mahmoudi E, Lee SY. The intersection of disability and healthcare disparities: a conceptual framework. Disabil Rehabil 2015;37(7):632–41.

49. Maddux AB, Pinto N, Fink EL, et al. Postdischarge Outcome Domains in Pediatric Critical Care and the Instruments Used to Evaluate Them: A Scoping Review. Crit Care Med 2020;48(12):e1313–21.

50. Jarvis JM, Roy J, Schmithorst V, et al. Limbic pathway vulnerability associates with neurologic outcome in children after cardiac arrest. Resuscitation 2022; 182:109634.

51. Madurski C, Jarvis JM, Beers SR, et al. Serum Biomarkers of Regeneration and Plasticity are Associated with Functional Outcome in Pediatric Neurocritical Illness: An Exploratory Study. Neurocrit Care 2021;35(2):457–67.

52. Badke CM, Marsillio LE, Carroll MS, et al. Development of a Heart Rate Variability Risk Score to Predict Organ Dysfunction and Death in Critically Ill Children. Pediatr Crit Care Med 2021;22(8):e437–47.

53. Royka M, Unit G. Promoting Psychosocial Adjustment in Pediatric Burn Patients Through Music Therapy and Child Life Therapy.

54. Morrison WE, Haas EC, Shaffner DH, et al. Noise, stress, and annoyance in a pediatric intensive care unit. Crit Care Med 2003;31(1):113–9.

55. Mazer BSE. Hospital Noise and the Patient Experience : Seven Ways to Create and Maintain a Quieter Environment.

56. Kawai Y, Weatherhead JR, Traube C, et al. Quality Improvement Initiative to Reduce Pediatric Intensive Care Unit Noise Pollution With the Use of a Pediatric Delirium Bundle. J Intensive Care Med 2019;34(5):383–90.

57. Spazzapan M, Vijayakumar B, Stewart CE. A bit about me: Bedside boards to create a culture of patient-centered care in pediatric intensive care units (PICUs). J Healthc Risk Manag 2020;39(3):11–9.

58. DeSanti RL, Brown DH, Srinivasan S, et al. Patient- and Family-Centered Video Rounds in the Pediatric Intensive Care Unit. Telehealth and Medicine Today 2020;1–14. https://doi.org/10.30953/tmt.v5.231.

59. Anand KJS, Sepanski RJ, Giles K, et al. Pediatric intensive care unit mortality among Latino children before and after a multilevel health care delivery intervention. JAMA Pediatr 2015;169(4):383–90.

60. Environments C, Briggs LP, Fontaine DK, et al. Designing Humanistic Critical Care Environments. Crit Care Nurse Q 2001;24(3):21–34.

61. Chlan L. Integrating nonpharmacological, adjunctive interventions into critical care practice: A means to humanize care. American journal of criti 2002; 11(1):14–6.

62. Ross-Driscoll K, Esper G, Kinlaw K, et al. Evaluating Approaches to Improve Equity in Critical Care Resource Allocation in the COVID-19 Pandemic. Am J Respir Crit Care Med 2021;204(12):1481–4.

63. Davidson JE, Aslakson RA, Long AC, et al. Guidelines for Family-Centered Care in the Neonatal, Pediatric, and Adult ICU. Crit Care Med 2017;45(1):103–28.

64. Curfman A, Hackell JM, Herendeen NE, et al. Telehealth: Opportunities to Improve Access, Quality, and Cost in Pediatric Care. Pediatrics 2022;149(3). https://doi.org/10.1542/peds.2021-056035.

65. Dale CM, Carbone S, Istanboulian L, et al. Support needs and health-related quality of life of family caregivers of patients requiring prolonged mechanical ventilation and admission to a specialised weaning centre: A qualitative longitudinal interview study. Intensive Crit Care Nurs 2020;58:102808.

66. DeLemos D, Chen M, Romer A, et al. Building trust through communication in the intensive care unit: HICCC. Pediatr Crit Care Med 2010;11(3):378–84.

67. Hall TA, Leonard S, Bradbury K, et al. Post-intensive care syndrome in a cohort of infants & young children receiving integrated care via a pediatric critical care & neurotrauma recovery program: A pilot investigation. Clin Neuropsychol 2022; 36(3):639–63.

68. Ista E, Redivo J, Kananur P, et al. ABCDEF Bundle Practices for Critically Ill Children: An International Survey of 161 PICUs in 18 Countries. Crit Care Med 2022; 50(1):114–25.

69. Ista E, Redivo J, Kananur P, et al. Assessing Pain, Both Spontaneous Awakening and Breathing Trials, Choice of Sedation, Delirium Monitoring/Management, Early Exercise/Mobility, and Family Engagement/Empowerment Bundle Practices for Critically Ill Children. Crit Care Med 2021;1–15. https://doi.org/10.1097/ccm. 0000000000005168.

70. Smith HAB, Besunder JB, Betters KA, et al. Society of Critical Care Medicine Clinical Practice Guidelines on Prevention and Management of Pain, Agitation, Neuromuscular Blockade, and Delirium in Critically Ill Pediatric Patients With Consideration of the ICU Environment and Early Mobility. Pediatr Crit Care Med 2022;23(2):e74–110.

71. Choong K, Awladthani S, Khawaji A, et al. Early Exercise in Critically Ill Youth and Children, a Preliminary Evaluation: The wEECYCLE Pilot Trial. Pediatr Crit Care Med 2017;18(11 PG-546–554):e546–54.

72. Treble-Barna A, Beers SR, Houtrow AJ, et al. PICU-Based Rehabilitation and Outcomes Assessment. Pediatr Crit Care Med 2019;20(6):1.

73. Patel Rv, Redivo J, Nelliot A, et al. Early Mobilization in a PICU: A Qualitative Sustainability Analysis of PICU Up!*. Pediatr Crit Care Med 2021;E233–42. https:// doi.org/10.1097/PCC.0000000000002619.

74. Hopkins RO, Choong K, Zebuhr CA, et al. Transforming PICU Culture to Facilitate Early Rehabilitation HHS Public Access. J Pediatr Intensive Care 2015;4(4): 204–11.

75. Wieczorek B, Ascenzi J, Kim Y, et al. PICU Up!: Impact of a quality improvement intervention to promote early mobilization in critically ill children. Pediatr Crit Care Med 2016;17(12):e559–66.

76. Fink EL, Beers SR, Houtrow AJ, et al. Early protocolized versus usual care rehabilitation for pediatric neurocritical care patients: A randomized controlled trial. Pediatr Crit Care Med 2019;20(6):540–50.

77. LaRosa JM, Nelliot A, Zaidi M, et al. Mobilization Safety of Critically Ill Children. Pediatrics 2022;149(4). https://doi.org/10.1542/peds.2021-053432.

78. Wang J, Ren D, Liu Y, et al. Effects of early mobilization on the prognosis of critically ill patients: A systematic review and meta-analysis. Int J Nurs Stud 2020; 110:103708.

79. Jarvis J, Choong K, Khetani M. Associations of participation-focused strategies and rehabilitation service use with caregiver stress after pediatric critical illness. Arch Phys Med Rehabil 2019;100(4):703–10.

80. Liu MH, Zhu LH, Peng JX, et al. Effect of personalized music intervention in mechanically ventilated children in the PICU: A pilot study. Pediatr Crit Care Med 2020;21(1):e8–14.

81. Bush HI, LaGasse AB, Collier EH, et al. Effect of Live Versus Recorded Music on Children Receiving Mechanical Ventilation and Sedation. Am J Crit Care 2021; 30(5):343–9.

82. Garcia Guerra G, Joffe AR, Sheppard C, et al. Music Use for Sedation in Critically ill Children (MUSiCC trial): a pilot randomized controlled trial. J Intensive Care 2021;9(1):1–9.

83. Gerber SM, Jeitziner MM, Wyss P, et al. Visuo-acoustic stimulation that helps you to relax: A virtual reality setup for patients in the intensive care unit. Sci Rep 2017; 7(1):1–10.

84. Lai B, Powell M, Clement AG, et al. Examining the feasibility of early mobilization with virtual reality gaming using head-mounted display and adaptive software with adolescents in the pediatric intensive care unit: Case report. JMIR Rehabil Assist Technol 2021;8(2):1–12.

85. Lee LA, Moss SJ, Martin DA, et al. Comfort-holding in critically ill children: a scoping review. Can J Anesth 2021;68(11):1695–704.

86. Reade MC, Finfer S. Sedation and delirium in the intensive care unit. N Engl J Med 2014;370(5):444–54.

87. Chlan LL, Weinert CR, Heiderscheit A, et al. Effects of patient-directed music intervention on anxiety and sedative exposure in critically Ill patients receiving mechanical ventilatory support: A randomized clinical trial. J Am Med Assoc 2013;309(22):2335–44.

88. Rennick JE, Stremler R, Horwood L, et al. A Pilot Randomized Controlled Trial of an Intervention to Promote Psychological Well-Being in Critically Ill Children. Pediatr Crit Care Med 2018;19(7):1.

89. Wang SH, Owens T, Johnson A, et al. Evaluating the Feasibility and Efficacy of a Pediatric Intensive Care Unit Diary. Crit Care Nurs Q 2022;45(1):88–97.

90. McIlroy PA, King RS, Garrouste-Orgeas M, et al. The Effect of ICU Diaries on Psychological Outcomes and Quality of Life of Survivors of Critical Illness and Their Relatives: A Systematic Review and Meta-Analysis. Crit Care Med 2019;47(2): 273–9.

91. Waak M, Harnischfeger J, Ferguson A, et al. Every child, every day, back to play: the PICUstars protocol - implementation of a nurse-led PICU liberation program. BMC Pediatr 2022;22(1). https://doi.org/10.1186/s12887-022-03232-2.

92. Hickey E, Johnson T, Kudchadkar SR, et al. Persistence Matters! Hurdles and High Points of PICU Follow-Up Clinic. Pediatr Crit Care Med 2022;23(8):397–9.

93. Samuel VM, Colville GA, Goodwin S, et al. The value of screening parents for their risk of developing psychological symptoms after PICU: A feasibility study evaluating a pediatric intensive care follow-up clinic. Pediatr Crit Care Med 2015;16(9): 808–13.

94. Ducharme-Crevier L, La KA, Francois T, et al. PICU Follow-Up Clinic: Patient and Family Outcomes 2 Months After Discharge. Pediatr Crit Care Med 2021;22(11): 935–43.

95. Butcher B, Eaton T, Montgomery-Yates A, et al. 2022 undefined. Meeting the Challenges of Establishing Intensive Care Unit Follow-up Clinics. Am J Crit Care 2022;31(4):324–8.

96. Anthony L, Hilder A, Newcomb D, et al. General practitioner perspectives on a shared-care model for paediatric patients post-intensive care: A cross-sectional survey. Aust Crit Care 2022. https://doi.org/10.1016/J.AUCC.2022. 07.007.

97. Madrigal V, Walter JK, Sachs E, et al. Pediatric continuity care intensivist: A randomized controlled trial. Contemp Clin Trials 2019;76(September 2018):72–8.

98. Leimanis Laurens M, Snyder K, Davis AT, et al. Racial/Ethnic Minority Children with Cancer Experience Higher Mortality on Admission to the ICU in the United States*. Pediatric Critical Care Medicine 2020;859–68. https://doi.org/10.1097/ PCC.0000000000002375.

68. ...

69. ...

70. ...

Rehabilitation Care of the Child with an Acute Severe Traumatic Brain Injury

Matthew J. McLaughlin, MD, MS[a,b,]*, Sathya Vadivelu, DO[a,b],
Kimberly C. Hartman, MD, MHPE[a,b]

KEYWORDS

- Pediatrics • Traumatic brain injury • Prognosis • Disorders of consciousness
- Paroxysmal sympathetic hyperactivity • Rehabilitation

KEY POINTS

- Pediatric patients with traumatic brain injury (TBI) may have a varied recovery depending on the age at the time of injury.[1]
- Rehabilitation of patients with a TBI should begin early during the acute care phase with the identification and management of comorbidities and continue well beyond discharge with the involvement of pediatric physiatrists.
- Complications after TBI require a thorough evaluation of potential causes, optimization of nonpharmacological management, and thoughtful use of medications as needed.
- Providing parental and caregiver education throughout the healing process of TBI allows for grieving to occur and planning for the long-term needs of the patient.

INTRODUCTION

Traumatic brain injury (TBI) is caused by an external force to the head or penetrating injury and results in disruption of the normal functioning of the brain. TBI is the leading cause of death and disability in children and adolescents worldwide.[1] Injury to the developing brain presents unique challenges in the pediatric population, including impact on the rapidly changing social, cognitive, and physical abilities of the child. Although acute medical care is crucial for stabilizing the child and minimizing secondary injury, provision of early rehabilitation management by a pediatric physiatrist for children with severe TBI is critical to minimize long-term sequelae and optimize recovery.

[a] Children's Mercy – Kansas City/University of Missouri, Kansas City School of Medicine, 2401 Gillham Road, Kansas City, MO 64108, USA; [b] Department of Physical Medicine and Rehabilitation, University of Kansas School of Medicine, 3901 Rainbow Blvd, Kansas City, KS 66160, USA
* Corresponding author. Children's Mercy - Kansas City, 2401 Gillham Road, Kansas City, MO 64108.
E-mail address: mjmclaughlin@cmh.edu

Pediatr Clin N Am 70 (2023) 415–428
https://doi.org/10.1016/j.pcl.2023.01.003
0031-3955/23/© 2023 Elsevier Inc. All rights reserved.
pediatric.theclinics.com

Epidemiology

Children and adolescents (birth to 17 years) with TBI accounted for over 640,000 emergency department (ED) visits in 2013.[2] This same group accounted for more than 16,000 hospitalizations in 2019 and nearly 3,000 deaths in 2020.[3] After adults $\geq$ 75 years, children 0 to 4 years and 15 to 24 years have the highest rates of TBI-related ED visits, hospitalizations, and deaths.[1]

Falls, being struck by/against an object, and motor vehicle collisions represent the most common mechanisms of injury in children.[4] Falls are the most common mechanism in younger children, with increasing incidence of sports- and motor vehicle-related injuries in older children.[5] In addition, in children under 12 months of age, abusive head trauma is an unfortunately common etiology of injury (22% of cases).[5] Assault, including firearms, accounts for 10% of TBI-related hospitalizations in adolescents over 15 years old.[5]

Classifying Brain Injury

Brain injury can be classified in several ways, including severity, level of arousal, and imaging findings. Glasgow Coma Scale (GCS), duration of loss of consciousness (LOC), and duration of post-traumatic amnesia (PTA) are used to assess severity as well as prognosis. GCS is used to evaluate the level of consciousness based on best verbal response, motor response, and eye opening. Traditionally, TBI severity is defined as mild (GCS 13 to 15), moderate (GCS 9 to 12), or severe (GCS 3 to 8). Use of GCS score can be confounded by medical comorbidities, variability in prehospital care, and timing of attainment, making it challenging to use in isolation.[6] Duration of LOC and PTA are also used to classify severity, particularly in mild TBI, and track recovery in severe TBI. LOC is defined as the inability to respond to the environment in a meaningful way. PTA is the time after injury in which the individual is unable to form new memories.[6,7]

Level of arousal or consciousness is used to classify clinical status and trajectory of recovery in TBI. Impaired consciousness in TBI is often described by the spectrum of disorders of consciousness (DOC). DOC include coma, unresponsive wakefulness syndrome (UWS; previously referred to as vegetative state), and minimally conscious state (MCS). Each phase is characterized by a certain degree of environmental awareness and functional/clinical features (**Fig. 1**).[8–10] Accurate diagnosis of DOC involves optimizing the environment, minimizing confounding variables, serial examinations, and use of standardized assessment tools.[8]

Outcomes and Prognosis

Given the complexity of the brain and unique details of each injury, predicting recovery remains challenging. Younger children (0 to 4 years), adolescents (15+ years), males, and those injured by suicide or homicide have higher rates of death related to TBI.[2] In addition, children injured at younger ages are at higher risk for worse overall cognitive outcomes.[1,11] Health disparities exist in historically marginalized communities with Black and Hispanic children having increased lengths of hospitalization, lower cognitive scores, and lower health-related quality of life after TBI.[11,12] Lower socioeconomic status has been associated with poorer family functioning and resultant worse outcomes for children with TBI.[13]

Several medical markers can be used to guide prognosis. Higher risk of mortality and severe disability is associated with hypoxia, hypotension, hypothermia, bradycardia, pupillary changes, and chest and abdominal wall injuries.[14,15] Laboratory abnormalities, including hyperglycemia, and coagulopathies are associated with

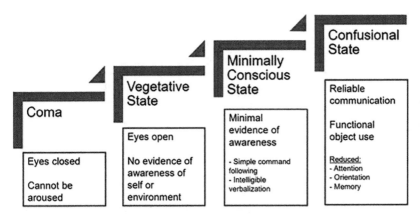

The neurologic stages of recovery progress from coma to posttraumatic confusional state with key

clinical features of each stage listed in the boxes below.

Fig. 1. Classification of disorders of consciousness. Data for this figure were collected from several sources.[8-10] (*Adapted from*: Giacino j, Katz D, Schiff N, Bodien Y. Assessment and Rehabilitation Management of Individuals with Disorders of Consciousness. In:Zasler N, Katz D,Zafonte R, eds. *Brain Injury Medicine: principles and practices*. Springer; 2022:Chap 30.)

worse outcomes.[16,17] Sustained elevations in intracranial pressure (ICP) and decreased cerebral perfusion pressure (CPP) $\leq$ 49 mm Hg lead to death or poorer outcomes.[18] On neuroimaging, deeper location of injury (particularly basal ganglia or brainstem), more severe DAI, and larger number and volume of lesions may predict worse outcomes in children with TBI.[19] Although new diagnostic studies (ie, blood biomarkers, genetic analyses, innovative neuroimaging techniques) show promise, they are not available for large-scale clinical application at this time.[20,21]

Classification of severity by GCS has some predictive value in terms of outcomes and prognosis. Of children with initial GCS 3 to 5, there are higher rates of death and a majority of survivors have a severe disability.[14] In addition, the 72-h motor score may be more predictive than the initial GCS when looking at the severity of disability, with motor scores of 1 to 3 leading to severe disability and scores of 4 to 6 having good recovery or moderate disability 74% of the time.[14,16]

Functional testing in the subacute phase is useful for prognostic discussions related to TBI. Time-to-follow commands (TFC) represent the time from injury until the individual can follow simple verbal commands twice in a 24-h period. In children, TFC > 26 days is associated with poor short- and long-term outcomes on the Glasgow Outcome Scale-Extended, Pediatric Revision (GOS-E Peds), a scale measuring functional independence, capacity for work/school, participation in social and leisure activities, and family and social interactions.[22] In conjunction with TFC, a longer duration of PTA is a strong predictor of outcomes on the GOS-E Peds.[6,22]

Acute Management of Severe Traumatic Brain Injury

Initial management of children with TBI has two primary goals: to stabilize the child quickly and to prevent secondary injury. Severe brain injuries are typically identified in the field and require rapid assessment, stabilization, and treatment of hypotension, hypoxia, and herniation.[23] Ensuring appropriate ventilation, oxygenation, and hemodynamic stability can improve outcomes. In children with severe brain injury, transport to a regional pediatric trauma center may improve survival and ultimately outcomes.[24,25]

After stabilization, critical and acute care management is directed at limiting the cascade of events leading to secondary injury, often in the pediatric intensive care unit (PICU). Guidelines for the management of pediatric severe TBI were updated in 2019 and research is ongoing into critical and acute care strategies (**Box 1**).[26]

Diagnoses and Management of Co-morbidities

Involving brain injury specialists, such as pediatric physiatrists, in the acute phase of recovery is beneficial. Early consultation of physiatry, within 48 h of admission, may lead to improved motor outcomes and significantly shorter acute lengths of stay.[27] Involvement of a brain injury physiatrist can also improve functional outcomes after discharge from rehabilitation and is associated with improved management of neuro-protective medication.[28] In addition, prolonged acute care stays with delayed admission to rehabilitation programs lead to worse functional recovery, highlighting the importance of early rehabilitation involvement for better outcomes.[29]

Given the nature of TBI, multiple neurologic sequalae can result, including posttraumatic seizures (PTS), posttraumatic hydrocephalus (PTH), and neuroendocrine dysfunction. Each comorbidity has symptoms that may overlap with other features of TBI. It is important to involve a brain injury specialist to help distinguish between expected and unexpected progression of symptoms. This will help facilitate early recognition and treatment of the following comorbidities that can arise in the acute phase of severe TBI.

Paroxysmal sympathetic hyperactivity

Paroxysmal sympathetic hyperactivity (PSH) is a common clinical finding during the early stages of acute TBI. Although known by many other names, such as storming, dysautonomia, autonomic instability, or paroxysmal autonomic instability with dysto-nia (PAID), there has been an increasing preference to term this condition PSH. Most frequently, these signs are observed within the first days to weeks after TBI. Chronic forms of PSH can develop, even with treatment.[30]

Key clinical findings of PSH include tachycardia, tachypnea, hypertension, hyper-thermia, diaphoresis, and posturing. PSH is associated with longer stay in the PICU

Box 1
Guidelines for acute management of pediatric severe traumatic brain injury[26]

Highlighted recommendations

Maintain ICP under 20 mm Hg

Maintain CPP between 40 and 50 mm Hg

Maintain normocapnia ($ETCO_2$ 35 to 40 mm Hg)

Avoid hyperventilation (unless significant concern for cerebral herniation)

Maintain systolic blood pressure $\geq$ 90 mm Hg (target of $\geq$ 110 mm Hg may be beneficial in older adolescent population)

Maintain normothermia

Initiate enteral nutrition within 72 h of injury

Abbreviations: CPP, cerebral perfusion pressure; $ETCO_2$, end-tidal carbon dioxide; ICP, intracra-nial pressure.

and higher likelihood of discharge to a rehabilitation setting.[31] As signs and symptoms may overlap, it is important to evaluate for other etiologies, such as seizures, sepsis, untreated pain, malignant hyperthermia, alcohol or sedative withdrawal, or neuroleptic malignant syndrome.

Managing environmental triggers and noxious stimuli can limit or decrease episodes of PSH. Environmental modifications may include decreasing external stimulation (ie, limiting visitors, keeping television off, dimming lights), clustering cares, and avoiding disruptions in sleep. Prompt identification and treatment of potential noxious stimuli, such as constipation, urinary retention, suctioning, and pain, may minimize PSH. Nursing interventions to modify stimuli should be individualized to the child and include the involvement of the family when possible.[32]

Pharmacologic options are frequently considered after environmental modifications. Abortive medications are typically used for severe symptoms and include antipyretics for hyperthermia, short-acting benzodiazepines for tone and posturing, pain medications for discomfort, and antihypertensive agents for hypertension. Medications should be selected based on symptoms and risk tolerance and in consultation with a pediatric brain injury specialist as there are limited studies in children.[33]

Nonselective beta-blockers (ie, propranolol) and alpha-2 agonists (ie, clonidine or dexmedetomidine) decrease catecholamine levels leading to improvements in sympathetic hyperactivity[34] and, in the case of propranolol use in adults with TBI, potentially improved survival.[33,35] Benzodiazepines are often considered for control of motor symptoms, such as posturing.[34] Midazolam, lorazepam, and diazepam are used most frequently because of their short-acting duration.[34] Unfortunately, their negative side effect profile and correlation with poor long-term outcomes limits use.[34] Other medications, such as baclofen, bromocriptine, gabapentin, and dantrolene may be used depending on the symptomatology of PSH and other comorbidities.[33,34] Additional studies are needed to determine the most effective management strategies for PSH, particularly in pediatric TBI.

Motor and tone deficits

Injury to the brain can result in a variety of motor concerns, including weakness, spasticity, dystonia, ataxia, and balance/coordination deficits. Early diagnosis and management can help prevent complications such as contractures, pain, and functional limitations. Weakness is best addressed by early mobility and consultation of physical and occupational therapy.

Spasticity, dystonia, rigidity, and other movement disorders are commonly seen after TBI although exact incidence is not known and hard to predict. The severity may evolve over the course of recovery (often beginning with flaccidity), therefore early and frequent involvement of pediatric physiatrists is beneficial to assess and prescribe appropriate interventions. Conservative measures, such as range of motion exercises, splinting or bracing, and physical and occupational involvement, have minimal adverse effects and should be initiated early to avoid contractures.

Oral baclofen is commonly used for spasticity and dystonia but can be sedating. Mid- or long-acting benzodiazepines are often considered, but risks of sedation and delayed recovery need to be weighed against the benefits. Dantrolene sodium is peripherally acting, thus minimizing potential sedation effects, but can have effects on hepatic function that may limit use. Clonidine and gabapentin also play a role in the management of hypertonicity and may have dual benefit for PSH, neuropathic pain, and arousal, respectively. Intrathecal baclofen and botulinum toxin injections have been used in refractory or global hypertonicity or when focal tone management is preferred. It is important to consider comorbidities when choosing a medication to minimize polypharmacy when able.

Agitation and behavioral concerns

As children progress through different stages of recovery after TBI, agitation may develop. Peak agitation may include motor restlessness or non-purposeful behavior, aggressive behavior, attempts to remove medical devices, increased impulsivity with poor safety awareness, and decreased attention span.

Although agitation after TBI may be unprovoked by external stimuli, it is important to consider iatrogenic contributions that may exacerbate symptoms. Medication or substance withdrawal, pain, and delirium may worsen agitation and should be addressed. In addition, medical complications such as infection or seizures may present with similar behavioral features as agitation. There is an association between altered sleep and agitation; therefore, improving sleep hygiene may help minimize agitation and behavioral concerns.[36–38]

As potential causes are addressed, it is important to keep the child and others safe during agitated episodes. Engage family and staff to provide frequent orientation, direct supervision, and redirection of behaviors. Minimize excessive visual, auditory, and tactile stimuli as able. If the child is not a danger to himself/herself or others, some degree of restlessness can be observed only. In the subacute setting, an enclosure bed may prevent falls. Restraints may be necessary for safety but should be used sparingly as these can worsen agitation. Consultation with a neuropsychologist for behavioral plans and caregiver/staff education may be beneficial.

Medications may be required to ensure safety of the child and others. Generally, medications used for PSH, such as propranolol or clonidine, can be considered for agitation. Antiepileptic agents, such as valproic acid, may reduce agitation symptoms. Antidepressants, including amitriptyline and selective serotonin reuptake inhibitors, may play a role in reducing behavioral concerns and should be considered based on symptoms and premorbid conditions.[33,39] Antipsychotic agents, such as ziprasidone, can be used sparingly and need should be reassessed regularly.[39,40] Benzodiazepines and haloperidol can negatively affect recovery from TBI.[33] Agitation and behavioral symptoms may change quickly during recovery, therefore it is important to engage brain injury experts when prescribing medications to limit potential detrimental effects and maximize outcomes.

Disorders of consciousness

For children with altered arousal and DOC, accurate assessment is critical before treatment strategies are deployed. The pediatric physiatrist starts by assessing and diagnosing stage of recovery (see **Fig. 1**). Standardized tools have been developed to assess DOC and monitor recovery, with the most evidence supporting the Coma Recovery Scale-Revised (CRS-R) in DOC programs.[41] Owing to variability in responsiveness, serial assessments are necessary for accurate diagnosis of DOC.[42] In addition, optimizing the environment, such as positioning the child upright, using adequate lighting, and limiting extraneous stimuli, can promote accurate assessment of arousal.[8]

Once accurate diagnosis is established, interventions can be initiated. Targeted sensory and motor stimulation has been used in treatment of DOC; however, evidence supporting this modality is limited.[43] Medications, such as amantadine, methylphenidate, carbidopa-levodopa, modafinil, and bromocriptine, have been used to promote arousal, albeit mainly off-label and with limited evidence in the pediatric population.[33] Of these, amantadine has the most supporting evidence to promote greater functional improvements in a shorter amount of time in adults with severe TBI.[44] Paradoxically, zolpidem has been shown to improve clinical response in approximately 5% of adults with TBI in a small randomized controlled trial.[45]

Posttraumatic seizures

Disturbance to the brain's architecture and chemical milieu increase the risk for seizures after TBI. A PTS is classified as immediate (within 24 h of injury), early (within 7 days of injury), or late (beyond 7 days postinjury).[46] Infants and children are particularly susceptible to seizures, with PTS confirmed in up to 70% with severe TBI.[26] Risk factors for PTS include younger age, penetrating injury (particularly with retained fragments of bone or metal), depressed skull fracture, cerebral contusions, subdural or epidural hematoma, location of lesion, and focal neurologic deficits.[26] Seizure activity can worsen secondary injury after TBI and is associated with poorer recovery,[47] therefore prophylaxis for 7 days is recommended.[26] Although there is limited evidence, levetiracetam or phenytoin/fosphenytoin are generally recommended for prophylaxis. It is important to note that early PTS is a risk factor for posttraumatic epilepsy (PTE), early prophylaxis does not prevent development of PTE, and children with TBI remain at higher risk for PTS/PTE long-term.[48] It is important to monitor for subclinical seizures, as symptoms may overlap with other neurologic sequalae of TBI.

Posttraumatic hydrocephalus

Ventricular enlargement, also known as ventriculomegaly, can be seen after severe TBI. Ventriculomegaly may be related to ex vacuo changes or hydrocephalus (**Fig. 2**). With ex vacuo changes, there is compensatory enlargement of the cerebrospinal fluid (CSF) due to loss of brain parenchyma secondary to TBI and imaging reveals large ventricles with diffuse cerebral atrophy and prominent sulci. No intervention is required for ex vacuo ventriculomegaly as there is no associated increase in ICP.

In contrast, hydrocephalus is ventricular enlargement associated with increased ICP. PTH requires acute intervention and occurs in approximately 1% of children hospitalized with TBI.[49] PTH may be caused by decreased CSF absorption or by

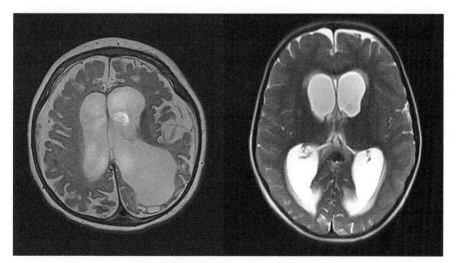

Fig. 2. Brain magnetic resonance imaging of hydrocephalus ex vacuo (left) compared with hydrocephalus. Note ex vacuo changes have deep sulci and brain atrophy compared with hydrocephalus, which is characterized by enlarged ventricles with transependymal flow.

obstruction of CSF flow. Symptoms of PTH in infants include bulging fontanelle, separation of cranial sutures, irritability, emesis, and headache. In older children with severe TBI, PTH should be suspected when there is regression or change in skills/progress, persistent PSH, or increase in muscle tone without explanation.[50] Acute management includes CSF diversion, typically via external ventricular drain or ventriculoperitoneal shunt.

Neuroendocrine disorders

Pituitary function may be disrupted in 5% to 61% of children with severe brain injury.[51,52] Problems can arise with acute and chronic endocrinopathies,[51] notably with growth hormone, gonadotropin, and Adrenocorticotropic Hormone (ACTH).[51] Close monitoring is required as symptoms may overlap with other common complications, such as fatigue, irritability, or abnormal weight gain. Although there are no consistent guidelines, symptom and laboratory monitoring is recommended acutely after injury, at 3 months, 6 months, and annually for 5 years after injury.[51] Clinical and laboratory monitoring help monitor for these problems (**Table 1**).[51]

Disorders of sodium regulation can be seen after TBI although exact incidence is unknown. Hyponatremia may have symptoms that are common in brain injury, such as confusion, headache, nausea, vomiting, or seizures. It can be caused by the syndrome of inappropriate diuretic hormone or cerebral salt wasting. Diagnoses can be made by serum sodium and hydration status. Diabetes insipidus presents with hypernatremia and increased urine output. Prompt diagnosis and treatment can minimize complications (**Table 2**).

Heterotopic ossification

Heterotopic ossification (HO) is the abnormal formation of bone in soft tissue and may be seen in up to 14% of children with severe TBI.[53] Older age (over 11 years), diffuse brain injury, longer duration of DOC, PSH, and spasticity are associated with higher risk for HO formation.[53–55] The hip is the most common location for HO after TBI followed by the knee, shoulder, and elbow.[53,54] Symptoms include warmth, tenderness, and swelling of the affected joint along with potential limitation in range of motion or wound of the overlying skin.[53] Triple-phase bone scan detects early HO, often before clinical symptoms seem.[56] Treatment involves range of motion, non-steroidal anti-inflammatory drugs, bisphosphonates, and potentially surgery and/or radiation to the site.[56]

Venous thromboembolism

Deep vein thrombosis (DVT) and pulmonary embolism (PE) are types of venous thromboembolism (VTE). Generally more common in adults, children with severe TBI are at

Table 1	
Assessment of neuroendocrine function after severe traumatic brain injury[51]	
Height	AM Cortisol
Weight	Free T4
Pubertal Staging	Thyroid Stimulating Hormone (TSH)
Thorough Review of systems	Insulin-like Growth Factor (IGF-1)
	Prolactin
	Follicle Stimulating Hormone (FSH)[a]
	Luteinizing Hormone (LH)[a]
	Testosterone or estradiol[b]

[a] In pubertal children.
[b] Based on gender.

Table 2
Common sodium abnormalities after traumatic brain injury

	DI	SIADH	CSW
Serum Na	Increased	Decreased	Decreased
Serumosmolality	Increased	Decreased	Decreased
Urine osmolality	Decreased	Increased	Increased or normal
Serum ADH	Decreased	Increased (inappropriately high)	Decreased
Extracellular volume	Normal or decreased	Normal	Decreased

Abbreviations: ADH, antidiuretic hormone; CSW, central salt wasting; DI, diabetes insipidus; Na, sodium; SIADH, syndrome of inappropriate antidiuretic hormone secretion.

risk for VTE.[57] Immobility, use of central venous catheters, mechanical ventilation, and acute traumatic coagulopathy are additional risk factors for VTE.[57] Children under 3 years of age or post-pubertal may be at higher risk along with those with abusive mechanisms of injury.[57]

Symptoms of DVT may include extremity swelling, erythema, and pain, whereas PE may present with shortness of breath, chest pain, cough, hemoptysis, tachypnea, or tachycardia.[58] Doppler venous ultrasound is used to diagnose DVT and computed tomography (CT) pulmonary angiogram can diagnose PE. Chemical prophylaxis is recommended in children with low risk of bleeding who are over 15 years old or post-pubertal and Injury Severity Score greater than 25.[59] Mechanical prophylaxis is generally recommended although has limited supporting evidence.[59] Treatment of VTE in children with TBI is similar to children without TBI and should be managed by a hematologist.

Gastrointestinal disorders
Children with TBI are at risk for gastrointestinal disorders, such as neurogenic bowel, constipation, and delayed motility, and may have concomitant bowel injuries.[60] Early nutrition is recommended for optimal recovery[26] and constipation or delayed motility may decrease tolerance to feeds. Swallow should be assessed by a speech or occupational therapist before initiating oral diet or liquids to ensure safety and avoid aspiration.[60] Finally, fecal incontinence is addressed as the child is cognitively able to participate or through a carefully timed bowel program.[60]

Genitourinary disorders
Children with TBI are also at risk for bladder dysfunction, including urinary retention and incontinence.[60] Often, an indwelling catheter may be necessary for fluid management and evidence of dysfunction may not present until after the catheter is removed. Urine output, including volume and time of void and post-void residual, should be monitored carefully until the child is consistently emptying spontaneously. Intermittent catheterization may be required to avoid urinary tract infections and overdistension of the bladder, which can trigger PSH and agitation. Timed voids may be necessary when working on continence.

Education and Support of the Family/Guardian
A severe TBI is life-changing for the child and family. Acutely, caregivers are often left with conflicting emotions of shock, hope, and denial.[61] Caregiver education and involvement in medical and rehabilitation care is critical for the grieving process and to better understand their child's current and future needs.[61] Given that pediatric

physiatrists provide care throughout the spectrum of recovery, they are uniquely positioned to provide education acutely and discuss subacute and long-term prognosis. Neuropsychologists, psychologists, family therapists, and social workers may also address some of these areas and provide support to the child and caregivers throughout the recovery process.[61]

Subacute and Long-Term Rehabilitation Management

The effects of TBI last well beyond the acute phase with heterogeneity in functional outcomes and recovery. An intensive inpatient rehabilitation program may be recommended to maximize function, address and minimize complications, and provide additional family education and support before discharging home.[62] It is important to consider programs that specialize in pediatric brain injury, which include a comprehensive team focused on the child and caregivers: pediatric physiatrists, nurses, pediatric therapists, neuropsychologists, teachers, child life specialists, social workers, care managers, and more. The child will participate in an average of 3 h or more of therapy daily, including physical, occupational, and speech therapy services. Once medically stable, children with DOC may benefit from intensive inpatient DOC-specific rehabilitation programs to optimize stimulation and medications as well as provide education, training, and equipment for ongoing needs. Depending on function and tolerance to therapy, outpatient or in-home therapy services may be recommended. The pediatric physiatrist can assist with appropriate disposition.

SUMMARY

Injury to the developing brain has global implications acutely and long-term. Children with severe TBI benefit from prompt stabilization and diligent acute care management to minimize the impact of secondary injury and maximize outcomes. Rehabilitation of the child with severe TBI begins after injury and includes assessing for and managing complications such as PSH, hypertonicity, agitation, and impaired arousal. In addition, the pediatric physiatrist is specially trained to recognize and prevent complications and provide robust family and patient education. Rehabilitation continues into the subacute and chronic phases of TBI and long-term follow-up is vital for optimizing function.

CLINICS CARE POINTS

- Including a pediatric physiatrist in the care of patients with traumatic brain injury (TBI) has been shown to improve clinical outcomes.[28]
- Although prognostication after TBI remains challenging, shorter time-to-follow commands and post-traumatic amnesia are favorable.[6]
- Managing paroxysmal sympathetic hyperactivity and agitation should start with removing potentially noxious stimuli.
- Long-term monitoring and management of complications help to facilitate the most optimal outcomes.

DISCLOSURE

The authors have nothing to disclose.

REFERENCES

1. Tavano A, Galbiati S, Recla M, et al. Cognitive recovery after severe traumatic brain injury in children/adolescents and adults: similar positive outcome but different underlying pathways? Brain Inj 2014;28(7):900–5.
2. Centers for Disease Control and Prevention. Report to congress: the management of traumatic brain injury in children. Atlanta, GA: National Center for Injury Prevention and Control; Division of Unintentional Injury Prevention; 2018.
3. CfDCa Prevention. TBI Data. Centers for Disease Control and Prevention. 2022. Available at: https://www.cdc.gov/traumaticbraininjury/data/. Updated March 21, 2022. Accessed October 16, 2022.
4. Taylor CA, Bell JM, Breiding MJ, et al. Traumatic Brain Injury-Related Emergency Department Visits, Hospitalizations, and Deaths - United States, 2007 and 2013. MMWR Surveill Summ 2017;66(9):1–16.
5. Thurman DJ. The Epidemiology of Traumatic Brain Injury in Children and Youths: A Review of Research since 1990. J Child Neurol 2016;31(1):20–7.
6. Suskauer SJ, Slomine BS, Inscore AB, et al. Injury severity variables as predictors of WeeFIM scores in pediatric TBI: Time to follow commands is best. J Pediatr Rehabil Med 2009;2(4):297–307.
7. Ewing-Cobbs L, Levin HS, Fletcher JM, et al. The Children's Orientation and Amnesia Test: relationship to severity of acute head injury and to recovery of memory. Neurosurgery 1990;27(5):683–91, discussion 691.
8. Giacino J, Katz D, Schiff N, et al. Assessment and Rehabilitation Management of Individuals with Disorders of Consciousness. In: Brain injury medicine: principles and practices. New York, NY: Springer; 2022. p. 30.
9. Multi-Society Task Force on PVS. Medical aspects of the persistent vegetative state (1). N Engl J Med 1994;330(21):1499–508.
10. Giacino JT, Ashwal S, Childs N, et al. The minimally conscious state: definition and diagnostic criteria. Neurology 2002;58(3):349–53.
11. Jimenez N, Ebel BE, Wang J, et al. Disparities in disability after traumatic brain injury among Hispanic children and adolescents. Pediatrics 2013;131(6): e1850–6.
12. Haider AH, Efron DT, Haut ER, et al. Black children experience worse clinical and functional outcomes after traumatic brain injury: an analysis of the National Pediatric Trauma Registry. J Trauma 2007;62(5):1259–62, discussion 1262-1263.
13. Anderson V, Godfrey C, Rosenfeld JV, et al. Predictors of cognitive function and recovery 10 years after traumatic brain injury in young children. Pediatrics 2012; 129(2):e254–61.
14. Michaud LJ, Rivara FP, Grady MS, et al. Predictors of survival and severity of disability after severe brain injury in children. Neurosurgery 1992;31(2):254–64.
15. Vavilala MS, Bowen A, Lam AM, et al. Blood pressure and outcome after severe pediatric traumatic brain injury. J Trauma 2003;55(6):1039–44.
16. Tude Melo JR, Rocco FD, Blanot S, et al. Mortality in Children With Severe Head Trauma: Predictive Factors and Proposal for a New Predictive Scale. Neurosurgery 2010;67(6):1542–7.
17. Elkon B, Cambrin JR, Hirshberg E, et al. Hyperglycemia: an independent risk factor for poor outcome in children with traumatic brain injury. Pediatr Crit Care Med 2014;15(7):623–31.
18. Carter BG, Butt W, Taylor A. ICP and CPP: excellent predictors of long term outcome in severely brain injured children. Child's Nerv Syst 2008;24(2):245–51.

19. Suskauer SJ, Huisman TA. Neuroimaging in pediatric traumatic brain injury: current and future predictors of functional outcome. Dev Disabil Res Rev 2009;15(2): 117–23.

20. Maas AIR, Menon DK, Adelson PD, et al. Traumatic brain injury: integrated approaches to improve prevention, clinical care, and research. Lancet Neurol 2017;16(12):987–1048.

21. Caliendo ET, Kim N, Edasery D, et al. Acute Imaging Findings Predict Recovery of Cognitive and Motor Function after Inpatient Rehabilitation for Pediatric Traumatic Brain Injury: A Pediatric Brain Injury Consortium Study. J Neurotrauma 2021;38(14):1961–8.

22. Davis KC, Slomine BS, Salorio CF, et al. Time to Follow Commands and Duration of Posttraumatic Amnesia Predict GOS-E Peds Scores 1 to 2 Years After TBI in Children Requiring Inpatient Rehabilitation. J Head Trauma Rehabil 2016;31(2): E39–47.

23. Viamonte M, Madikians A, Giza C. Pediatric neurocritical care: special considerations. In: Zasler N, editor. Brain injury medicine principles and practice. 3rd edition. New York, NY: Demos Medical; 2021.

24. Potoka DA, Schall LC, Gardner MJ, et al. Impact of pediatric trauma centers on mortality in a statewide system. J Trauma 2000;49(2):237–45.

25. Bardes JM, Benjamin E, Escalante AA, et al. Severe traumatic brain injuries in children: Does the type of trauma center matter? J Pediatr Surg 2018;53(8): 1523–5.

26. Kochanek PM, Tasker RC, Carney N, et al. Guidelines for the management of pediatric severe traumatic brain injury, Third Edition: Update of the Brain Trauma Foundation Guidelines. Pediatr Crit Care Med 2019;20(3S Suppl 1):S1–82.

27. Wagner AK, Fabio T, Zafonte RD, et al. Physical medicine and rehabilitation consultation: relationships with acute functional outcome, length of stay, and discharge planning after traumatic brain injury. Am J Phys Med Rehabil 2003; 82(7):526–36.

28. Greiss C, Yonclas PP, Jasey N, et al. Presence of a dedicated trauma center physiatrist improves functional outcomes following traumatic brain injury. J Trauma Acute Care Surg 2016;80(1):70–5.

29. Tepas JJ 3rd, Leaphart CL, Pieper P, et al. The effect of delay in rehabilitation on outcome of severe traumatic brain injury. J Pediatr Surg 2009;44(2):368–72.

30. Baguley IJ, Perkes IE, Fernandez-Ortega JF, et al. Paroxysmal sympathetic hyperactivity after acquired brain injury: consensus on conceptual definition, nomenclature, and diagnostic criteria. J Neurotrauma 2014;31(17):1515–20.

31. Alofisan TO, Algarni YA, Alharfi IM, et al. Paroxysmal Sympathetic Hyperactivity After Severe Traumatic Brain Injury in Children: Prevalence, Risk Factors, and Outcome. Pediatr Crit Care Med 2019;20(3):252–8.

32. Letzkus L, Keim-Malpass J, Anderson J, et al. Paroxysmal Sympathetic Hyperactivity in Children: An Exploratory Evaluation of Nursing Interventions. J Pediatr Nurs 2017;34:e17–21.

33. Pangilinan PH, Giacoletti-Argento A, Shellhaas R, et al. Neuropharmacology in pediatric brain injury: a review. PM & 2010;2(12):1127–40.

34. Pozzi M, Conti V, Locatelli F, et al. Paroxysmal Sympathetic Hyperactivity in Pediatric Rehabilitation: Pathological Features and Scheduled Pharmacological Therapies. J Head Trauma Rehabil 2017;32(2):117–24.

35. Cotton BA, Snodgrass KB, Fleming SB, et al. Beta-blocker exposure is associated with improved survival after severe traumatic brain injury. J Trauma 2007; 62(1):26–33 ; discussion 33-35.

36. Stocker RPJ, Khan H, Henry L, et al. Effects of Sleep Loss on Subjective Complaints and Objective Neurocognitive Performance as Measured by the Immediate Post-Concussion Assessment and Cognitive Testing. Arch Clin Neuropsychol 2017;32(3):349–68.

37. Nguyen S, McKay A, Wong D, et al. Cognitive Behavior Therapy to Treat Sleep Disturbance and Fatigue After Traumatic Brain Injury: A Pilot Randomized Controlled Trial. Archives of Physical Medicine and Rehabilitation 2017;98(8): 1508–1517 e2.

38. Sullivan KA, Blaine H, Kaye SA, et al. A Systematic Review of Psychological Interventions for Sleep and Fatigue after Mild Traumatic Brain Injury. J Neurotrauma 2018;35(2):195–209.

39. Luaute J, Plantier D, Wiart L, et al. Care management of the agitation or aggressiveness crisis in patients with TBI. Systematic review of the literature and practice recommendations. Annals of Physical and Rehabilitation Medicine 2016; 59(1):58–67.

40. Hicks AJ, Clay FJ, Hopwood M, et al. Efficacy and Harms of Pharmacological Interventions for Neurobehavioral Symptoms in Post-Traumatic Amnesia after Traumatic Brain Injury: A Systematic Review. J Neurotrauma 2018;35(23):2755–75.

41. American Congress of Rehabilitation Medicine BI-ISIGDoCTF, Seel RT, Sherer M, et al. Assessment scales for disorders of consciousness: evidence-based recommendations for clinical practice and research. Archives of Physical Medicine and Rehabilitation 2010;91(12):1795–813.

42. Giacino JT, Katz DI, Schiff ND, et al. Practice guideline update recommendations summary: Disorders of consciousness: Report of the Guideline Development, Dissemination, and Implementation Subcommittee of the American Academy of Neurology; the American Congress of Rehabilitation Medicine; and the National Institute on Disability, Independent Living, and Rehabilitation Research. Neurology 2018;91(10):450–60.

43. Lombardi F, Taricco M, De Tanti A, et al. Sensory stimulation of brain-injured individuals in coma or vegetative state: results of a Cochrane systematic review. Clin Rehabil 2002;16(5):464–72.

44. Giacino JT, Whyte J, Bagiella E, et al. Placebo-controlled trial of amantadine for severe traumatic brain injury. N Engl J Med 2012;366(9):819–26.

45. Whyte J, Rajan R, Rosenbaum A, et al. Zolpidem and restoration of consciousness. American Journal of Physical Medicine & Rehabilitation 2014;93(2):101–13.

46. Yablon SA. Posttraumatic seizures. Archives of Physical Medicine and Rehabilitation 1993;74(9):983–1001.

47. Ates O, Ondul S, Onal C, et al. Post-traumatic early epilepsy in pediatric age group with emphasis on influential factors. Child's Nervous System 2006;22(3): 279–84.

48. Tanaka T, Litofsky NS. Anti-epileptic drugs in pediatric traumatic brain injury. Expert Rev Neurother 2016;16(10):1229–34.

49. Rumalla K, Letchuman V, Smith KA, et al. Hydrocephalus in Pediatric Traumatic Brain Injury: National Incidence, Risk Factors, and Outcomes in 124,444 Hospitalized Patients. Pediatr Neurol 2018;80:70–6.

50. Weintraub AH, Gerber DJ, Kowalski RG. Posttraumatic Hydrocephalus as a Confounding Influence on Brain Injury Rehabilitation: Incidence, Clinical Characteristics, and Outcomes. Archives of Physical Medicine and Rehabilitation 2017;98(2): 312–9.

51. Reifschneider K, Auble BA, Rose SR. Update of Endocrine Dysfunction following Pediatric Traumatic Brain Injury. J Clin Med 2015;4(8):1536–60.

52. Casano-Sancho P. Pituitary dysfunction after traumatic brain injury: are there definitive data in children? Arch Dis Child 2017;102(6):572–7.
53. Hurvitz EA, Mandac BR, Davidoff G, et al. Risk factors for heterotopic ossification in children and adolescents with severe traumatic brain injury. Archives of Physical Medicine and Rehabilitation 1992;73(5):459–62.
54. Kluger G, Kochs A, Holthausen H. Heterotopic ossification in childhood and adolescence. J Child Neurol 2000;15(6):406–13.
55. Bargellesi S, Cavasin L, Scarponi F, et al. Occurrence and predictive factors of heterotopic ossification in severe acquired brain injured patients during rehabilitation stay: cross-sectional survey. Clin Rehabil 2018;32(2):255–62.
56. Brady RD, Shultz SR, McDonald SJ, et al. Neurological heterotopic ossification: Current understanding and future directions. Bone 2018;109:35–42.
57. Leeper CM, Vissa M, Cooper JD, et al. Venous thromboembolism in pediatric trauma patients: Ten-year experience and long-term follow-up in a tertiary care center. Pediatr Blood Cancer 2017;64(8). https://doi.org/10.1002/pbc.26415.
58. Radulescu VC, D'Orazio JA. Venous Thromboembolic Disease in Children and Adolescents. Advances in experimental medicine and biology 2017;906:149–65.
59. Mahajerin A, Petty JK, Hanson SJ, et al. Prophylaxis against venous thromboembolism in pediatric trauma: A practice management guideline from the Eastern Association for the Surgery of Trauma and the Pediatric Trauma Society. J Trauma Acute Care Surg 2017;82(3):627–36.
60. Evanson N, Babcock L, Kurowski B. Pediatric traumatic brain injury: special considerations. In: Zasler N, editor. Brain injury medicine: principles and practices. 3rd edition. New York, NY: Demos Medical; 2021.
61. Gan C, Depompei R. Pediatric traumatic brain injury: special considerations. In: Zasler N, editor. Brain injury medicine: principles and practices. 3rd edition. New York, NY: Demos Medical; 2021.
62. Gao S, Treble-Barna A, Fabio A, et al. Effects of inpatient rehabilitation after acute care on functional and quality-of-life outcomes in children with severe traumatic brain injury. Brain Inj 2022;1–8. https://doi.org/10.1080/02699052.2022.2120211.

Evaluation, Treatment, and Outcomes of Viral and Autoimmune Encephalitis in Children

Joshua A. Vova, MD[a,b,c,*], Robyn A. Howarth, PhD[b,c]

KEYWORDS

- Encephalitis • Viral encephalitis • Autoimmune encephalitis
- Anti-NMDA receptor body encephalitis • Acute disseminated encephalomyelitis
- Outcomes • Rehabilitation • Treatment

KEY POINTS

- Viruses are the most common cause of infectious encephalitis; however, autoimmune encephalitis occurs nearly as frequently and our ability to identify new autoantibodies is constantly expanding.
- Identification of the cause of an encephalitis is a combination of laboratory results, clinical history, as well as systemic and neurologic symptoms.
- Early identification and treatment of autoimmune encephalitides may help improve outcomes.
- Encephalitis in childhood is associated with an increased risk for acute and long-term neurologic and cognitive sequelae.

INTRODUCTION

Encephalitis is an inflammation of the brain parenchyma that results in a clinical syndrome and associated neurologic dysfunction.[1] Although encephalitis is commonly viral or autoimmune in origin, it can also be caused by other pathogens, such as bacteria or fungi.[2] Viral encephalitis is the most common type of encephalitis in children and adolescents, with a high rate of both morbidity and mortality.[3] The incidence of viral encephalitis in children is approximately 7 per 100,000 per year in the United States,[4] increasing to 16 per 100,000 children worldwide.[5] Autoimmune encephalitis

a Department of Physical Medicine and Rehabilitation, Children's Healthcare of Atlanta, 1001 Johnson Ferry Road Northeast, Atlanta, GA 30342, USA; b Department of Neuropsychology, Children's Healthcare of Atlanta, 5461 Meridian Mark Road NE, Atlanta, GA 30342, USA; c Department of Pediatrics, Division of Neurology, Emory University School of Medicine
* Corresponding author. Department of Neuropsychology, Children's Healthcare of Atlanta, 5461 Meridian Mark Road NE, Atlanta, GA 30342.
E-mail address: Joshua.Vova@CHOA.org

Pediatr Clin N Am 70 (2023) 429–444
https://doi.org/10.1016/j.pcl.2023.01.007
0031-3955/23/© 2023 Elsevier Inc. All rights reserved.

(AE) is often triggered by a viral central nervous system (CNS) infection[6,7] and at 11.6 per 100, 000[8] has nearly the same prevalence in children as infectious encephalitis. If the leptomeninges and the brain parenchyma are both involved, this is known as a meningoencephalitis. Parainfectious encephalitis occurs when a systemic viral infection causes a febrile encephalopathy.[7] In this case, there may be inflammation of the cerebral spinal fluid (CSF) but no direct invasion of virus into the brain.[7] Regardless of type or origin, encephalitis is a significantly debilitating neurologic disorder that can have long-lasting repercussions on patients and their families.

General Clinical Presentation of Viral Encephalitis

The classic presentation for an encephalitis starts with a "flu-like" prodrome that is followed by severe headaches, nausea, vomiting, and altered consciousness. Other common symptoms include seizures, cranial neuropathies, cognitive changes, and movement disorders.[9,10] One factor that helps distinguish viral encephalitis from other pathogens is that it tends to present acutely or subacutely.[10] Viral encephalitis also may start with a systemic presentation such as a fever or rash. In 2013, the International Encephalitis Consortium published criteria for diagnosis of a viral encephalitis to assist in early recognition[9] (**Box 1**).

Pathophysiology

A viral encephalitis will occur as an uncommon complication of a common infection, such as herpes virus or as a characteristic complication of a rare virus, such as rabies.[10] When the virus reaches the brain parenchyma, the cells such as neurons, astrocytes, and microglia, may become infected, promoting the secretion of proinflammatory molecules and the subsequent immune cell infiltration that leads to brain injury, seizures, and behavioral changes.[11] After resolving the viral infection, the local immune response can remain active, contributing to long-term neuropsychiatric disorders, neurocognitive impairment, and degenerative diseases.[12]

Diagnosis of encephalitis

A diagnosis of viral encephalitis is confirmed by a combination of CSF, electroencephalogram (EEG), and brain MRI. The International Encephalitis Consortium has suggested an algorithm for an initial encephalitis workup[9] (**Box 2**). CSF will demonstrate pleocytosis and high protein levels with normal glucose.[13] CSF cultures and polymerase chain reaction (PCR) assays are useful in trying to determine the

---

Box 1
International Encephalitis Consortium Diagnosis Criteria for Encephalitis

Major criteria (required).
  Altered mental status at the time of presentation lasting greater than 24 h. Altered mental status defined as lethargy, personality change or altered level of consciousness. No alternative cause of mental status change identified

Minor criteria (2 for possible and 3 or greater for probable or confirmed encephalitis).
  Fever of greater than 38° that occurred 72 h prior or after presentation
  New focal neurologic findings
  New seizures not attributed to an earlier seizure disorder
  CSF contains at least 5 or more WBC per cubic millimeter
  New abnormality on electroencephalograph that is consistent with encephalitis
  Neuroimaging that demonstrates an abnormality in the brain parenchyma consistent with encephalitis

Reference:[9]

Box 2
Routine studies

CSF
    Obtain opening pressure, WBC with differential, RBC, protein, glucose
    Send for Gram Stain and bacterial Culture
    HSV-1/2 PCR, consider HSV IgG and IgM
    Enterovirus PCR
    Oligoclonal bands
    Additional tests based on clinical signs, eg, autoimmune encephalitis if neuropsychiatric
    signs, VZV if vesicular rash or arbovirus based on season and possible exposures
    Collect at least 5 mL of CSF and freeze unused portion

Serum
    Routine blood cultures
    EBV serology (viral capsid antigen antibody [VCA IgG] and IgM and epstein barr virus nuclear
    antigen antibody [EBNA IgG])
    Mycoplasma pneumonia IgM and IgG
    Hold acute serum and collect convalescent serum for paired antibody testing

Imaging
    MRI

EEG
    Mycoplasma PCR from throat
    Enterovirus PCR and/or culture from throat and stool
    Other tissue biopsy of skin lesions, bronchoalveolar lavage and/or endobronchial biopsy in
    those with pneumonia/pulmonary lesions, throat swab PCR/culture in those with upper
    respiratory illness; stool culture in those with diarrhea

Reference:[9]

---

causative agent. However, a specific virus is implicated less than 50% of the time.[14] Although mentioned in the 2013 International Encephalitis Consortium, autoimmune encephalitis was not recognized as prevalent but, based on current information, it should also be considered in initial workup based on symptomology. In contrast to viral encephalitis, less than 50% of patients with autoimmune encephalitis will have an elevated white blood cell count in their CSF.[8] Based on clinical symptomology, consider testing for commonly recognized autoimmune antibodies to N-methyl-D-aspartate receptor (NMDA), gamma-aminobutyric acid (GABA) A and B, alpha-amino-3-hydroxy-5-methyl-4-isoxazoleprponic acid (AMPAR) or dopamine −2 (D2) receptor antibodies.[8,15] It is advisable to freeze an additional initial sample should initial testing be unrevealing and new information or a broader clinical workup is warranted.[10]

Neuroimaging is used in the initial diagnostic workup for patients with encephalitis, with MRI being more sensitive and specific compared with CT; however, initial neuroimaging may be normal or even remain normal throughout the disease course despite clinical symptoms and/or functional deficits. Although neuroimaging may not always assist with identifying a specific cause, some characteristic neuroimaging patterns are associated with specific viral agents (eg, herpes simplex virus [HSV], acute disseminated encephalomyelitis [ADEM], enterovirus). Brain MRIs may show characteristic findings specific to viruses or autoimmune encephalitis (**Table 1**). In the absence of MRI findings or inflammatory markers in the CSF, a patient may be diagnosed with encephalitis.[9] The presence of an initial or concurrent infection and clinical signs of encephalopathy with focal neurologic deficits raises the possibility of an immune-mediated encephalopathy affecting the brain.[16]

Table 1
MRI characteristics of common viral encephalitis

Virus	MRI Findings
HSV	Asymmetric abnormalities in the medial temporal lobe, cingulate gyrus, orbital surface of frontal lobes. May have associated edema, restricted diffusion or hemorrhage
Japanese Encephalitis (JEV)	Thalamus, substantia nigra, basal ganglia
Varicella Zoster virus (VZV)	Lesions in brainstem, cerebellum, and or temporal lobes. May have ischemic or hemorrhagic lesions in white matter or gray–white junction
Enterovirus	Typically normal or have brainstem abnormalities EV 71: Dorsal pons, medulla, midbrain, dentate nucleus of cerebellum May also show demyelination and necrosis
HHV-6	Medial temporal lobes, thalamus, hippocampus. Cerebral edema
Influenza	Usually normal but can manifest as an acute necrotizing encephalopathy with bilateral thalamic regions. May also show lesions on splenium of corpus callosum
Respiratory Syncytial virus	Diffuse cerebral edema; infarctions, or hemorrhage
Arbovirus (WNV, Eastern equine encephalitis, St Louis encephalitis, and so forth)	Brainstem involvement; basal ganglia and/or thalamus. Also has leptomeningeal involvement
Zika virus	Cortical edema and hyperintense T2 lesions in the cortical and subcortical white matter
ADEM	Multifocal abnormalities in the subcortical white matter, involvement may be seen in brain stem, thalamus, or basal ganglia
ANMADRE	Increased signal on T2-weighted flair in the medial aspect of the temporal lobes

References.[1,9,10,23–25]

Electroencephalography (EEG) may be important in the evaluation of patients with encephalitis, both in clinical treatment and identification of a causative agent.[13] Seizures in children with encephalitis may be subtle or masked by movement disorders. Uncontrolled seizures can lead to an increase in intracranial pressure (ICP) directly or indirectly by increasing metabolic activity, acidosis, or vasodilation.[2] In approximately 80% of patients with viral encephalitis, the EEG will be abnormal. Some forms of encephalitis may have more characteristic EEG findings. For example, delta brush may be associated with anti-NMDA receptor encephalitis (ANMDARE),[17,18] and periodic lateralizing epileptiform discharges in the temporal lobes are associated with HSV encephalitis[19]; however, these findings are considered suggestive not diagnostic. EEG may also be predictive of outcomes. A study by Mohammad and colleagues found that nonreactive EEG background was predictive of a poor outcome and shifting focal seizure patterns was more predictive of a drug refractory epilepsy in children with viral meningitis.[20]

Causes of viral encephalitis
There are various causes of viral encephalitis. HSV is the most common cause of viral encephalitis, occurring globally in 2 to 4 cases per million people each year.[12] In the

United States, HSV remains the most common cause of viral encephalitis followed by West Nile virus and enteroviruses.[21] Other notable viral etiologic agents include Epstein-Barr virus (EBV), cytomegalovirus (CMV), varicella-zoster virus (VZV), measles virus, mumps virus, rubella virus, and human herpes virus (HHV)-6 and HHV-7.[21] Arboviruses, more endemic to the United States, also include Eastern equine, Western equine, St. Louis, Venezuelan equine, Zika, and West Nile.[21] In addition, new viruses are constantly emerging and spreading as evidenced by recent outbreaks such as West Nile virus, Zika virus, and severe acute respiratory syndrome coronavirus 2 (SARS-CoV-2).

The epidemiology of a virus may be related to patient risk factors, seasonal occurrence, animal exposure, and/or geographic location, especially with arboviruses and enterovirus.[7,10] Often findings on history and physical examination may provide clues to the possible cause of the encephalitis (see **Table 1**; **Table 2**). Enteroviruses, mumps, and rabies may demonstrate a clinical picture of brainstem abnormalities or lower cranial neuropathies.[2,13] In children with movement disorders, consider viruses that are likely to infect the basal ganglia such as arboviruses, Japanese encephalitis, or West Nile virus (WNV).[2] If the patient has a movement disorder, which is also associated with psychiatric symptoms or oral facial dyskinesias, consider anti-NMDA receptor body encephalitis or a limbic encephalitis.[2,22] Focal limb weakness that accompanies an encephalitis may be associated with enteroviruses or ADEM.[10] Focal deficits may be a sign of a stroke due to inflammatory monocytes from HSV or WNV,[23] AE,[22] or from a hypercoagulable state that follows SARS-CoV-2[24] **(Table 3)**.

Immune-Mediated Encephalitis

Immune-mediated encephalitis can present similarly to viral encephalitis and can be triggered by an initial viral infection.[8] Immune-mediated encephalopathy occurs when neuronal autoantibodies bind to proteins in the brain that are crucial for normal function. The most described pediatric immune-mediated encephalitides are AE and ADEM. If the synaptic proteins are affected, then the patient will present with neurologic and with neuropsychological symptoms such as movement disorders, psychiatric symptoms, and seizures, such as in ANMARE.[11] ADEM occurs when the antibodies are directed against myelin and myelin-associated proteins.[11]

Postviral infections can cause neuronal injury and the release of intracellular antigens and debris. This excess debris may be due to poor clearance of apoptotic debris,

Table 2	
Viral encephalitis based on clinical presentation	
Symptoms	**Possible Viral Agent**
Cranial nerve involvement	HSV, EBV
Ataxia	VZV, EBV, mumps
Dementia	Measles, HIV
Polio-like flaccid myelitis	Polio, enterovirus, JEV, WNV
Movement disorders	JEV, WNV
Retinitis	CMV, WNV,
Rash	VZV, HHV-6, WNV, rubella, HIV, enterovirus, SARS-CoV-2
Respiratory	Influenza, SARS-CoV-2
Parotitis	Mumps
Lymphadenopathy	HIV, EBV, CMV, measles rubella, WNV

References.[6,10,26,27]

Table 3
Clinical Symptoms Associated with Viral Eitiology

Virus Type	Example	Clinical Symptoms
Arbovirus	WNV, Zika	Headache, high fevers, muscle aches, confusion, seizures, poor coordination, coma
Rhabdovirus	Rabies	Fever, hypersalivation, swallowing difficulty, throat pain, organ failure, coma
Enterovirus	EV-71	Fever, headaches, respiratory, vomiting diarrhea, autonomic dysfunction, cardiopulmonary failure
Herpesvirus	HSV 1 and 2	Fever, headaches, seizures, focal neurologic deficits
Orthomyxovirus	Influenza	Febrile seizures, ataxia
Orthopneumovirus	HHV	Headache, dizziness, confusion, loss of taste and smell
Coronavirus	SARS-CoV-1 and 2	Headache, dizziness, loss of taste and smell

References.[6,10,26,27]

inflammation-mediated modification of self-antigen, or cross-reactivity between foreign and self-antigens.[25] As a result, the created autoantibodies are brain-restricted "neoantigens."[15] These antigens are antibody-specific B cells in the lymph nodes that then mature into plasma cells.[15] This inflammatory response may be nonspecific, which is why autoantibodies are found not only in NMDA but $GABA_A$, $GABA_B$, AMPAR, and D_2 at the same time.[15] Although antibodies against the N-methyl-D-aspartate receptor (NMDAR) are the most prevalent and well known, the list of known AE-associated antibodies is constantly growing. Amange and colleagues demonstrated that autoimmune encephalitis occurred in 27% of patients with herpes simplex encephalitis.[12] Of the patients identified with an AE, 64% had ANMDARE, with one patient having a coexisting $GABA_A$ receptor antibody, and the remaining 36% were unidentified. An expert consensus proposed a criteria to help clinicians determine a clinical diagnosis and consider treatment options before the results of antibody testing[22] (**Box 3**). Unlike viral encephalitis, AE has available treatments to reduce

Box 3
Diagnostic Criteria for Autoimmune Encepahlitis

Diagnostic criteria for autoimmune encephalitis:

All 3 criteria must be met.

1. Subacute onset, rapid progression of less than 3 mo of working memory deficits, altered level of consciousness, lethargy, personality change of psychiatric symptoms

2. At least 1 of the following
   a. New focal CNS findings
   b. CSF pleocytosis (WBC >5 cells/mm³)
   c. New onset seizures
   d. MRI suggestive of encephalitis

3. Reasonable exclusion of other causes

Reference.[28]

symptoms and lessen sequelae. Early recognition and treatment of AE is important in maximizing potential recovery.[8,16,26]

Anti-N-Methyl-ᴅ-Aspartate Receptor Encephalitis

The most recognized AE is ANMDARE. ANMDARE is widely identified as the most common AE in children and occurs more than 4 times more frequently than HSV-1, VZV, or VZV.[27,28] Similar to viral encephalitis, ANMDARE typically begins with a "flu-like" syndrome that includes fever, nausea, vomiting, headache, and fatigue.[29] After the prodrome, 87% of patients will demonstrate neuropsychiatric and autonomic symptoms.[30] Symptoms include seizures, movement disorders, behavior and speech problems, disorders of consciousness, hypoventilation, and autonomic instability.[31] Common neuropsychiatric features include irritability, mutism, behavioral regression, hallucinations, aggression, agitation, and depression. It is estimated that between 50% and 75% of patients are initially seen by a psychiatrist,[29,32–34] and 40% of patients were first hospitalized in a psychiatric facility.[35]

Treatment is primarily with immunotherapies such as corticosteroids, intravenous immunoglobulins, plasmapheresis (PLEX), rituximab, and cyclophospha-mide.[30,31,36,37] Often second-line treatments are needed, as it has been documented that first-line treatment was unsuccessful in 44% to 69% of patients.[30,38] In pediatric patients who have relapsing symptoms, choreoathetosis is most common.[15]

Acute Disseminated Encephalomyelitis

ADEM is considered a postinfectious, monophasic inflammatory demyelinating disease that affects the brain, optic nerves, and spinal cord with acute encephalopathy at onset as well as associated cognitive deficits.[39–41] ADEM is predominantly a pediatric disorder that presents with a mean age of onset ranging from 5 to 8 years.[40] ADEM is distinguished from other demyelinating diseases in that it is a first episode with no new signs, symptoms, or MRI findings 3 months after onset.[41] ADEM occurs days to weeks after an acute febrile illness or respiratory tract infection. Patients with more than 1 ADEM-like event have ongoing autoimmunity, consistent with antibodies against myelin oligodendrocyte glycoprotein antibodies, which differentiate them from classic ADEM.[41] Recently, there have been case studies associated with SARS-CoV-2.[42,43]

ADEM typically presents with behavioral changes, altered mental status, fever, vomiting, and headaches. There may also be focal neurologic defects that are related to the areas in the brain that correspond to the demyelinating lesions. Common deficits include movement disorders, hemiparesis, ataxia, dysphagia, visual changes, and cranial neuropathies.[44,45] About 25% of patients may have spinal cord involvement as well.[44]

CSF in patients with ADEM can be normal or show increased lymphocytic pleocytosis and/or increased proteins. It is the absence of oligoclonal bands, which is important in distinguishing it from multiple sclerosis.[45] An MRI of the brain is crucial in identifying T2-hyperintense lesions that are multifocal, irregular, and poorly margin-ated. The lesions typically involve the subcortical and central white matter throughout the brain and are predominately found in the frontal and temporal lobes.[45] Treatment of ADEM consists of high-dose steroids, intravenous immunoglobulin, and plasma exchange.[41,44] Other medications such as cyclophosphamide have been used in refractory cases.[44]

Although AE and ADEM have similar initial presenting symptoms and treatment strategies, patients with AE tend to require second-line immunotherapy more often, have longer hospital stays, and have a higher percentage of neurologic disability at hospital discharge.[46] When discharged from the hospital, 26% patients with ADEM and 30.8% of patients with AE were sent to an inpatient rehabilitation program. However, 47.8% of patients with ADEM and 30.8% of patients with AE were discharged to an outpatient rehabilitation program.[46]

Treatment

Initial treatment in treating encephalitis is with a broad-spectrum antibiotic until bacterial causes can be ruled out completely. Children who have lethargy, seizures, mucocutaneous vessels, CSF pleocytosis, hepatomegaly, thrombocytopenia, ascites, and/or elevated transaminases should be carefully monitored.[47] Furthermore, HSV PCR may have a false-negative, especially in early disease and in children.[9] If HSV is still suspected, based on clinical findings, the HSV PCR can be repeated in 3 to 7 days.[9] It is recommended that in all cases of sporadic viral encephalitis, acyclovir be started immediately.[1] Acyclovir should be completed until HSV is ruled out or another diagnosis is established. When started early, acyclovir has been shown to significantly decrease mortality and morbidity and limit the severity of long-term behavioral and cognitive impairments.[21]

Increased ICP is a common cause of mortality in children with encephalitis. Patients with a Glasgow Coma Scale (GCS) score less than 8, in status epilepticus, or having clinical signs of increased ICP, such as tonic posturing, should be treated in the intensive care unit (ICU). Close monitoring of acid–base and electrolytes as well as measures to decrease ICP, such as mannitol, hypertonic saline and seizure management should be instituted.[48] Hatachi and colleagues performed a retrospective cohort study on 9386 children with acute encephalitis to determine prognostic factors.[49] They identified the following factors as unfavorable outcomes: patients aged 12 to 18 years, congenital anomalies, epilepsy, lower levels of consciousness, 2 or more intravenous antiepileptic drugs, mechanical ventilation, vasoactive agents, steroid therapy, and immunoglobulin use.[49] However, they found that HSV infection, influenza virus, and mannitol/glycerol use were associated with favorable outcomes.[49]

The sequalae of encephalitis can result in functional declines in motor skills, self-care skills, and cognition. Once the patient is stabilized, initial issues that should be addressed include feeding, prevention of venous thrombosis, sleep hygiene, and early mobilization.[44] The introduction of a rehabilitation team consisting of a pediatric physiatrist in conjunction with the physical therapist, occupational therapist, and speech language pathologist may improve outcomes. Early introduction of a physiatrist into a trauma service significantly reduced medical complications such as pressure injury, joint contracture, deep venous thrombosis, urinary tract infections, delirium, and pneumonia.[50] Due to the degree of illness and immobility in children with encephalitis, early intervention with a pediatric physiatrist may be able to help prevent medical complications, optimize reintroduction of mobility and function, as well as addressing movement disorders and neuropsychiatric symptoms.

One of the challenging medical aspects of managing pediatric patients with encephalitis is the accompanying neuropsychiatric symptoms. The pediatric physiatrist is often challenged with the task of managing behavior while not further disrupting the patient's cognitive processes. In patients who have autoimmune encephalitis, pathways crucial for normal function are inhibited, creating the neurologic and neurophysiological symptoms.[11] As a result, pharmacologic treatment of symptoms may result in deleterious outcomes. Patients with ANDMARE are at risk for developing fever, rigidity, and autonomic instability that may mimic neuroleptic malignant syndrome.[20,51–53] One study found that 58% of children with ANMDARE who received antipsychotics had adverse reactions.[20] As previously noted, autoantibodies from viral encephalopathies can cause disruption not only in NMDA but also in $GABA_A$, $GABA_B$, AMPAR, and D_2. It may be more advantageous to rely less on psychotropics, and minimizing polypharmacy may provide a more useful strategy to manage behavior and allow for more meaningful interactions with their rehabilitation program.[51] Agitation is the most common reason for the use of polypharmacy.[20,38] Two separate studies cited that an average of 8 medications were used for symptom management, with agitation being the problem most needing treatment.[20,38] Before the use of chemical restraints, the focus should be on strategies useful for patients with brain injuries, such as reducing overstimulation, clustering care, reducing physical restraints, focusing on sleep hygiene, and environment evaluation.[51,54,55] It is important to recognize that patients with encephalitis often have erratic behavior that may compel the use of chemical restraints in the critical care setting to deliver necessary care. It is necessary to recognize the potentially deleterious effects some medications may play in the recovery from encephalopathies.

Rehabilitation

The goal of the pediatric physiatrist is to work collaboratively with other medical subspecialties and the physical, speech, and occupational therapists to improve functional outcomes. There are challenges in creating therapy protocols due to the significant heterogeneity in the population, relative infrequency of these patients in rehabilitation programs, and variability in the level of impairment.[56–58] An experienced rehabilitation team that focuses on family-centered, goal-directed care to patients and their families will be able to determine appropriate rehabilitation goals and treatment plans. Pediatric patients with encephalitis commonly require inpatient rehabilitation due to cognitive-linguistic, motor, and/or functional deficits.

In a previous case series examining the functional status of children with various forms of encephalitis in an inpatient rehabilitation setting, Tailor and colleagues concluded that patients demonstrated significant improvement in functional gains throughout admission but there was a wide range in patients' degree of recovery.[58] A more recent review of long-term outcomes from childhood encephalitis revealed long-term deficits in approximately half of children, particularly with regard to developmental delays, abnormal behavior, motor dysfunction, and seizures.[59] A retrospective review of 99 pediatric patients who had suspected encephalitis were followed for an average of 29 months. Approximately 50% of these patients developed neurologic sequelae. In that cohort of patients, 47.9% were found to have learning problems, 39.6% had developmental delay, 20.8% had behavioral problems but only 4% had motor deficits.[60] There was a correction with children who were readmitted after their acute illness and those who developed epilepsy and the development of neurologic sequelae. A retrospective study of 93 children admitted to the hospital in Stockholm, Sweden, between 2000 and 2004 demonstrated that 60% of patients had sequelae at discharge from hospital.[61] Some of these were mild symptoms such as fatigue but in 24% of cases, symptoms included cognitive impairment, dysphasia, motor impairment, ataxia, or epilepsy.[61] Long-term complications include dystonia, spasticity, epilepsy, ataxia, neurocognitive, and behavioral problems, some of which are not recognized until after the acute phase of the illness subsided.[61]

Similar to viral encephalitis, patients with AE have similar patterns in recovery. Findings revealed good progress during inpatient rehabilitation for pediatric patients with ANMDARE, despite functional deficits at discharge.[62–64] Younger age at disease onset, the presence of seizures, and higher number of treatments received were associated with poorer functioning during the initial months of recovery following inpatient rehabilitation.[63] Results showed that a minority of these patients demonstrated minimal to no functional gains early in recovery. Faster improvements may be seen in mobility and self-care skills compared with cognition during the acute phase of recovery. Recently, a case series reported on the rehabilitation of 6 children with ANMDARE. All these children made progress during inpatient rehabilitation but all demonstrated persistent functional deficits at the time of discharge. Similarly in ADEM, motor symptoms are the predominant focus but tend to recover well; however, it is the social and cognitive deficits that persist.[65]

Broad Outcomes

In general, viral encephalitis produces inflammation of the brain that tends to diffusely affect the white matter. Cognitive, motor, and functional deficits will vary based on the location and extent of brain disruption. Brain injury may be caused by the virus itself or secondary to an immune-mediated response elicited by a virus, immunization, or other antigens. Some viruses tend to impact certain brain regions Two separate studies identified risk factors for more severe and/or persistent cognitive deficits include younger age at onset, seizures at presentation, ICU admission, focal signs on neurologic examination, abnormal neuroimaging, confirmed infectious cause, and/or longer length of admission.[66,67] Given the fastest rate of recovery is often seen within the first 6 to 12 months, previous research suggests the benefit of ongoing monitoring for at least the first year following diagnosis to monitor the manifestation of sequalae at different developmental stages.[66,67] Severity of impairments in pediatric patients tends to be greatest in infants aged younger than 1 year, with an increased risk of cognitive impairment compared with other causes. HSV encephalitis is associated with a higher incidence of personality and/or emotional disturbance in early recovery as well as long-term behavioral difficulties and personality changes. Children with a history of encephalitis are more likely to display increased risk for developmental delays, behavior problems, and/or neurologic sequelae, such as seizures.[59] Younger age at diagnosis, seizures and lethargy at onset, abnormal neuroimaging or EEG findings, and delayed initiation of acyclovir treatment have been shown to be associated with poorer outcomes over time.[68,69] Persistent weakness, motor difficulties, swallowing problems, academic issues, intellectual disability, impaired language, vision problems, developmental delay, behavioral and sleep difficulties highlight the need for continued follow-up from the rehabilitation team once they are discharged from the hospital.[59,66,70,71]

Long-term outcomes are similar in immune-mediated encephalitis. In a recent systematic review of both adult and pediatric patients, cognitive deficits were identified in a majority of cases ($\sim$80%), with higher rates of dysfunction noted earlier in the disease course.[72] Younger age at disease onset, the presence of seizures, and higher number of treatments received were associated with poorer functioning during the initial months of recovery following inpatient rehabilitation.[63] Results showed that a minority of these patients demonstrated minimal to no functional gains early in recovery. Faster improvements may be seen in mobility and self-care skills compared with cognition, particularly during the acute phase of recovery.

The most commonly reported core deficits are in the areas of executive functioning and memory, with deficits being cited in attention/working memory, language, fine motor speed, emotional–behavioral functioning, and social cognition.[29,72–76] Persistent deficits were recently reported in sustained attention and fatigue, with associated academic performance problems and reduced quality of life.[27] Younger age at onset has been shown to be associated with worse outcomes over time. A recent study found that infants and toddlers (aged younger than 3 years) clinically present with movement disorders, developmental regression, and/or abnormal behaviors.[77] Younger patients diagnosed with ANMDARE were found to have a higher rate of cooccurring viral encephalitis, which was a risk factor for poor outcome. Compared with patients who were aged older than 3 years at the time of onset, infants and toddlers displayed poorer outcomes at long-term follow-up.[77] In addition to younger age, risk factors associated with poor clinical outcome have included abnormal neuroimaging findings, seizures, and/or sensorimotor deficit at onset as well as delayed diagnosis and/or initiation of treatment.[74,78,79] Despite overall favorable clinical outcomes, cognitive problems may persist in pediatric anti-NMDARE, particularly in the areas of executive functioning, memory, language, and behavioral-emotional functioning.

Despite limited research, previous studies suggest that pediatric patients with ADEM are at risk for cognitive deficits, with varying rates of impairment being reported.[80–83] Despite limited studies, the most common cognitive deficits have been found in the areas of processing speed, attention/executive functioning, and (short-term) memory with associated deficits in academic performance particularly for children with a younger age at onset.[84,85] Other difficulties have been reported with aspects of language (expressive vocabulary, verbal retrieval, and naming), visuomotor integration, and visual matching.[80,86] A wide range of cognitive deficits may be observed, with more notable risks reported for processing speed and attention. With the recent coronavirus disease 2019 pandemic, emerging research is now examining outcomes for ADEM associated with SARS-CoV-2 infection. A recent review of patients (~20% were aged younger than 18 years) found that patients with SARS-CoV-2-ADEM may have a longer duration to symptom onset, be older in age, display a slower rate and extent of recovery as well as a higher risk of poor outcome compared with classic ADEM.[43]

SUMMARY

Encephalitis in childhood is associated with an increased risk for acute and long-term neurologic and cognitive sequelae based on a variety of factors. The fastest rate of recovery tends to be seen early in the disease course, although patients may still display functional deficits, even after inpatient rehabilitation. Cognitive domains that tend to be most affected include processing speed, attention/executive functioning, and memory. Additional deficits have been reported with aspects of language, fine motor functioning, and emotional–behavioral functioning in addition to deficits associated with neuroimaging findings. Risk factors for poor outcomes, regardless of cause, include younger age at onset, the presence of complicating medical factors (eg, seizures, abnormal neuroimaging, or EEG findings), and delayed initiation of treatment. The fact that many children have persistent deficits indicates the need for ongoing rehabilitative services to maximize functional skills, make adaptations for functional deficits, and assist with community integration. The existing literature highlights the importance of ongoing monitoring of patients over time to better understand the trajectory of recovery as well as to identify appropriate interventions.

CLINICS CARE POINTS

- Recognition of viral and autoimmune encephalitis have increased in recent years. A thoughtful clinical evaluation is crucial to determining the cause of the encephalitis and guiding further diagnostic work-up.

- Empiric treatment with acyclovir should be considered in all cases until HSV or VZV are eliminated from the differential.

- Autoimmune encephalitides have available treatments and early recognition is imperative to reduce symptoms, and sequalae as well maximizing recovery.

- Although gross motor recovery tends to be favorable, there is a significant risk of fine motor, cognitive, and neuropsychiatric symptoms that persist after a viral or autoimmune encephalitis infection. This may result in a need for persistent rehabilitation services to maximize outcomes.

DECLARATION OF INTERESTS

The authors declare no competing interests.

REFERENCES

1. Tunkel AR, Glaser CA, Bloch KC, et al. The management of encephalitis: Clinical practice guidelines by the Infectious Diseases Society of America. Clin Infect Dis 2008;47(3):303–27.
2. Thompson C, Kneen R, Riordan A, et al. Encephalitis in children. Arch Dis Child 2012;97(2):150–61.
3. Costa BK da, Sato DK. Viral encephalitis: a practical review on diagnostic approach and treatment. J Pediatr 2020;96:12–9.
4. Vora NM, Holman RC, Mehal JM, et al. Burden of encephalitis-associated hospitalizations in the United States , 1998 – 2010. Neurology 2014;82(5):443–51.
5. Johnson RT. Acute Encephalitis. Clin Infect Dis. 1996;23(2):219–24.
6. Bohmwald K, Andrade CA, Gálvez NMS, et al. The Causes and Long-Term Consequences of Viral Encephalitis. Front Cell Neurosci 2021;15(11):1–19.
7. Aksamit AJ. Treatment of Viral Encephalitis. Neurol Clin 2021;39(1):197–207.
8. Dubey D, Toledano M, Mckeon A. Clinical presentation of autoimmune and viral encephalitides 2018;24(2):80–90.
9. Venkatesan A, Tunkel AR, Bloch KC, et al. Case definitions, diagnostic algorithms, and priorities in encephalitis: Consensus statement of the international encephalitis consortium. Clin Infect Dis 2013;57(8):1114–28.
10. Venkatesan A, Murphy OC. Viral Encephalitis. Neurol Clin 2018;36(4):705–24.
11. Wright SK, Wood AG. Neurodevelopmental outcomes in paediatric immune-mediated and autoimmune epileptic encephalopathy. Eur J Paediatr Neurol 2020;24:53–7.
12. Armangue T, Spatola M, Vlagea A, et al. Frequency, symptoms, risk factors, and outcomes of autoimmune encephalitis after herpes simplex encephalitis: a prospective observational study and retrospective analysis. Lancet Neurol 2018; 17(9):760–72.
13. Kneen R, Michael BD, Menson E, et al. Management of suspected viral encephalitis in children - Association of British Neurologists and British Paediatric Allergy, Immunology and Infection Group National Guidelines. J Infect 2012;64(5): 449–77.
14. Singh TD, Fugate JE, Rabinstein AA. The spectrum of acute encephalitis: Causes, management, and predictors of outcome. Neurology 2015;84(4): 359–66.
15. Prüss H. Postviral autoimmune encephalitis: Manifestations in children and adults. Curr Opin Neurol 2017;30(3):327–33.
16. Dale RC, Gorman MP, Lim M. Autoimmune encephalitis in children: Clinical phenomenology, therapeutics, and emerging challenges. Curr Opin Neurol 2017; 30(3):334–44.

17. Schmitt SE, Pargeon K, Frechette ES, et al. Extreme Delta Brush :A unique EEG pattern in adults with anti-NMDA receptor encephalitis. Neurology 2012;79: 1094–100.
18. Baykan B, Gungor Tuncer O, Vanli-Yavuz EN, et al. Delta Brush Pattern Is Not Unique to NMDAR Encephalitis: Evaluation of Two Independent Long-Term EEG Cohorts. Clin EEG Neurosci 2018;49(4):278–84.
19. Kennedy PGE. Viral encephalitis: Causes, differential diagnosis, and management. Neurol Pract 2004;75(Suppl-1). https://doi.org/10.1136/jnnp.2003.034280.
20. Mohammad SS, Jones H, Hong M, et al. Symptomatic treatment of children with anti-NMDAR encephalitis. Dev Med Child Neurol 2016;58(4):376–84.
21. Said S, Kang M. Viral encephalitis. StatPearls; 2022. Available at: https://www.ncbi.nlm.nih.gov/books/NBK470162/.
22. Graus F, Titulaer MJ, Balu R, et al. A clinical approach to diagnosis of autoimmune encephalitis. Lancet Neurol 2016;15(4):391–404.
23. Terry RL, Getts DR, Deffrasnes C, et al. Inflammatory monocytes and the pathogenesis of viral encephalitis. J Neuroinflammation 2012;9(1):1.
24. Ray STJ, Abdel-mannan O, Sa M, et al. Neurological manifestations of SARS-CoV-2 infection in hospitalised children and adolescents in the UK : a prospective national cohort study. Lancet Child Adoolesc Heal 2021;5:631–41.
25. Suurmond J, Diamond B. Autoantibodies in systemic autoimmune diseases : specificity and pathogenicity. J Clin Invest 2015;125(6). https://doi.org/10.1172/JCI78084.but.
26. Broadley J, Seneviratne U, Beech P, et al. Prognosticating autoimmune encephalitis: A systematic review. J Autoimmun 2018;96(October 2018):24–34.
27. De Bruijn MAAM, Bruijstens AL, Bastiaansen AEM, et al. Pediatric autoimmune encephalitis. Neurol Neuroimmunol Neuroinflamm 2020;7:e682.
28. Gable MS, Sheriff H, Dalmau J, et al. The frequency of autoimmune N-methyl-D-aspartate receptor encephalitis surpasses that of individual viral etiologies in young individuals enrolled in the california encephalitis project. Clin Infect Dis 2012;54(7):899–904.
29. Dalmau J, Gleichman AJ, Hughes EG, et al. Anti-NMDA-receptor encephalitic: case series and analysis of the effects of antibodies. Lancet Neurol 2008;7(12): 1091–8.
30. Titulaer MJ, McCracken L, Gabilondo I, et al. Treatment and prognostic factors for long-term outcome in patients with anti-NMDA receptor encephalitis: An observational cohort study. Lancet Neurol 2013;12(2):157–65.
31. Bartolini L, Muscal E. Differences in treatment of anti-NMDA receptor encephalitis: results of a worldwide survey. J Neurol 2017;264(4):647–53.
32. Maat P, De Graaff E, Van Beveren NM, et al. Psychiatric phenomena as initial manifestation of encephalitis by anti-NMDAR antibodies. Acta Neuropsychiatr 2013;25(3):128–36.
33. Gibson LL, Pollak TA, Blackman G, et al. The Psychiatric Phenotype of Anti-NMDA Receptor Encephalitis. J Neuropsychiatry Clin Neurosci 2019;31(1):70–9.
34. Zhang M, Li W, Zhou S, et al. Clinical features, treatment, and outcomes among Chinese children with anti-methyl-d-aspartate receptor (Anti-NMDAR) encephalitis. Front Neurol 2019;10(JUN):1–9.
35. Lejuste F, Thomas L, Picard G, et al. Neuroleptic intolerance in patients with anti-NMDAR encephalitis. Neurol - Neuroimmunol Neuroinflammation 2016;3(5):e280.
36. Ryan N. Anti-N-Methyl-d-Aspartate Receptor-Mediated Encephalitis: Recent Advances in Diagnosis and Treatment in Children. Curr Probl Pediatr Adolesc Health Care 2016;46(2):58–61.

37. Sartori S, Nosadini M, Cesaroni E, et al. Paediatric anti-N-methyl-d-aspartate receptor encephalitis: The first Italian multicenter case series. Eur J Paediatr Neurol 2015;19(4):453–63.
38. Alvarez G, Krentzel A, Vova J, et al. Pharmacologic Treatment and Early Rehabilitation Outcomes in Pediatric Patients With Anti-NMDA Receptor Encephalitis. Arch Phys Med Rehabil 2021;102(3):406–12.
39. Tenembaum SN. 3rd edition. Acute Disseminated Encephalomyelitis, 112. Amsterdam: Elsevier B.V; 2013.
40. Pohl D, Tenembaum S. Treatment of acute disseminated encephalomyelitis. Curr Treat Options Neurol 2012;14(3):264–75.
41. Pohl D, Aloer G, Van Haren K, et al. Acute disseminated encephalomyelitis: Updates on an inflammatory CNS syndrome. Neurology 2016;87(Suppl 2):S38–45.
42. Siracusa L, Cascio A, Giordano S, et al. Neurological complications in pediatric patients with SARS-CoV-2 infection: a systematic review of the literature. Ital J Pediatr 2021;47(1). https://doi.org/10.1186/s13052-021-01066-9.
43. Wang Y, Wang Y, Huo L, et al. SARS - CoV - 2 - associated acute disseminated encephalomyelitis : a systematic review of the literature. J Neurol 2022;269(3): 1071–92.
44. Massa S, Fracchiolla A, Neglia C, et al. Update on acute disseminated encephalomyelitis in children and adolescents. Children 2021;8(280):1–17.
45. Esposito S, Di Pietro GM, Madini B, et al. A spectrum of inflammation and demyelination in acute disseminated encephalomyelitis (ADEM) of children. Autoimmun Rev 2015;14(10):923–9.
46. Mcgetrick ME, Varughese NA, Miles DK, et al. Pediatric Neurology Clinical Features , Treatment Strategies , and Outcomes in Hospitalized Children With Immune-Mediated Encephalopathies. Pediatr Neurol 2021;116:20–6.
47. Autore G, Bernardi L, Perrone S, et al. Update on viral infections involving the central nervous system in pediatric patients. Children 2021;8(9):1–13.
48. Aneja S, Sharma S. Diagnosis and Management of Acute Encephalitis in Children. Indian J Pediatr 2019;86(1):70–5.
49. Hatachi T, Michihata N, Inata Y, et al. Prognostic Factors among Children with Acute Encephalitis/Encephalopathy Associated with Viral and Other Pathogens. Clin Infect Dis 2021;73(1):76–82.
50. Robinson LR, Tam AKHH, MacDonald SL, et al. The Impact of Introducing a Physical Medicine and Rehabilitation Trauma Consultation Service to an Academic Level I Trauma Center. Am J Phys Med Rehabil 2018;98(1):1.
51. Vova JA. A narrative review of pharmacologic approaches to symptom management of pediatric patients diagnosed with anti-NMDA receptor encephalitis. J Pediatr Rehabil Med 2021;14(3):333–43.
52. Wang J, Zhang B, Zhang M, et al. Comparisons between Psychiatric Symptoms of Patients with Anti-NMDAR Encephalitis and New-Onset Psychiatric Patients. Neuropsychobiology 2018;75(2):72–80.
53. Dalmau J, Lancaster E, Martinez-Hernandez E, et al. Clinical experience and laboratory investigations in patients with anti-NMDAR encephalitis. Lancet Neurol 2011;10(1):63–74.
54. Luauté J, Plantier D, Wiart L, et al. Care management of the agitation or aggressiveness crisis in patients with TBI. Systematic review of the literature and practice recommendations. Ann Phys Rehabil Med 2016;59(1):58–67.
55. Plantier D, Hamonet J, Wiart L, et al. Non pharmacological treatments for psychological and behavioural disorders following traumatic brain injury (TBI). A

systematic literature review and expert opinion leading to recommendations. Ann Phys Rehabil Med 2016;59(1):31–41.

56. Christie S, Chan V, Mollayeva T, et al. Rehabilitation interventions in children and adults with infectious encephalitis: A systematic review protocol. BMJ Open 2016;6(3):1–5.

57. Moorthi S, Schneider WN, Dombovy ML, et al. Rehabilitation outcomes in encephalitis - a retrospective study 1990-1997. Brain Inj 2009;13(2):139–46.

58. Tailor Y, Suskauer SJ, Sepeta LN, et al. Functional status of children with encephalitis in an inpatient rehabilitation setting: A case series. J Pediatr Rehabil Med 2014;6(3):163–73.

59. Khandaker G, Jung J, Britton PN, et al. Long-term outcomes of infective encephalitis in children : a systematic review and meta-analysis. Dev Med Child Neurol 2016;58:1108–15.

60. Rismanchi N, Gold JJ, Sattar S, et al. Neurological outcomes after presumed childhood encephalitis. Pediatr Neurol 2015;53(3):200–6.

61. Fowler Å, Stödberg T, Eriksson M, et al. Childhood encephalitis in Sweden: Etiology, clinical presentation and outcome. Eur J Paediatr Neurol 2008;12(6):484–90.

62. Houtrow A, BHANDAL M, Prantini N, et al. The Rehabilitation of Children with AntiYN-methyl-D-aspartateYReceptor Encephalitis:A Case Series. Am J Phys Med Rehabil 2012;91(5):435–41.

63. Howarth RA, Vova J, Blackwell LS. Early Functional Outcomes for Pediatric Patients Diagnosed with Anti-NMDA Receptor Encephalitis during Inpatient Rehabilitation. Am J Phys Med Rehabil 2018;98(7):529–35.

64. Zelada-Ríos L, Pacheco-Barrios K, Galecio-Castillo M, et al. Acute disseminated encephalomyelitis and COVID-19: A systematic synthesis of worldwide cases. J Neuroimmunol 2021;359(July).

65. Sunnerhagen KS, Johansson K, Ekholm S. Rehabilitation problems after acute disseminated encephalomyelitis: Four cases. J Rehabil Med 2003;35(1):20–5.

66. Fowler Å, Stödberg T, Eriksson M, et al. Long-term outcomes of acute encephalitis in childhood. Pediatrics 2010;126(4):e828–35.

67. Michaeli O, Kassis I, Shachor-Meyouhas Y, et al. Long-term motor and cognitive outcome of acute encephalitis. Pediatrics 2014;133(3):e546–52.

68. Hsieh W Bin, Chiu NC, Hu KC, et al. Outcome of herpes simplex encephalitis in children. J Microbiol Immunol Infect 2007;40(1):34–8.

69. Genc H, Yalc EU, Öncel S, et al. Clinical outcomes in children with herpes simplex encephalitis receiving steroid therapy. J Clin Virol 2016;80:87–92.

70. Rao S, Elkon B, Flett KB, et al. Long-term outcomes and risk factors associated with acute encephalitis in children. J Pediatric Infect Dis Soc 2017;6(1):20–7.

71. Chow C, Dehority W. Long-Term Outcomes in Children Surviving Tropical Arboviral Encephalitis: A Systematic Review. J Trop Pediatr 2021;67(2):1–10.

72. McKeon GL, Robinson GA, Ryan AE, et al. Cognitive outcomes following anti-N-methyl-D-aspartate receptor encephalitis: A systematic review. J Clin Exp Neuropsychol 2018;40(3):234–52.

73. Peery HE, Day GS, Dunn S, et al. Anti-NMDA receptor encephalitis. The disorder, the diagnosis and the immunobiology. Autoimmun Rev 2012;11(12):863–72.

74. Finke C, Kopp UA, Prüss H, et al. Cognitive deficits following anti-NMDA receptor encephalitis. J Neurol Neurosurg Psychiatry 2012;83(2):195–8.

75. De Bruijn MAAM, Aarsen FK, Van Oosterhout MP, et al. Long-term neuropsychological outcome following pediatric anti-NMDAR encephalitis. Neurology 2018; 90(22):e1997–2005.

76. Wilkinson-Smith A, Blackwell LS, Howarth RA. Neuropsychological outcomes in children and adolescents following anti-NMDA receptor encephalitis. Child Neuropsychol 2022;28(2):212–23.
77. Ren C, Zhang W, Ren X, et al. Clinical Features and Outcomes of Anti-N-Methyl-D-Aspartate Receptor Encephalitis in Infants and Toddlers. Pediatr Neurol 2021; 119(2021):27–33.
78. Raja P, Shamick B, Nitish LK, et al. Clinical characteristics, treatment and long-term prognosis in patients with anti-NMDAR encephalitis. Neurol Sci 2021; 42(11):4683–96.
79. Bartels F, Krohn S, Nikolaus M, et al. Clinical and Magnetic Resonance Imaging Outcome Predictors in Pediatric Anti – N-Methyl-D-Aspartate Receptor Encephalitis. Ann Neurol 2020;88(1):148–59.
80. Kuni BJ, Banwell BL, Till C, et al. Cognitive and Behavioral Outcomes in Individuals With a History of Acute Disseminated Encephalomyelitis (ADEM) Cognitive and Behavioral Outcomes in Individuals With a History of Acute Disseminated Encephalomyelitis (ADEM). Dev Neuropsychol 2012;37(8):682–96.
81. Suppiej A, Cainelli E, Casara G, et al. Pediatric Neurology Long-Term Neurocognitive Outcome and Quality of Life in Pediatric Acute Disseminated Encephalomyelitis. Pediatr Neurol 2014;50(4):363–7.
82. Kanmaz S, Köse S, Eraslan C, et al. Neuropsychological outcome in cases with acute disseminated encephalomyelitis. Turk J Pediatr 2020;62(4):594–605.
83. Beatty C, Bowler RA, Farooq O, et al. Pediatric Neurology Long-Term Neurocognitive , Psychosocial , and Magnetic Resonance Imaging Outcomes in Pediatric-Onset Acute Disseminated Encephalomyelitis. Pediatr Neurol 2016;57:64–73.
84. Tan A, Hague C, Greenberg BM, et al. Neuropsychological outcomes of pediatric demyelinating diseases: a review. Child Neuropsychol 2018;24(5):575–97.
85. Hahn CD, Miles BS, Macgregor DL, et al. Neurocognitive Outcome After Acute Disseminated Encephalomyelitis. Pediatr Neurol 2003;8994(03):117–23.
86. Elbin RJ, Beatty A, Covassin T, et al. A preliminary examination of neurocognitive performance and symptoms following a bout of soccer heading in athletes wearing protective soccer headbands. Res Sport Med 2015;23(2):203–14.

Return to Learn After Traumatic Brain Injury

Michael Dichiaro, MD*, David Baker, PsyD, ABPP-CN, Sarah J. Tlustos, PhD, ABPP-CN

KEYWORDS

- Traumatic brain injury • Pediatric • Concussion • Learn • School • Educational

KEY POINTS

- Preparing a child or teen and the school for a successful return to the educational setting after traumatic brain injury (TBI) is an important aspect of the management of pediatric brain injury and has been shown to impact functional outcomes.
- The nature and severity of the TBI, as well as age at onset, has implications for recovery and both short- and long-term educational needs.
- Educational supports may range from temporary, informal adjustments to accommodations and interventions formalized through 504 plans or Individualized Education Programs (IEPs).
- Familiarity with educational law, processes, and mechanisms for securing various educational interventions and supports is important for the pediatrician or primary care provider to guide families in accessing free and appropriate educational resources to improve outcomes and increase equity in resource access.

BACKGROUND

When a child suffers a brain injury, the pediatrician is often tasked with managing the impacts of the brain injury, including how to return the child to their normal activities. A key part of this is facilitating the return to school process, which is critical for the child's recovery and ongoing development. Acquired brain injury is common in children with trauma as the most common cause, although other causes include infection, hypoxia/ischemia, surgery, cancer, and immunologic/inflammatory conditions. There are approximately 1.7 million pediatric traumatic brain injuries (TBIs) per year leading to 474,000 pediatric Emergency Department visits, 35,000 hospitalizations, and approximately 2200 deaths per year.[1] On the milder end of the TBI spectrum, concussions represent the most prevelant form of TBI. The actual prevalence of concussion in children and teens is difficult to determine. Some estimates indicate a yearly incidence of approximately 1.5 to 2 million youth concussions in the United States[2] with other epidemiologic studies estimating a concussion prevalence of approximately 3.6% to 7.0% for children ages 3 to 17 years and from 6.5% to 18.3% for adolescents 13 to 17 years.[3]

Department of Rehabilitation, University of Colorado School of Medicine, Children's Hospital Colorado, 13123 East 13th Avenue B 285, Aurora, CO, USA
* Corresponding author.
E-mail address: mike.dichiaro@childrenscolorado.org

Pediatr Clin N Am 70 (2023) 445–460
https://doi.org/10.1016/j.pcl.2023.01.004
0031-3955/23/© 2023 Elsevier Inc. All rights reserved.
pediatric.theclinics.com

There are several characteristics of the child's TBI that can help inform the child's prognosis and return to school. Initially, after the injury, the mechanism and severity of the injury are important. Duration of loss of consciousness, Glasgow Coma Scale/Pediatric GCS, duration of post-traumatic amnesia,[4] and time to follow commands[5] are commonly used to categorize the severity of the injury. The child's initial clinical course (including the need for intensive care, intubation, seizures, neurosurgical interventions, etc.), advanced imaging findings, and the rate of initial functional improvement is also important. Younger age and greater severity of TBI have been shown to be indicators of more severe cognitive deficits.[6,7]

Educational Law and Available Supports

There are various tiers of support available for students with an acquired brain injury (**Table 1**). Informal school adjustments are often implemented for those with milder injuries who might only require short-lived and minor accommodations or supports. However, with more significant or lasting injuries, a formal education plan often is warranted. The two major types of formalized education plans come from different aspects of federal law and offer different supports (**Table 2**). A 504 plan is derived from the Rehabilitation Act (1973) and Americans with Disabilities Act (1990). This plan is primarily meant to ensure appropriate physical accessibility to the school and classroom through various accommodations, so that the child has the opportunity to access the educational curriculum (additional information is available at https://www2.ed.gov/about/offices/list/ocr/504faq.html). An individualized education program (IEP) is derived from the Individuals with Disabilities Education Act (IDEA 1997). This states that children with disabilities have the right to a free and appropriate public education (FAPE) in the least restrictive environment. There are 13 qualifying diagnoses for an IEP (**Table 3**). IDEA intends that children with disabilities will receive modifications and specialized interventions tailored to their learning needs. Least restrictive environment informs the setting in which a child is educated (traditional classroom, specialized classes, specialized school, etc.) so that the child with a disability has their appropriate education and learning needs met alongside peers without disabilities as much as possible (additional information is available at https://www2.ed.gov/parents/needs/speced/iepguide/index.html). These varying levels of educational support are characterized as follows.

Table 1
Tiered levels of academic support for children with traumatic brain injury

Tiered Academic Support	What It is and Commonly Named	Reason It Might be Implemented in Context of TBI
Informal school adjustments	concussion protocol	Concussion or other temporary (non-disabling) injuries
Formal school accommodations	504 Plan	Brain injuries with lasting disability but without need for specific academic modifications or interventions. Accommodations are provided within the general education setting
Formal special education modifications and interventions	Individualized education program (IEP)	Brain injuries with lasting disability and need for academic modifications and specific interventions

Table 2
Comparison of 504 and individualized education program

	504	IEP
Aspect of Federal Law	Rehabilitation Act (1973) Americans with Disabilities Act (ADA) (1990)	Individuals with Disabilities Education Act (IDEA) (1997)
Age	No limitation	Ages 3 through 21
Curriculum	No modifications	Modified to best fit learning needs and goals of child
Therapy/services	None	Available as needed (physical, occupational, speech therapy, etc.)
Eligibility	Any impairment that substantially limits a major life activity related to a qualifying medical or psychological diagnosis	Qualifies for at least 1 of 13 specific diagnoses
Parents	Must provide permission for evaluation	Required to participate in process, sign final plan
Documentation	Recommended but not required	Written, includes goals and accommodations
Reevaluation	Not required, reviewed yearly	Reviewed yearly, reevaluated every 3 y

- *Accommodation*: a change to the environment to support the student's ability to complete the standard, grade-level assignments (eg, time extensions; use of technology; printed lecture notes; taking tests in alternative locations; access to a scribe; ramp or elevator access)
- *Modification*: changes in what students are expected to learn or assignments to complete, based on their individual abilities (eg, use of a lower reading level, shortened assignments, multiple choice instead of essay examinations)
- *Intervention*: Targeted instruction and resources to teach academic and behavioral strategies to obtain new skills. Helps the student to make progress toward the modified benchmark (eg, small-group reading instruction; speech-language therapy)

Public primary and secondary schools are required to identify and evaluate children who will likely benefit from an IEP. After a TBI, communication between a child's medical team, family, and school is critical to define the child's injury and how it might impede the child's academic progress. The child's parents or guardians must formally request an

Table 3
Individuals with disabilities education act disability categories

IDEA Disability Categories	
Specific learning disability	Hearing impairment
Other health impairment	Deaf-blindness
Autism spectrum disorder	Orthopedic impairment (ie, CP)
Emotional disturbance	Intellectual disability
Speech or language impairment	Traumatic brain Injury
Visual impairment including blindness	Multiple disabilities
Deafness	

evaluation be completed by the school team to determine eligibility. A clearly communicated letter from the medical provider with the medical diagnosis and functional impact of the condition is important to assist with qualifying a student for an IEP. By law, the school is required to respond within a specific time period, which may vary slightly across states, and conduct an assessment on the student to determine the scope of supports, interventions, and/or accommodations needed. Assessments completed outside of school (eg, by an independent neuropsychologist, developmental psychologist, speech-language pathologist, etc.) to further evaluate cognitive, linguistic, emotional, and behavioral functioning can also be used by the school to develop the educational program. The school must have an initial meeting with parents/guardians to discuss the proposed education plan. Once finalized, the plan will be signed by the school and the parents/guardians and is a legal and binding document. The school is required to review the IEP annually to ensure goals and supports are appropriate. The school must also have a more formal tri-annual (every 3 years) evaluation to reassess eligibility, program goals, services, and accommodations. The Wrightslaw website provides information on a wealth of topics for families navigating this process.

Most colleges and universities offer learning services for those with documented learning challenges or disabilities, but typically these are in the form of accommodations as opposed to modifications and interventions. In contrast to public primary and secondary education, colleges and universities are not required to identify a student with special learning needs, and instead the student must seek out services and provide appropriate documentation. A growing number of colleges are offering certificate or non-degree programs for students with intellectual disabilities. These inclusive programs focus on varying degrees of life, vocational and academic skills while still facilitating a typical college experience.

Return to School Considerations After Brain Injury

Mild traumatic brain injury/concussion

Mild TBI or concussion is a common presenting condition to many pediatric medical facilities and primary care clinics. Therefore, it is frequently the pediatrician or primary care provider who is tasked with making concussion management decisions including when and how to safely return the youth back to normal activities. Although there have been fairly well-established and published protocols for returning concussed athletes to their respective sports,[8,9] there has been much less consensus on returning youth back to school or learning.[10] Ultimately, how best to transition children to school after concussion lacks consistent evidentiary support but below, we offer several best practices based on available literature.

Concussion often results in a range of nonspecific physical, cognitive, and emotional symptoms, which could certainly impact school attendance and learning for a period of time.[11,12] Fortunately, in a majority of uncomplicated mild TBI or concussion cases, youth will recover quickly and completely without persisting or permanent sequelae.[7,13–15] Thus, more often than not, school-based supports following concussion are fairly short-lived and able to be implemented informally through tailored student-focused adjustments. Often it is in the acute period following concussion that academic adjustments are critical as symptoms are apt to be most pronounced.[16,17] Below we highlight several key school-related considerations often faced by health care professionals in managing the return to learn process following concussion.

School attendance

Often the matter of school attendance is one of the first decisions students, parents, and pediatricians must make following concussion. Unfortunately, there is very limited empirical evidence to guide this particular return-to-school decision and often it is determined on a case-by-case basis. However, the matter of cognitive rest (and subsequently returning to school) has received a modest degree of attention in the pediatric literature over the past decade. Although rest often is the first treatment recommendation for most concussions, the degree of rest has been routinely scrutinized with "complete" or "absolute" rest being particularly controversial.[18] At this point, the preponderance of empirical data supports an initial period of rest following concussion (eg, 24–72 hours) but with the importance of gradual resumption of safe, daily routines and activities in the days following concussion.[19,20] In fact, with regard to school in particular, studies have found that returning to normal activities such as school can actually have a positive impact on recovery while keeping students out of school too long after concussion could be detrimental and potentially iatrogenic.[21,22]

Consistent with the prevailing empirical evidence regarding cognitive rest, many students who are held out of school for multiple days to weeks following concussion are at increased risk to develop challenges largely unrelated to the concussion but more related to factors associated with social isolation, increased anxiety, disruption in normal routines, and falling behind in their school work.[23,24] Thus, although it is appropriate for some students to miss a few days of school, most should resume school attendance at partial or normal levels fairly quickly after their concussion. With proper communication to the school and school adjustments in place, most students are able to tolerate school even while symptomatic.

Informal versus formal school accommodations
In most of the concussion cases, informal or temporary school adjustments are sufficient in providing academic relief. Informal concussion school adjustments often are able to be implemented relatively quickly, with minimal complexity or paperwork, and can fluidly be adjusted or eliminated for many of the transitory symptoms a student might experience after a concussion. Because outcomes after concussion are favorable overall, very few children should need longer-lasting or formal educational supports such as those provided in a Section 504 Plan or an IEP. In fact, it is very rare that a formal 504 Plan and especially an IEP need to be created for a student based solely on an uncomplicated concussion.

Tailored school adjustments or accommodations
Implementing tailored school adjustments or accommodations soon after concussion seems to be a crucial component to concussion management in youth.[25] Often implementation of these school adjustments or accommodations requires medical documentation from a treating medical provider and delays in such documentation can often impact initiation of important school supports and could subsequently prolong concussion recovery.[26] Therefore, it is important very soon after concussion that school personnel should be notified of the injury by parents and medical personnel with clearly outlined recommendations for school attendance and tailored adjustments/accommodations. Because every concussion recovery and symptom profile are likely to differ, tailored or student-specific adjustments/accommodations are important (**Table 4**). In addition to clear medical documentation of the injury and recommendations for school adjustments, another critical aspect of most return-to-learn plans seems to be identifying a "point person" or identified school personnel. This person can help facilitate the immediate implementation of adjustments/accommodations and also monitor the student's status and progress during their recovery. A signed release of information from the student's parents is important in allowing free communication between the school's "point person" and the medical provider.

Table 4
Common concussion symptoms and possible school adjustments

Common Mild TBI/Concussion Symptoms	Possible School Adjustments
Physical symptoms	
Headache	• Allow brief breaks, as needed • Allow water bottle to promote hydration • Allow access to over-the-counter medicine as directed by physician
Fatigue	• Modified or partial days might be helpful initially • Allow rest breaks during the school day • Reduce classwork and homework load, as needed
Vision changes	• Preferential seating • Enlarged materials or computer font • Print computer work
Noise and light sensitivity	• Allow brief breaks in quiet, dark room • Minimize screen time and/or print computer material on paper
Dizziness/balance difficulties	• Allow student to leave class early to avoid busy hallways • Allow use of elevator if available • Assign a hallway "buddy" to assist with walking to and from class
Cognitive symptoms	
Difficulties concentrating	• Allow preferential seating to facilitate close monitoring and focused attention • Provide copies of teachers' or peers' notes • Provide more opportunity for individualized after-class or after-school follow-up to ensure successful learning • Chunk instructions or assignments
Memory difficulties	• Reschedule examinations if student is highly symptomatic or coordinate examinations to avoid multiple tests in 1 day • Allow the student to take tests in a distraction-free environment • Allow open-notes for tests/quizzes • Formula sheet for math equations
Slowed thinking	• Grant additional time for homework, examinations, and assignments • Reduce classwork and homework load, as needed • Allow extra time for responses
Emotional symptoms	
Irritability and moodiness	• Allow breaks during the school day • Allow increased access and frequent check-ins by school counselor
Heightened anxiety and stress	• Excuse missed work to reduce anxiety/stress • Create a reasonable plan/schedule for completion of make-up work

Prolonged post-concussion symptoms

As previously mentioned, a majority of youth with uncomplicated concussions (ie, no skull fracture or abnormal imaging findings) should recover completely and fairly quickly from their concussion (eg, within a few days to weeks). However, for some youth, the recovery from concussion is not as swift or predicable and is often complicated by a variety of injury and noninjury factors.[14,15,27] Recent Centers for Disease Control and Prevention (CDC) mild TBI systematic review and guidelines[27] noted several important risk factors for prolonged recovery including more severe initial symptom presentation, premorbid histories of concussion/mild TBI, comorbid neurologic or psychiatric disorder, learning difficulties, elevated pre-injury symptoms, older adolescents, Hispanic race/culture, low SES, as well as family and social stressors. These guidelines propose that those who have not recovered after 4 to 6 weeks and/or are at higher risk for persisting concussion recovery be referred for more specialized concussion evaluation and management. Protracted recovery from concussion can often lead to more prolonged school disruption and could extend the need for school adjustments/accommodations.

In the event of a longer-than-expected recovery and ongoing school disruption, more specialized evaluation and concussion management are likely to be required including the involvement of a pediatric neuropsychologist and physician with expertise in brain injury.[14]

Moderate and severe brain injury

In contrast to uncomplicated mild TBI/concussion, moderate and severe brain injury can result in a multitude of well-documented physical, cognitive, emotional, and behavioral long-term effects, which are strongly related to injury severity. The steepest part of the recovery curve of physical, cognitive, and functional abilities is typically seen primarily within the first 3 to 6 months after injury, though research suggests recovery may continue for 1 to 2 years or more.[28] Persistent cognitive and social-emotional deficits thereafter are especially common, particularly with more severe injury.[6] As such, children and adolescents who have sustained a moderate to severe brain injury are much more likely to require formalized academic support, particularly during the initial transition back to school, as they are continuing to recover.

Acute recovery and school reintegration

During the acute recovery phase (first 3 to 6 months) after a moderate to severe brain injury, injury-related symptoms, impairments, and associated levels of need are expected to change and evolve, sometimes rapidly. Common injury-related challenges during this phase include sensory-motor impairments, acute cognitive and communication deficits, and significant emotional-behavioral changes. Fatigue and somatic symptoms also remain common during this phase (**Table 5**). Many children who sustain injuries of this severity will have extended hospital stays and may require inpatient and/or outpatient rehabilitation, including intensive physical, occupational, and speech-language therapies. This is important because the length of hospital admission, insurance status, and access to outpatient rehabilitation services also seem to impact functional outcomes after pediatric brain injury, though the specific factors that contribute to this difference remain unclear.[29] Thus, much post-injury rehabilitation and support is now expected to occur within the educational system. Research clearly shows that children with severe TBI who come from lower SES social environments are at particularly high risk for poor outcomes.[30] As such, school systems can help to mitigate some of these risk factors associated with lower SES after TBI, by ensuring access to free and appropriate educational interventions, therapies, and social supports.

Thus, once cleared from a medical perspective, it is important that children and adolescents return to school during this recovery period, rather than wait for recovery to be "complete." Supportive, tailored school reintegration, access to peer interactions and typical routines of childhood are important for cognitive, social-emotional, and adaptive functioning after brain injury. Unfortunately, research has shown that a

Table 5
Common symptoms of moderate and severe traumatic brain injury and associated school supports

Common Moderate/Severe TBI Acute and/or Chronic Symptoms	Possible School Adjustments that May Require IEP or 504 Plan
Physical symptoms	
Motor weakness (paresis) of trunk or lower body	• May need equipment (wheelchair, walker, etc) to move around school setting • Physical assistance for transfers and/or self-cares, including toileting • Stand-by assistance and/or adult supervision when moving around for balance or motor coordination problems • Paraprofessional support • Physical therapy
Motor weakness (paresis) of one or both upper extremities	• Assistance with writing, including scribe and access to notes • Reduced emphasis on written work with alternative assessment options • Assistive technology, such as use of tables and computer keyboards and speech-to-text software • Assistance carrying materials • Occupational therapy
Ataxia/tremors/involuntary movements	• Stand-by assistance and/or adult supervision when moving around for balance or motor coordination problems • Reduced emphasis on written work with modified assignments and alternative assessment options • Assistive technology, such as use of tables and computer keyboards and speech-to-text software • Assistance carrying materials
Hearing impairment	• Preferential seating near the instruction • Amplification devices/FM system • Reduced distractions • Support from Deaf and Hard of Hearing teams
Double vision or visual field deficit	• Assistive technology and/or support from visual impairment specialists • Preferential seating, with instruction presented on side with better vision • Visual anchors to support "scanning" to non-preferred side • Support from Low Vision specialists
Feeding and swallowing	• Supervision and/or nursing support for specialized diet needs (eg, thickened liquids, pacing, g-tube feeds)
Cognitive symptoms	
Difficulties concentrating/paying attention	• Scheduled breaks • Alternating preferred and non-preferred activities • Allow preferential seating to facilitate close monitoring and focused attention

(continued on next page)

Table 5 (continued)	
Common Moderate/Severe TBI Acute and/or Chronic Symptoms	**Possible School Adjustments that May Require IEP or 504 Plan**
	• Provide copies of teachers' or peers' notes • Chunking tasks and assignments • Provide more opportunities for individualized after-class or after-school follow-up to ensure successful learning
Memory impairments	• Individualized instruction emphasizing supportive learning strategies (eg, mnemonics, "chunking," "chaining," frequent repetition and review, relating to previously learned material) • Errorless learning for severe memory impairments • Use of memory aids, such as planners, alarms, calendars, and reference materials • Allow the student to take tests in a distraction-free environment • Allow open notes for tests/quizzes
Slowed thinking	• Grant additional time for homework, examinations, and assignments • Reduce classwork and homework load, as needed • Extra time for responses
Language comprehension difficulties	• Breaking down instructions • Pair verbal with written and/or visual instructions and cues • Visual models, diagrams to supplement verbal and written information
Communication impairments	• Allow extra time for responses • Allow for alternative response formats • Provide cues and starter phrases to facilitate word recall • Multiple choice/recognition over free-recall for tests and assignments • Alternative/augmentative communication supports • Speech-language therapy
Problems with starting, organizing, planning, and carrying out tasks	• Consistent routines • Use of external structures, such as outlines, checklists, and diagrams to break tasks down and provide steps • Frequent check-ins and supports to get started, ensure understanding, and prompt to keep going
Global cognitive and adaptive impairments	• Functional academic curriculum • Adaptive skills training • Transition programming through age 21
Emotional-behavioral symptoms	

(continued on next page)

Table 5
(continued)

Common Moderate/Severe TBI Acute and/or Chronic Symptoms	Possible School Adjustments that May Require IEP or 504 Plan
Impulsive behaviors, "acting out"	• Proactive behavioral supports/antecedent management, emphasizing supervision and prevention of triggers (for more information about antecedent management: www.projectlearnet.org) • Individualized behavior intervention plan with or without functional behavioral assessment (FBA) • Breaks and downtime for "mental calming" • Avoiding overstimulation and prevention of fatigue • Use of sensory room
Irritability and moodiness	• Allow breaks during the school day • Allow increased access and frequent check-ins by school counselor
Heightened anxiety and stress	• Modified instruction tailored to the student's current level and needs • Excuse missed work to reduce anxiety/stress • Create a reasonable plan/schedule for completion of makeup work • Use of sensory room

very small proportion of children who have sustained a TBI receive individualized accommodations or services through the school, despite showing cognitive and academic impairments.[31] Children showing physical impairments ("visible" impairments) related to their injury may initially receive supports, and these may be tapered off as their physical functioning improves with recovery; it is commonly observed that cognitive and social-emotional recovery after brain injury lags behind physical recovery and these impairments ("invisible" deficits) may be less likely to be identified.[32]

Communication from hospital to school system has been identified as an important factor for increasing the initial identification of students with TBI for formal and informal educational supports.[33] Education for school teams and teachers on TBI is also believed to be an important factor in a successful school re-entry program.[34] As such, certain states have developed centralized resources for school districts to access to support school reintegration after brain injury. The BrainSTEPS program in Pennsylvania and Colorado is one such example.

Although return to school is therefore highly encouraged during the acute recovery period after brain injury, energy management is also important during this initial transition. Fatigue is a very common symptom of brain injury and can linger even past apparent recovery of most physical and cognitive symptoms.[35] Further, children may show increased sensitivities to environmental stimulation, including noise and activity level. As such, one must account for the overall activity "load" (physical, cognitive, sensory, social, emotional) when determining the most appropriate level and type of activities for each child (eg, as depicted by an "energy pie" for each activity, **Fig. 1**), and ensuring adequate supports and breaks to accommodate for more energy-intensive activities. A supported and gradual return to school, starting on a part-time basis and gradually building up to full-time, is generally recommended.

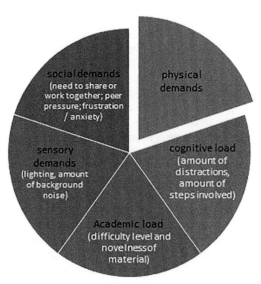

Fig. 1. "Energy Pie": hypothetical depiction of division of energy demands for any particular task.

Long-term academic support needs for children with moderate/severe brain injury
Research on long-term outcomes after moderate to severe TBI has indicated significant variability in cognitive, social-emotional, adaptive, and academic functioning. In general, more severe TBI is associated with greater cognitive problems.[6,7] In addition to injury severity, age is an important factor. For children who sustain injuries during the infancy or preschool years, the impact on IQ is fairly global, and they tend to show a slower rate of cognitive development over time.[36] As age at injury increases, however, the effects on IQ become more varied. Overlearned or "crystallized" skills such as vocabulary and other basic linguistic skills may be relatively spared, whereas those that rely on more distributed neural networks (eg, attention, processing speed, learning, and memory, problem-solving, abstract reasoning) or "fluid" skills are more vulnerable to insult.[7] Furthermore, weaknesses in various aspects of executive functioning, including working memory, self-regulation, inhibition or impulse control, planning, and concept formation likely contribute to significant challenges with academic achievement, adaptive functioning, social and emotional-behavioral functioning.[37] Problems with executive functioning may increase over the course of childhood as expected environmental expectations naturally grow more demanding with age,[38] and the impact on processing speed and goal-setting seem to be most chronic.[37] A recent study indicates that weaknesses in fluid reasoning and cognitive flexibility in children who sustained brain injuries in early childhood (between the ages of 3 and 7) remain a significant predictor of educational need at long-term follow-up (average of 7-year post-TBI).[39]

Pediatric brain injury increases the risk for a variety of psychosocial problems as well, including depressive and anxious symptoms, disruptive behavior disorders such as oppositional defiant disorder (ODD), and "secondary" attention-deficit/hyperactivity disorder (S-ADHD), which has been found to develop in approximately 15% to 20% of children with TBI who did not display premorbid ADHD.[38,40] In general, more severe injury and younger age at injury are related to higher levels of post-injury ADHD and behavior problems, with evidence for latent or emerging behavior problems over time for those injured at younger ages.[28,40,41] Older age at injury, by contrast, seems to place individuals at higher risk for internalizing problems, including depression and anxiety.[40] Children with TBI tend to also have worse social cognition and social competence, which places them at risk for peer rejection and victimization,[42] disruptive behavior, social maladjustment, and educational underachievement.[43] Persistent functional deficits[28] and reduced health-related quality of life are also common after severe TBI[44]; injury during early childhood may lead to increasing adaptive functioning problems over time.

These potential long-term cognitive, psychosocial, and adaptive functioning impairments have significant implications for long-term academic functioning. Research has highlighted low academic achievement after pediatric TBI, which again is affected both by injury severity as well as age at injury.[45] Children injured during infancy or the preschool years are at risk for difficulties in the acquisition of a broad range of academic skills including reading difficulties, poor academic achievement overall, and are more likely to be placed in self-contained classrooms.[46] Cognitive functioning is strongly related to academic performance, with better verbal story memory and inhibitory control being particularly associated with kindergarten readiness and early reading, spelling, and math.[47] Weaknesses in fluid reasoning, processing speed, and executive functions may be particularly predictive of later academic challenges.[39] Although children who sustain TBIs early in development have an increased risk for needing academic services, a significant number still have unmet academic needs.[38,40]

By contrast, individuals who sustain TBI in later childhood or adolescence are more likely to show age-appropriate basic academic achievement (eg, on standardized tests of reading and calculation), likely reflecting the fact that certain core academic skills, such as those underpinning reading (decoding, phonological processing) are fairly well-established earlier in childhood and rely on less widely-distributed neural networks.[45] When specific skill-based deficits do occur, reduced mathematics is particularly common.[45] Despite the potential for retained academic skills, children injured at any age often display remarkably poor everyday classroom functioning, such that achievement may be lower than anticipated based on ability.[48] Further, factors such as male gender, lower SES, more severe injury, and earlier age at injury have been shown to impact the likelihood of post-high school educational and vocational attainment.[49]

Despite this expansive empirical evidence of long-term deficits and educational impact after moderate and severe brain injury, a recent study showed that less than half of all children with TBI were receiving formal educational services through an IEP at 1-year post injury.[32] Children with more severe TBI, males, and those whose parents reported domain-specific concerns (eg, memory) seem to be most likely to be receiving services. This study highlighted that females and those with less obvious or later-appearing deficits were least likely to obtain services.

Further, quality research examining specific educational interventions after pediatric TBI is strikingly absent, perhaps in part because of the significant variability in the needs and settings of each child. A recent systematic review and meta-analysis identified only three qualifying studies published between 1980 and 2017; no statistically significant effects of educational interventions were identified.[50] Given the lack of direct empirical support, at this point, school intervention following brain injury must rely on indirect studies conducted with populations who may display similar manifest problems (eg, ADHD). Luckily, when children with TBI are viewed in terms of their individualized strengths and areas of functional impairment, there are a wealth of educational interventions to inform specialized interventions for these areas of need.[34] The website www.brainline.org/kids-tbi/school-education provides many useful resources for return to learn after moderate and severe TBI.

SUMMARY

Returning a child or teen back to school after brain injury is an important aspect of the management of pediatric brain injury. Regardless of the severity of the injury, returning to school is often an important aspect in improving recovery and functional outcomes. Often temporary informal school adjustments suffice in supporting children returning to school after concussion. For those with more significant brain injuries, often formal school supports and interventions, such as those implemented through an IEP or 504 Plan, are important. Given the resiliency and recovery often seen after pediatric brain injury, close monitoring, serial evaluations, and fluid supports are important in accurately identifying what specific sequelae require support in the school setting.

CLINICS CARE POINTS

- Early return to school after brain injury has many important benefits for youth regardless of severity
- Following concussion, youth often can return quickly and safely back to school with some temporary adjustments
- Very rarely would formalized school supports (504 Plan or IEP) need to be created for a youth who has sustained a concussion as informal temporary adjustments should suffice
- Often formalized school supports (504 Plan or IEP) are critical after more serious brain injury (ie, moderate to severe brain injury) where cognitive, academic, and emotional-behavioral challenges are likely to persist
- Children who sustain more severe brain injuries at a younger age are at the greatest risk for diffuse academic challenges
- Academic under-achievement is common in children with moderate and severe TBI injured at any age, and may translate into reduced educational and vocational attainment

DISCLOSURES

The authors have nothing to disclose.

REFERENCES

1. Faul M, Xu L, Wald MM, et al. Traumatic brain injury in the United States: emergency department visits, hospitalizations and deaths 2002–2006. Atlanta (GA): Centers for Disease Control and Prevention, National Center for Injury Prevention and Control; 2010.
2. Bryan MA, Rowhani-Rahbar A, Comstock RD, et al. Seattle Sports Concussion Research Collaborative. Sports- and Recreation-Related Concussions in US Youth. Pediatrics 2016;138(1):e20154635.
3. Haarbauer-Krupa J, Lebrun-Harris LA, Black LI, et al. Comparing prevalence estimates of concussion/head injury in U.S. children and adolescents in national surveys. Ann Epidemiol 2021;54:11–20.
4. McDonald CM, Jaffe KM, Fay GC, et al. Comparison of indices of traumatic brain injury severity as predictors of neurobehavioral outcome in children. Arch Phys Med Rehabil 1994;75(3):328–37.

5. Davis KC, Slomine BS, Salorio CF, et al. Time to Follow Commands and Duration of Posttraumatic Amnesia Predict GOS-E Peds Scores 1 to 2 Years After TBI in Children Requiring Inpatient Rehabilitation. J Head Trauma Rehabil 2016;31(2): E39–47.

6. Anderson VA, Catroppa C, Haritou F, et al. Identifying factors contributing to child and family outcome 30 months after traumatic brain injury in children. J Neurol Neurosurg Psychiatry 2005;76(3):401–8.

7. Babikian T, Asarnow R. Neurocognitive outcomes and recovery after pediatric TBI: meta-analytic review of the literature. Neuropsychology 2009;23(3):283–96.

8. Davis GA, Ellenbogen RG, Bailes J, et al. The Berlin International Consensus Meeting on Concussion in Sport. Neurosurgery 2018;82(2):232–6.

9. McCrory P, Meeuwisse W, Dvořák J, et al. Consensus statement on concussion in sport-the 5th international conference on concussion in sport held in Berlin, October 2016. Br J Sports Med 2017;51(11):838–47.

10. DeMatteo C, McCauley D, Stazyk K, et al. Post-concussion return to play and return to school guidelines for children and youth: a scoping methodology. Disabil Rehabil 2015;37(12):1107–12.

11. Ransom DM, Vaughan CG, Pratson L, et al. Academic effects of concussion in children and adolescents. Pediatrics 2015;135(6):1043–50.

12. Holmes A, Chen Z, Yahng L, et al. Return to Learn: Academic Effects of Concussion in High School and College Student-Athletes. Front Pediatr 2020;8:57.

13. Peloso PM, Carroll LJ, Cassidy JD, et al. Critical evaluation of the existing guidelines on mild traumatic brain injury. J Rehabil Med 2004;43(Suppl):106–12.

14. Kirkwood MW, Yeates KO, Taylor HG, et al. Management of pediatric mild traumatic brain injury: a neuropsychological review from injury through recovery. Clin Neuropsychol 2008;22(5):769–800.

15. Yeates KO, Taylor HG, Rusin J, et al. Longitudinal trajectories of postconcussive symptoms in children with mild traumatic brain injuries and their relationship to acute clinical status. Pediatrics 2009;123(3):735–43.

16. Broglio SP, Puetz TW. The effect of sport concussion on neurocognitive function, self-report symptoms and postural control : a meta-analysis. Sports Med 2008; 38(1):53–67.

17. Williams RM, Puetz TW, Giza CC, et al. Concussion recovery time among high school and collegiate athletes: a systematic review and meta-analysis. Sports Med 2015;45(6):893–903.

18. Kirkwood MW, Randolph C, Yeates KO. Sport-related concussion: a call for evidence and perspective amidst the alarms. Clin J Sport Med 2012;22(5):383–4.

19. Schneider KJ, Leddy JJ, Guskiewicz KM, et al. Rest and treatment/rehabilitation following sport-related concussion: a systematic review. Br J Sports Med 2017; 51(12):930–4.

20. DiFazio M, Silverberg ND, Kirkwood MW, et al. Prolonged Activity Restriction After Concussion: Are We Worsening Outcomes? Clin Pediatr (Phila) 2016;55(5): 443–51.

21. Thomas DG, Apps JN, Hoffmann RG, et al. Benefits of strict rest after acute concussion: a randomized controlled trial. Pediatrics 2015;135(2):213–23.

22. Majerske CW, Mihalik JP, Ren D, et al. Concussion in sports: postconcussive activity levels, symptoms, and neurocognitive performance. J Athl Train 2008; 43(3):265–74.

23. Kirkwood MW, Howell DR, Brooks BL, et al. The Nocebo Effect and Pediatric Concussion. J Sport Rehabil 2021;30(6):837–43.

24. Ponsford J, Cameron P, Fitzgerald M, et al. Predictors of postconcussive symptoms 3 months after mild traumatic brain injury. Neuropsychology 2012;26(3): 304–13.

25. Purcell LK, Davis GA, Gioia GA. What factors must be considered in 'return to school' following concussion and what strategies or accommodations should be followed? A systematic review. Br J Sports Med 2019;53(4):250.

26. Arbogast KB, McGinley AD, Master CL, et al. Cognitive rest and school-based recommendations following pediatric concussion: the need for primary care support tools. Clin Pediatr (Phila) 2013;52(5):397–402.

27. Lumba-Brown A, Yeates KO, Sarmiento K, et al. Centers for Disease Control and Prevention Guideline on the Diagnosis and Management of Mild Traumatic Brain Injury Among Children [published correction appears in JAMA Pediatr. 2018 Nov 1;172(11):1104]. JAMA Pediatr 2018;172(11):e182853.

28. Fay TB, Yeates KO, Wade SL, et al. Predicting longitudinal patterns of functional deficits in children with traumatic brain injury. Neuropsychology 2009;23(3): 271–82.

29. Juliano AC, Lequerica AH, Marino C, et al. Inpatient length of stay moderates the relationship between payer source and functional outcomes in pediatric brain injury. Brain Inj 2020;34(10):1395–400.

30. Gerring JP, Wade S. The essential role of psychosocial risk and protective factors in pediatric traumatic brain injury research. J Neurotrauma 2012;29(4):621–8.

31. Hawley CA, Ward AB, Magnay AR, et al. Return to school after brain injury. Arch Dis Child 2004;89(2):136–42.

32. Lundine JP, Todis B, Gau JM, et al. Return to School Following TBI: Educational Services Received 1 Year After Injury. J Head Trauma Rehabil 2021;36(2): E89–96.

33. Glang A, Todis B, Thomas CW, et al. Return to school following childhood TBI: who gets services? NeuroRehabilitation 2008;23(6):477–86.

34. Ylvisaker M, Todis B, Glang A, et al. Educating students with TBI: themes and recommendations. J Head Trauma Rehabil 2001;16(1):76–93.

35. Bogdanov S, Brookes N, Epps A, et al. Fatigue in Children With Moderate or Severe Traumatic Brain Injury Compared With Children With Orthopedic Injury: Characteristics and Associated Factors. J Head Trauma Rehabil 2021;36(2): E108–17.

36. Anderson V, Godfrey C, Rosenfeld JV, et al. Predictors of cognitive function and recovery 10 years after traumatic brain injury in young children. Pediatrics 2012; 129(2):e254–61.

37. Beauchamp M, Catroppa C, Godfrey C, et al. Selective changes in executive functioning ten years after severe childhood traumatic brain injury. Dev Neuropsychol 2011;36(5):578–95.

38. Petranovich CL, Smith-Paine J, Wade SL, et al. From Early Childhood to Adolescence: Lessons About Traumatic Brain Injury From the Ohio Head Injury Outcomes Study. J Head Trauma Rehabil 2020;35(3):226–39.

39. Treble-Barna A, Schultz H, Minich N, et al. Long-term classroom functioning and its association with neuropsychological and academic performance following traumatic brain injury during early childhood. Neuropsychology 2017;31(5): 486–98.

40. Wade SL, Kaizar EE, Narad ME, et al. Behavior Problems Following Childhood TBI: The Role of Sex, Age, and Time Since Injury. J Head Trauma Rehabil 2020;35(5):E393–404.

41. Karver CL, Wade SL, Cassedy A, et al. Age at injury and long-term behavior problems after traumatic brain injury in young children. Rehabil Psychol 2012; 57(3):256–65.

42. Yeates KO, Gerhardt CA, Bigler ED, et al. Peer relationships of children with traumatic brain injury. J Int Neuropsychol Soc 2013;19(5):518–27.

43. Derosier ME, Lloyd SW. The Impact of Children's Social Adjustment on Academic Outcomes. Read Writ Q 2011;27(1):25–47.

44. McCarthy ML, MacKenzie EJ, Durbin DR, et al. Health-related quality of life during the first year after traumatic brain injury. Arch Pediatr Adolesc Med 2006; 160(3):252–60.

45. Catroppa C, Anderson VA, Morse SA, et al. Outcome and predictors of functional recovery 5 years following pediatric traumatic brain injury (TBI). J Pediatr Psychol 2008;33(7):707–18.

46. Ewing-Cobbs L, Prasad MR, Kramer L, et al. Late intellectual and academic outcomes following traumatic brain injury sustained during early childhood. J Neurosurg 2006;105(4 Suppl):287–96.

47. Fulton JB, Yeates KO, Taylor HG, et al. Cognitive predictors of academic achievement in young children 1 year after traumatic brain injury. Neuropsychology 2012; 26(3):314–22.

48. Ewing-Cobbs L, Barnes M, Fletcher JM, et al. Modeling of longitudinal academic achievement scores after pediatric traumatic brain injury. Dev Neuropsychol 2004;25(1–2):107–33.

49. Todis B, Glang A, Bullis M, et al. Longitudinal investigation of the post-high school transition experiences of adolescents with traumatic brain injury. J Head Trauma Rehabil 2011;26(2):138–49.

50. Linden MA, Glang AE, McKinlay A. A systematic review and meta-analysis of educational interventions for children and adolescents with acquired brain injury. NeuroRehabilitation 2018;42(3):311–23.

Congenital and Acquired Spinal Cord Injury and Dysfunction

Loren T. Davidson, MD*, Maya C. Evans, MD

KEYWORDS

- Pediatric spinal cord injury • Myelomeningocele • Neurogenic bowel
- Neurogenic bladder

KEY POINTS

- Optimal care of children with congenital spinal defects and acquired spinal cord injury is multidisciplinary and the pediatrician plays an essential role.
- Prognosis for walking is a big concern for families at the time of diagnosis. A pediatric physiatrist can provide anticipatory guidance.
- Proper bowel and bladder management protects renal health and improves the quality of life.

Pediatric spinal cord injury and dysfunction (SCI/D) can result from atypical embryologic development or be acquired as the result of trauma, infection, autoimmune conditions, and tumors. The age of onset and causal mechanism of SCI/D has dramatic implications for function and risk of comorbidities throughout the lifespan. Optimal care of children with SCI/D is multidisciplinary and the pediatrician is a very important member of this team. Specialized interdisciplinary care is usually organized at a regional children's hospital with experts from multiple disciplines collaborating together often under the leadership of a pediatric physiatrist who helps direct care to maximize function and mitigate the negative consequences of SCI/D on the child's health and well-being. This review highlights functional prognosis and important health maintenance issues to prevent complications and maximize independence. It is intended to assist the pediatrician in the care of this unique patient population.

Dysfunction of the spinal cord can cause the complete or partial motor and sensory loss below the lesion level. The terms upper motor neuron (UMN) and lower motor neuron (LMN) lesions are frequent and helpful descriptors. UMN lesions are proximal

Physical Medicine and Rehabilitation, UC Davis Department of Physical Medicine and Rehabilitation, University of California, Davis and Shriners Children's Northern California, 4860 Y Street, Suite 3850, Sacramento, CA 95817, USA
* Corresponding author.
E-mail address: ldavidson@ucdavis.edu

Pediatr Clin N Am 70 (2023) 461–481
https://doi.org/10.1016/j.pcl.2023.01.017
0031-3955/23/© 2023 Elsevier Inc. All rights reserved.

to the anterior horn cell and are associated with exaggerated muscle stretch reflexes and spasticity. LMN lesions are at or distal to the level of the anterior horn cell and are associated with flaccid paralysis, muscle atrophy, and absent reflexes. Congenital SCI/D is typically LMN and can develop UMN features during periods of rapid growth due to tethered cord. Acquired SCI/D can be either UMN or LMN predominant depending on the etiology and area of the spinal cord that is injured. For example, acute flaccid myelitis and injuries to the cauda equina are LMN and traumatic injuries to descending motor tracts of the spinal cord lead to UMN.

CONGENITAL SPINAL CORD INJURY AND DYSFUNCTION

Congenital malformations of the spinal cord may be large and diagnosed easily pre or postnatally as in the case of myelomeningocele (MMC), or they can be harder to detect as in conditions such as fibrolipoma of the filum terminale. Regardless of size, these conditions known as spinal dysraphisms are the result of caudal neural tube defects (NTDs). Dysraphisms are divided into closed and open states (**Table 1**). Closed spinal dysraphisms are covered by skin and fat and depending on the defect may require neurosurgical treatment in infancy or in later years due to the development of tethered cord. In open dysraphisms, the neural elements are exposed, and surgical treatment is needed before or shortly after birth to prevent life-threatening infection.

MMC is the most common open spinal dysraphism. People with MMC have an often-asymptomatic Chiari II malformation and a high rate of hydrocephalus, which frequently requires neurosurgical intervention. Historically approximately 80% of people with MMC had ventriculoperitoneal (VP) shunts placed for hydrocephalus, but this percentage is decreasing due to fetal surgery and changing practice patterns.[1] MMC is commonly referred to as spina bifida; however, it is important to distinguish this condition from spina bifida occulta, which is an incidental finding and is very rarely associated with neurologic symptoms. In the United States, 3000 pregnancies are affected by NTDs and 1400 babies with MMC are born each year.[2] NTDs are caused by a variety of factors including genetic and environmental causes.

ACQUIRED SPINAL CORD INJURY AND DYSFUNCTION

Acquired SCI/D can have traumatic and nontraumatic causes such as infection, autoimmune conditions, and neoplasm. Anatomical differences such as those seen in children with Down syndrome, skeletal dysplasias, and inflammatory conditions such as juvenile rheumatoid arthritis can predispose to spinal stenosis and associated SCI/D. Similarly, infants and young children are particularly vulnerable to traumatic SCI because of their proportionally large heads, weak neck muscles, and increased flexibility of the spine. Owing to the latter, children may have SCI without radiographic

Table 1 Open and closed spinal dysraphisms		
Open	**Closed with Subcutaneous Mass**	**Closed Without Subcutaneous Mass**
Myelomeningocele	Lipomyelomingocele	Caudal regression syndrome
Hemimyelomeningocele	Meningocele	Diastematomyelia
Myelocele	Myelocystocele	Intradural lipoma
Hemimyelocele		Tight filum terminale
Myeloschisis		

abnormality (SCIWORA), associated with a sudden stretch of the spinal cord in which x-rays and computed tomography (CT) of the spine are normal. MRI identifies an abnormality of the spinal cord in the majority of SCIWORA injuries, thus it is important to check advanced imaging if there is a sufficient concern for SCI/D even with normal x-rays and CT.[3]

The annual incidence of pediatric SCI in the United States is estimated to be 1.99 cases per 100,000 children.[4] More than 95% of these cases are teens. In adolescents, as in adults, males outnumber females by a ratio of 4:1.[5] The most common cause of SCI in children and adolescents is motor vehicle crashes (MVCs), followed by violence and sports.[5]

Traumatic spinal injuries may be associated with vertebral instability and require surgical fusion. This intervention halts the growth of the fused region and has long-term implications on the height and mobility of the spine. Oncologic spinal disease may require surgical debulking as well as radiation, which can also damage the spinal cord. Children with autoimmune and infectious Spinal Cord Dysfunction (SCD) receive treatment to quiet inflammation and treat the infectious organism. These medical and surgical interventions, as in the surgical closure of MMC, aim to stop the progression of injury to the spinal cord. Neurologic recovery following injury to the spinal cord is variable and depends on the injury type and severity. Research is ongoing, but currently there are no approved therapies to regenerate the damaged spinal cord. Permanent neurologic deficits are common and impact future growth and development.

PROGNOSTICATION AND CLASSIFICATION OF PEDIATRIC SPINAL CORD INJURY AND DYSFUNCTION

When a diagnosis of SCI/D is made, one of the first questions families ask is whether the child will be able to walk. Engaging a pediatric rehabilitation medicine specialist (pediatric physiatrist) in this discussion will provide the best quality information and long-term care for a child with SCI/D. Although there are many factors that contribute to the ability to ambulate, the minimal motor function needed for community ambulation is bilateral hip flexion against gravity and knee extension against gravity on at least one side. This information is clinically communicated through a classification score. In acquired SCI/D a physiatrist will perform the American Spinal Injury Association (ASIA) International Standards for Neurological Classification of SCI (ISNCSCI) examination. This highly standardized examination evaluates light touch and pinprick sensation bilaterally at each dermatome and motor strength in key muscle groups of the upper and lower limbs to determine the neuroanatomic level of injury. From a prognostic standpoint motor complete lesions (AIS A) and sensory incomplete lesions (AIS B) are least likely to have motor improvement. Motor incomplete lesions AIS C and AIS D are likely to have a motor improvement in the first year, with the most dramatic improvement within the first 6 months.

Classification of congenital SCI/D is complicated by the fact that atypical embryologic development affects neurosegmentation, because of this, scales tend to use broad terms to describe patterns of strength (**Table 2**). In MMC community ambulation is often possible for persons with a lesion level of midlumbar or lower.

People with SCI/D mobilize in a variety of ways depending on intrinsic and environmental factors. There are a variety of assistive devices, such as braces, walkers, crutches, and manual and power wheelchairs. The child's pediatric physiatrist and physical/occupational therapist will recommend developmentally appropriate devices to maximize independence and access while decreasing the potential for overuse injury. Power mobility may be needed if there is limited upper extremity strength or

Table 2
Spina bifida motor function classification

Motor Level	Leg Function
Thoracic	Flaccid lower limbs
High lumbar	Hip flexion against gravity
Mid lumbar	Knee extension against gravity
Low lumbar	Ankle dorsiflexion against gravity
Sacral	Presence of ankle plantar flexion

limited endurance. These devices are often very heavy and require a wheelchair-accessible van for transportation, which can significantly limit their utility.

The ability of a child with SCI/D to live independently in adulthood and actively participate in the community is dependent on a variety of factors including neurologic level of injury, socioeconomic resources, and accessibility of the environment. Driving improves community reintegration, odds of employment, and life satisfaction. There are a variety of vehicle modifications that enable safe driving for individuals with lower and or upper extremity weakness. An occupational and/or physical therapist with additional certification as a driver rehabilitation specialist will determine what, if any modifications are needed.

CARE DELIVERY

In children with congenital SCI/D care often starts with prenatal consultation and after delivery is ideally delivered at regular intervals through multidisciplinary clinics, with providers from disciplines including pediatric rehabilitation, urology, neurosurgery, and orthopedics.[6,7] Care coordination has been identified as one of the most important functions of these clinics.[8] Referral to early intervention services and regular evaluations of therapy needs and school accommodations are important in maximizing function and independence.

After the acute care hospitalization for the inciting injury or illness, children and adolescents with acquired SCI/D may benefit from acute inpatient rehabilitation. This intensive program provides 3 h of developmentally appropriate therapy 6 days a week and maximizes patient function, provides caregiver education, and assists with a successful transition to home and school. After discharge, outpatient therapies assist with the continued acquisition of developmentally appropriate skills, also known as habilitation. Unfortunately, pediatric resources such as acute inpatient rehabilitation, adaptive sports, and peer support are often hard to find in more rural areas due to the relatively low incidence of SCI in children.

Nervous System Dysfunction

Children and adolescents with congenital and acquired SCI/D are at risk for a variety of neurologic conditions. Proper management of these conditions promotes optimal function and prevents potentially life-threatening medical complications.

All children and adolescents with congenital SCI/D are at risk of clinically significant tethered cord. In this condition, the motion of the distal spinal cord in the spinal canal is limited due to a tight tissue attachment. This is noted on MRI of the spine in most children who have had neurosurgical treatment of spinal dysraphism. During periods of rapid growth children can develop significant symptoms such as ascending weakness, spasticity, pain, scoliosis, and changes in bowel and bladder. Close monitoring by a neurosurgeon and judicious use of surgical untethering may prevent further decline.

People with MMC are monitored closely for uncompensated hydrocephalus, which can present with headaches, vomiting, seizures, and a decline in grades. Neurosurgical treatment of hydrocephalus includes VP shunts, endoscopic third ventriculostomy, and choroid plexus coagulation. Owing to structural differences in the brain, people with MMC have a unique pattern of cognitive strengths and weaknesses. Rote learning is a relative strength and extrapolation is a relative weakness.[9] This may affect school performance and individuals with higher anatomic lesion levels tend to have more challenges. In addition, teens with MMC typically have a 2- to 5-year delay in the acquisition of self-care skills.[9] Keeping this in mind when setting expectations for a teen with MMC can limit parent and teacher frustration and set the teen up for success.

Acquired SCI at or above the level of T6 affects the autonomic nervous system, which predisposes to autonomic dysreflexia (AD) and hypo/hyperthermia. In AD, blood pressure rises 20 to 40 mm Hg above baseline in response to a noxious stimulus below T6. Bladder distention is the most common irritant. More than half of children with complete injuries above T6 experience AD. Clinicians, parents, and other caregivers need to know the child's baseline blood pressure and watch for signs of AD. Timely intervention to relieve the noxious stimulus will abort the episode and prevent serious complications, such as stroke.[10] Initial management includes sitting the person up, loosening tight clothing, and catheterizing the bladder. Education on AD is an important part of acute inpatient rehabilitation and ongoing evaluation and management will be provided in the SCI clinic.

In acquired SCI/D thermoregulatory centers do not receive typical signals from the peripheral nervous system and response to an external temperature below the level of injury may be impaired due to distal sympathetic nervous system dysfunction. As a result, people with complete SCI/D may quickly become hypothermic in cold environments and hyperthermic in hot environments. This condition is known as poikilothermia.[11,12] People who have an acute SCI and young children are particularly susceptible to this complication.

As noted earlier, spasticity is a component of the UMN syndrome. It is characterized by velocity-dependent resistance to passive stretch due to increased muscle stretch reflexes.[13] In acquired SCI/D spasticity develops gradually over the weeks to months following injury.[3] Congenital SCI/D is typically described as LMN resulting in a flaccid paralysis. However, people with congenital SCI/D may develop spasticity during periods of rapid growth due to tethered cords and require monitoring for this.

Spasticity may be beneficial as it can help to maintain muscle mass and bone mineral density and be used to assist in certain functional tasks. By contrast, it can also cause pain, deformity, and limit function. A pediatric physiatrist can provide comprehensive spasticity management if the tone is bothersome.[14] It is important to keep in mind that acute pain and illness can exacerbate spasticity. Treating these conditions is an important first step before initiating or advancing anti-spasticity medications. Spasticity management often progresses from least to most invasive. It is reasonable to start with stretching exercises and splinting. A variety of oral medications treat generalized spasticity (**Table 3**). Baclofen is the most commonly used medication. Sedation and muscle weakness are common side effects and can be avoided by starting with a low dose and titrating to effect. Spasticity in select muscle groups can be treated with intramuscular botulinum toxin (BTX) injections and phenol/alcohol neurolysis by a specialist, such as a pediatric physiatrist who is well-versed in localization and pediatric dosing.

Table 3
Dosing guidelines, pharmacologic actions, and adverse event profile of commonly prescribed oral antispasmodic medications for children

Oral Medication (Dose/Freq., Age/Weight Range)	Mode of Action	Adverse Events/Precautions
Baclofen (0.125 to 1 mg/kg/day) *Dosing guideline 2 to 7 years* 2.5 to 10 mg tid-qid (10 to 40 mg/day) *8 to 12 years* 5 mg –15 mg tid-qid (15 to 60 mg/day) *12 to 16 years* 5 to 20 mg tid-qid (20 to 80 mg/day) Note: Caution advised with renal impairment, consider reducing the dose.	Centrally acting, structural analog of GABA, binds to GABA$_B$ receptors causing presynaptic inhibition of mono/polysynaptic spinal reflexes. Rapid absorption, blood level peaks in 1 h, half-life 5.5 h. Renal (70% to 80% unchanged) and hepatic (15%) excretion.	CNS depression (sedation, drowsiness, fatigue), nausea, headache, dizziness, confusion, euphoria, hallucinations, hypotonia, ataxia, paraesthesiae. Note: *Abrupt withdrawal* may cause seizures, hallucinations, rebound muscle spasms, and hyperpyrexia.
Diazepam (0.12 to 0.8 mg/kg/day) *Dosing guideline* *6 mo to 12 years* 0.12 to 0.8 mg/kg/day PO divided q 6 to 8h *>12 years* 2 to 10 mg PO bid-qid Note: Prescription of a *qhs* dose only or proportionately larger dose at bedtime may limit excessive daytime sedation.	Centrally acting, binds to GABA$_A$ receptors mediating presynaptic inhibition in brain stem reticular formation and spinal polysynaptic pathways. Rapid absorption, blood level peaks in 1 h, with half-life of 30 to 60 h.	CNS depression (sedation, impaired memory, and attention), ataxia. Dependence/potential for substance abuse/overdose. Withdrawal syndrome (including anxiety, agitation, irritability, tremor, muscle twitching, nausea, insomnia, seizures, and hyperpyrexia). Increased potential for adverse effects with low albumin levels due to being 98% protein bound.
Dantrolene sodium (3 to 12 mg/day) *Dosing guideline (for children >5 years old)* *6 to 8 mg/kg/d PO divided bid-qid* Start 0.5 mg/kg qd-bid for 7 days, then 0.5 mg/kg tid for 7 days, then 1 mg/kg tid for 7 days, then 2 mg/kg tid to a maximum of 12 mg/kg/d or 400 mg/day.	Peripheral action, blocking release of calcium from sarcoplasmic reticulum with uncoupling of nerve excitation and skeletal muscle contraction. Blood level peaks in 3 to 6 h (active metabolite 4 to 8 h), with half-life of approx. 15 h	Malaise, fatigue, nausea, vomiting, diarrhea, muscle weakness with high dose. Note: Hepatotoxicity (baseline liver function tests MUST be checked before starting dantrolene, tested weekly during dose titration, and regularly every 1 to 2 months thereafter). Drug *should be discontinued* promptly if liver enzymes become elevated.

Tizanidine
Dosing guideline
In children <10 years: Commence 1 mg orally at bedtime initially, increasing to 0.3 to 0.5 mg/kg in 4 divided doses.
In children >10 years: Commence 2 mg orally at bedtime initially, increased according to response, maximum 24 mg/day in 3 to 4 divided doses.

Centrally acting, alpha-2 adrenoceptor agonist activity at both spinal and supraspinal sites. Prevents release of excitatory amino acids, facilitating presynaptic inhibition. Good oral absorption, blood level peaks in 1 to 2 h, with a half-life of 2.5 h

Dry mouth, drowsiness, tiredness, headache, dizziness, insomnia, anxiety, aggression, mood swings, visual hallucinations, risk of hypotension (although 10 times less anti-hypertensive potency than clonidine), nausea, vomiting, and constipation. Liver function tests should be monitored: baseline and 1 month after main dose achieved.

Surgical options include tendon lengthening and intrathecal baclofen (ITB). Tendon lengthening may be considered when conservative management fails and is very effective in spasticity of spinal origin.[15] Baclofen delivered to the intrathecal space via an implanted pump maximizes the drug's efficacy and minimizes sedative effects. However, potential complications of ITB are severe and include central nervous system infections, respiratory depression, and life-threatening withdrawal.

RESPIRATORY

During the acute phase, respiratory complications in acquired SCI/D cause significant morbidity and mortality.[16] Weakness of the diaphragm, intercostal and abdominal musculature limits the ability to inhale an adequate tidal volume and expectorate secretions. Children with injuries at or below C4 may be weaned from ventilatory support during the acute hospitalization or subsequent inpatient rehabilitation.[16] Children who are unable to wean require mechanical ventilation full-time or in some cases a phrenic pacer (**Fig. 1**) and intermittent mechanical ventilation to prevent atelectasis may be used. In either case, a tracheostomy is typically maintained and effective cough assistance is essential to prevent infection.

In MMC, Chiari II malformation is commonly associated with delayed advancement of food textures in infants and toddlers as well as an increased frequency of sleep-disordered breathing in people of all ages. Moderate to severe obstructive sleep apnea affects approximately 30% of people with MMC.[17] Symptomatic Chiari II malformation is typically treated surgically by addressing hydrocephalus or via Chiari decompression. In severe cases, dysphagia, stridor, and apnea may prompt tracheostomy and gastrostomy tube placement. Although decompression surgery is more frequently required with higher level lesions, tracheostomy after Chiari decompression is related to younger age at the time of surgery.[18]

Neurogenic Bladder

Bladder function is affected in the majority of patients with SCI/D. Urine will leak from the urethra resulting in wet diapers; however, the lack of coordination between bladder contraction and sphincter relaxation often results in incomplete bladder

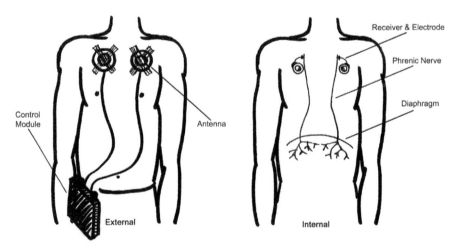

Fig. 1. Phrenic pacer.

emptying and increases the risk of urinary tract infection (UTI). If there is vesicoureteral reflux, renal scarring and failure can occur. Proper medical management preserves renal function and provides social continence.[19] A pediatric physiatrist can initiate a bladder management and renal monitoring program. A pediatric urologist versed in the care of children with neurogenic bladder provides surgical management when indicated.

In acquired SCI/D, Clinical Practice Guidelines from the Consortium of Spinal Cord Medicine recommends the use of clean intermittent urinary self-catheterization (CIC) as the standard of care. It is typically initiated shortly after diagnosis, even in children younger than the typical potty-training age.[20] In congenital SCI/D, the likelihood of neurogenic bladder is determined by the type of dysraphism and the optimal time to start CIC is being studied.[21] Some centers advocate for early CIC, whereas others will initiate CIC after there is evidence of hydronephrosis. The initiation of CIC does not decrease the potential for a child to develop bladder control and starting in infancy may increase cooperation with CIC in toddler and early school-age children.

Kidney health is monitored with a combination of imaging studies, functional assessments, and bloodwork (Table 4). In all cases of neurogenic bladder, dimercaptosuccinic acid (DMSA) scans can evaluate renal scaring and the relative contribution of each kidney. Early referral to pediatric nephrology should be considered in children with evidence of upper tract changes.

Pediatricians often evaluate children for UTIs. Bacteriuria is expected in all persons who perform CIC and should not be mistaken for a UTI. Strong-smelling urine alone is not concerning in this population and can be managed with increased fluid intake and increased CIC frequency. Testing for a UTI should be reserved for patients with constitutional symptoms such as fever or abdominal pain. Providers should check a urinalysis with microscopic evaluation and a culture with sensitivities, rather than a urine dipstick. Patients with a UTI will have pyuria >25 White Blood Cells (per high power field) (WBC) and colony-forming units of 50,000 to 100,000.[3,21] Antibiotic treatment should be tailored to sensitivities. It is important for families and patients to be educated on this issue to assure proper treatment. The use of prophylactic antibiotics in patients with neurogenic bladder is discouraged and should be done in consultation with a urologist or nephrologist if deemed necessary.

By the age of 3 years of children should be introduced to the idea of self-CIC. Dolls and storybooks can help to normalize the process and make learning about CIC fun. In acquired SCI/D complete independence by 7 to 8 years of age is typical. However, children with MMC tend to gain independence between the ages of 9 and 14 years.[23] Children with quadriplegia who do not have sufficient hand function to catheterize should instead develop autonomy through the direction of caregivers.

Social continence, or being dry between CIC, promotes self-esteem and societal integration.[24] Bladder continence requires sufficient bladder size and bladder neck or outlet resistance to store urine between CIC. Urodynamic testing is helpful to understand the bladder characteristics and indicate potential treatments. Anticholinergic medications, detrusor BTX injections, and bladder augmentation may be required to increase bladder storage capacity.[25,26]

An open bladder neck or weak urinary sphincter can be treated with urethral bulking injection, an artificial urinary sphincter, or a bladder reconstruction. In some cases, the bladder neck is surgically closed and a continent catheterizable urinary diversion, such as Mitrofanoff (Fig. 2) is created for CIC. This procedure can also improve independence with CIC in persons with limited hand function or hip range of motion to access the urethra, or females with difficulty mobilizing to the toilet.[22,27]

Table 4
Recommended frequency of bladder and kidney surveillance

	MMC	Acquired SCI/D
Kidney and bladder ultrasound	≤2 years: every 6 months >2 years: annually or more frequently if there are abnormalities or clinical concerns	Annually or more frequently if there are abnormalities or clinical concerns
Urodynamic testing	≤3 years: annually >4 years: if there are abnormalities on ultrasounds or clinical concerns	If there are abnormalities on ultrasounds or clinical concerns
Blood work • Creatinine in most cases • Consider cystatin C in the case of low muscle mass	<1 year: once <6 years: annually if upper tract changes ≥6 years: annually	If there are abnormalities on ultrasounds or clinical concerns

Data from Refs.[22,22]

Neurogenic Bowel

Bowel function is affected in the majority of patients with SCI/D.[19] There are two typical patterns of bowel dysfunction; upper and LMNs. In UMN bowel dysfunction the external anal sphincter and colon are spastic and spinal reflexes are intact. In LMN bowel dysfunction the anal sphincter is flaccid and the colon is areflexic. Both patterns are seen in acquired SCI/D. However, most individuals with congenital SCI/D have LMN bowel dysfunction.

Regardless of the etiology or type of dysfunction, the goal of neurogenic bowel management is controlled evacuation of stool in the toilet and avoiding constipation.[19] In UMN bowel dysfunction, it is reasonable to try conservative measures such as sitting on the toilet after eating to promote evacuation via the gastrocolic reflex. However, more than 80% of children with acquired SCI/D require oral medication, rectal stimulation/medication, or a combination (**Table 5**).[28] In LMN oral and rectal medications are often ineffective in creating social continence and scheduled use of large-volume enemas or manual disimpaction of the hard stool are eventually needed.

Preventing constipation is important at all ages because it leads to megacolon and UTIs. In congenital SCI/D constipation often starts when infants transition to food. Dietary modifications and medication should be started as soon as possible. Bowel programs that target a single bowel movement a day are introduced around 2 to 4 years of age. In LMN bowel, such as congenital SCI/D, medications are trialed first and if not effective, large volume flushes are often needed to gain social continence. Retrograde irrigation systems such as cone enemas or transanal irrigation systems are often effective but difficult to perform independently. If these are not successful, children may benefit from anterograde enemas such as those delivered through a cecostomy or anterograde continence enema (ACE) procedure, where a stoma is made from the abdomen to the proximal colon (**Fig. 3**).[29] ACE is well tolerated, has minimal side effects, and is generally quite effective.[30,31]

The ability to achieve complete independence with the performance of a bowel program depends on the neurologic level of injury, method of bowel elimination, and the motivation and emotional maturity of the child. Please see **Table 6** for a description of the level of independence that is possible based on the neurologic level of injury in acquired SCI/D.[32]

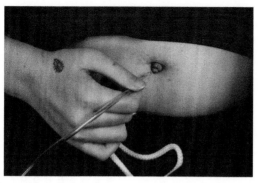

Fig. 2. Mitrofanoff.

Orthopedic

Almost every child who has an acquired SCI/D before age 12 will develop scoliosis and approximately 2/3 of these children will eventually require surgery regardless of the level of injury or gender.[33,34] Bracing with a thoraco-lumbar-sacral orthotic (TLSO) slows curve progression and increases the age at which surgery is performed.[35] However, many children and teens do not tolerate these braces because they are bulky and limit mobility.[36] Curves greater than 40°, age greater than 10 years, and a rapidly progressing curve are indications for surgery in a growing child. Impaired function or pain are indications for surgery in a skeletally mature patient.

In congenital SCI/D scoliosis and kyphosis can be due to rib or vertebral malformations and/or neuromuscular weakness. Early kyphectomy is indicated in children with congenital gibbus malformation to prevent skin breakdown. Unlike acquired SCI/D the benefits of bracing neuromuscular scoliosis in congenital SCI/D is unclear and indication for surgery and recommendations for specific surgical interventions have not been defined. In addition, tethered cords may be associated with rapidly progressive curves. Therefore, a case-by-case approach is recommended.

More than 90% of children with acquired SCI/D develop hip subluxation or dislocation before age 10 years.[37] This appears to be independent of spasticity, unlike cerebral palsy (CP).[38] An unstable hip maybe become painful in sensate patients and limit the ability to do passive standing or functional electrical stimulation biking. Some authors recommend close x-ray surveillance of hips and an aggressive approach to surgical management, but there are no consensus guidelines.[38]

In contrast to acquired SCI/D and CP, surveillance hip imaging and surgery are rarely recommended for congenital SCI/D. In children with low lumbar/sacral level lesions with impaired function due to hip instability who fail conservative management, hip reconstruction surgery can be considered but is not yet the standard of care.[39]

Children with SCI/D have lower bone density than age and gender-matched controls, especially those that use wheelchairs for mobility.[40,41] Bone fragility, increased activity, and risk-taking behavior may predispose children and teens with SCI/D to insufficiency fracture. These fractures are frequently painless due to sensory deficits and are associated with erythema and swelling. Patient education, passive standing, and optimizing calcium and vitamin D can help prevent fractures.

In congenital SCI/D, foot deformities may be visible on prenatal ultrasound. Gentle stretching is recommended after birth. In clubfoot and congenital vertical talus, the process of casting and/or tendon release is usually begun during the first year of life. Similarly, children and teens with MMC and lipomyelomeningocele may develop

Table 5
Bowel meds

Dosing Guideline, Pharmacologic Actions, and Side Effect Profile of Commonly Prescribed Neurogenic Bowel Medication for Children

Class	Medication (Dose/Frequency, Age/Weight Range)	Mode of Action	Side Effects/Precautions
Bulk forming	Psyllium (eg, Metamucil, Fibercon, Citrucel) Dosing guidelines <6 y: Safety and efficacy not established 6 to 12 y: 1.25 to 15 g/d orally in 227.3 mL (8 oz) of water in divided doses >12 y: 2.5 to 7.5 g in 227.3 mL (8 oz) of water orally, ≤ 30 g/d in divided doses	Absorbs water to create stool bulk	Bloating, flatulence, abdominal cramps, gastrointestinal obstruction, and constipation
Stool softeners	Docusate (Colace and Surfak) Dosing guidelines Children 2 to 11 y: dose: 50 to 150 mg/d orally divided daily, twice a day ≥ 12 y: 50 to 300 mg/d orally divided daily twice a day	Emulsifies stool fat and water, allowing mixture Metabolism is unknown	Diarrhea, abdominal cramps, rash, throat irritation, liquid form tastes bitter, and is poorly tolerated
Hyperosmolar	Lactulose (1 mL/kg orally daily, twice a day) Dosing guidelines: maximum: 60 mL/d Note: response may require 24 to 48h	Draw fluid into intestines increasing stool water content; it can also increase stool acidity, trapping NH4 ions Metabolized by colon; colon with < 3% systemic absorption	Flatulence, intestinal cramps, abdominal distension, nausea, and vomiting May cause electrolyte disorders or metabolic acidosis with excessive doses
	Sorbitol (25 g/120 mL, 50 g/240 mL) Dosing guidelines: 1 to 12 y: 25 to 50 g orally once within 1 h of ingestion Note: not recommended for multiple-dose treatment	Draws excessive water into the colon, promoting evacuation Not metabolized, because it is not absorbed systemically	Vomiting, constipation, black stools, and diarrhea May cause electrolyte imbalance, fecal impaction, and bronchiolitis obliterans
	Miralax (0.8 g/kg orally daily) Dosing guidelines: children < 17 y: commence with 4 grams and progress to maximum of 17 grams fully dissolved in 113.6 to 227.3 mL (4 to 8 oz) of liquid before administration daily	Causes water retention in stool, producing a laxative effect Not metabolized, because it is not absorbed systemically	Cramping, flatulence, nausea, abdominal distention, and urticarial May cause electrolyte disturbance with prolonged and excessive use

Stimulants	Senna (Senokot) Dosing guidelines 2 to 5 y: 1 tab orally every night at bedtime as needed; start: half a tab every night at bedtime; maximum; 1 tab twice a day 6 to 11 y: 2 tabs orally every night at bedtime as needed; Start: 1 tab every night at bedtime; maximum: 2 tabs twice a day > 12 y: 2 to 4 tabs orally every night at bedtime; start: 2 tabs every night at bedtime; maximum: 4 tabs twice a day	Increases intestinal motility by stimulating peristalsis Liver metabolism, although minimal systemic uptake. Takes 6 to 12 h to work	Nausea, abdominal distension, cramps, flatulence, diarrhea, and urine discoloration
	Bisacodyl (Dulcolax) Dosing guidelines 6 to 11 y: 1 tab orally daily as needed; do not cut/crush/chew >12 y: 1 to 3 tabs orally daily as needed; do not cut/crush/chew	Increases intestinal motility Metabolized by liver with 15% systemic absorption	Diarrhea, cramping, rectal sensation burning, and vomiting nausea
	Magnesium citrate Dosing guidelines 2 to 5 y: 2 to 4 mL/kg/d orally divided daily, twice a day; maximum: 60 to 90 mL/d 6 to 12 y: 100 to 150 mL/d orally divided daily, twice a day: maximum: 150 mL/d > 12 y: 150 to 300 mL/d orally divided daily, twice a day: maximum: 300 mL/d	Stimulates colonic motility, used for complete bowel evacuation	Large volume, poor taste, electrolyte imbalance, hypotension, diarrhea, and flatulence
	Milk of magnesia Dosing guidelines 6 mo to 1 y: 40 mg/kg orally daily 2 to 5 y: 400 to 1200 mg orally daily 6 to 11 y: 1200 to 2400 mg orally daily >12 y: 2400 to 4800 mg orally daily	Neutralizes gastric acidity, which causes water retention in the stool Not metabolized, with 15% to 30% systemic absorption	Diarrhea, abdominal pain, nausea, dehydration, and vomiting

(continued on next page)

Table 5
(continued)

Dosing Guideline, Pharmacologic Actions, and Side Effect Profile of Commonly Prescribed Neurogenic Bowel Medication for Children

Class	Medication (Dose/Frequency, Age/Weight Range)	Mode of Action	Side Effects/Precautions
Enemas	Saline Dosing guidelines 2 to 12 y: 6 mL/kg (approximately 118 mL rectum) daily >12 y: 1 bottle (118 mL) by rectum daily	Hyperosmotic effect of sodium draws excess water into the colon, promoting evacuation Minimal systemic absorption	Abdominal distension, nausea, discomfort, electrolyte imbalance, and metabolic acidosis Do not use in renal failure
	Mineral Oil Dosing guidelines 2 to 11 y: 1/2 bottle by rectum daily >12 y: 1 bottle by rectum daily	Softens and lubricates stool Unknown metabolism with minimal systemic absorption	Diarrhea, abdominal cramps, and pruritus
Suppositories	Bisacodyl (Dulcolax) Dosing guidelines 6 to 11 y: half a suppository by rectum daily >12 y: 1 suppository by rectum daily	Causes increased peristalsis mild colonic irritation Liver metabolized, with 15% systemic absorption	Diarrhea, abdominal pain, nausea, dehydration, vomiting, and electrolyte imbalance
	Glycerin Dosing guidelines <2 y: half infant/pediatric suppository by rectum daily 2 to 5 y: 1 infant/pediatric suppository by rectum daily >6 y: adult suppository by rectum daily	Irritates mucosa, increasing peristalsis; increases stool water content Liver metabolized with poor rectal absorption	Diarrhea, headache, nausea, and rectal irritation

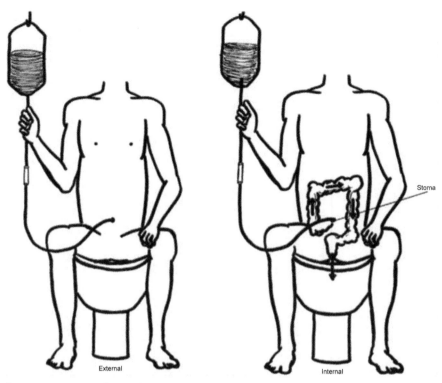

Fig. 3. An anterograde continence enema.

in-toeing, out-toeing or progressive foot deformities as a consequence of tethered cord or the effect of paralysis. Regardless of age, the goal of orthopedic treatment is to create a braceable plantigrade foot for shoe wear and weightbearing.

Skin

Owing to the lack of protective sensation for pressure/sheer and temperature, children with all types of SCI/D are at risk for skin breakdown. The most common sites of skin breakdown are on the feet for ambulators and over the ischial tuberosities or coccyx for wheelchair users. Prevention is key and maintaining the appropriate fit of wheelchair/cushion and orthoses, as well as preventing incontinence and ensuring proper nutrition are important for skin preservation.[42] Frequent skin checks catch the early signs of skin breakdown, such as blanchable erythema over bony prominences. Once a wound is present, weight-bearing area to the area should be avoided and a wound-care specialists should be consulted. Wound debridement and Vacuum Assisted Closure may be required for larger wounds and if conservative measures fail a myocutaneous flap may be needed.

Obesity/Metabolic Syndrome

Obese adolescents with congenital and acquired SCI/D have an increased risk of metabolic syndrome and cardiovascular disease because of decreased aerobic fitness, muscular strength, decreased lean mass, and increased fat mass.[43] Health care providers can stress the importance of physical activity, and use of goal setting

Table 6
Potential functional performance and adaptive equipment by the level of injury

Level of Injury	Potential Functional Performance Outcome for Bowel Care[a]	Bathroom Equipment Options	Assistive Device Options[b]
C1-5	Independent in providing verbal instruction; dependent on performance of bowel care; dependent on transfers	• Padded, tilt-in-space roll-in shower/commode chair with positioning/safety accessories • Padded, upright roll-in shower/commode chair • Perform in bed	• Mechanical lift and sling • Transfer board
C6	Independent in providing verbal instruction; assistance with clothing; modified independent performance of bowel care; possibly independent with transfers	• Padded, upright roll-in shower/commode chair with perianal cutout • Padded, elevated toilet seat • Grab bar • Perform in bed	• Digital stimulator • Suppository inserter • Adaptive equipment for clothing management • Transfer board • Mechanical lift • Mirror
C7	Modified independent with all components	• Padded upright roll-in shower/commode chair with perianal cutout • Padded, elevated toilet seat • Grab bar • Perform, in bed	• Digital stimulator • Suppository inserter • Adaptive equipment for clothing management • Transfer board • Mirror
C8-T1	Modified independent to independent with all components	• Padded upright roll-in shower/commode chair with perianal cutout • Padded, elevated toilet seat • Grab bar • Perform, in bed	• Digital stimulator • Suppository inserter • Transfer board • Mirror

T2-T6	Independent with all components	• Padded upright roll-in shower/commode chair with perianal cutout • Padded, elevated toilet seat • Grab bar • Perform, in bed	• Transfer board
T7-1.2	Independent with all components	• Padded upright roll-in shower/commode chair with perianal cutout • Padded, elevated toilet seat • Grab bar • Perform, in bed	• Transfer board

[a] Potential functional performance outcomes are considered to be optimal functional outcomes by level of injury. However, completeness of injury; other physical, cognitive, and environmental factors; and the amount of time, energy, and resources available to complete bowel care may limit or enhance the achievement of performance outcomes.

[b] Additional supplies for bowel care (individuals may not require every item listed): gloves, suppository, water-soluble lubricant, plastic-lined pads, and washcloths or wipes for cleanup.

Reprinted with permission from topics in spinal cord injury rehabilitation.

to monitor progress. A physiatrist and/or recreational therapist, with knowledge of community resources, can help address barriers to physical activity.

Precocious Puberty

Central precocious puberty affects approximately 50% of girls and between 10% and 30% of boys with MMC.[44] Hydrocephalus is thought to lead to disruption of the hypothalamic–pituitary–gonadal axis and pubertal changes before age 8 years in girls or 9 years in boys. Endocrinology evaluation is recommended, and treatment may include long-acting gonadotropin-releasing hormone analogs.

Sexuality

Sexual function is altered in SCI/D. In males, sexual function and fertility is often affected and a urologist with special training in erectile dysfunction can be helpful. In females, less is known about sexual function but fertility is typically unaffected. Women with MMC, women who have had a child with MMC, and women whose partners have MMC should be encouraged to take a high dose of folic acid, 4 mg as opposed to 0.4 mg, starting 3 months before becoming pregnant and continued through the first trimester to decrease the risk of having a child with MMC.

SUMMARY

Although there is currently no cure for SCI/D, there are many areas of active research. The field of stem cell research continues to make strides in identifying potential restorative treatments.[45] Although some stem cell studies in SCI/D exclude children due to safety concerns, research on the use of mesenchymal stem cells during intrauterine closure for MMC is underway. There are several exciting medical technology devices such as exoskeleton orthoses, brain–machine interfaces (BMI), and limb reanimation through a variety of stimulation paradigms. The potential to have novel treatments for congenital and acquired SCI/D in the near future is quite exciting, but as outlined in this review the importance of comprehensive multidisciplinary care led by a pediatric physiatrist cannot be overstated.

CLINICS CARE POINTS

- The relative risk of upper urinary tract disease such as hydronephrosis is higher with congenital spinal cord injury and dysfunction (SCI/D) and requires more frequent monitoring of renal and bladder function.
- Urinary tract infections are defined and treated differently in children with neurogenic bladder.
- Regardless of injury level, 90% of children younger than 12 years of age with acquired spinal cord injury develop scoliosis, and most will require surgery.
- Unlike acquired SCI/D, rapidly progressive scoliosis and back pain in congenital SCI/D may be indicative of spinal cord tethering.
- Treatment of skin breakdown in children with SCI/D includes removing all pressure from the area, alleviating the inciting force, optimizing nutrition, and proper wound care.

DISCLOSURE

The authors have nothing to disclose.

REFERENCES

1. Association SB. Guidelines for the care of people with spina bifida, Available at: http://www.spinabifidaassociation.org/guidelines/. Accessed December 05, 2022.
2. Centers for Disease Control (CDC) Website. Data and Statistics on Spina Bifida. Available at: https://www.cdc.gov/ncbddd/spinabifida/data.html.
3. Kirshblum S, Lin VW, editors. Spinal cord medicine. 3rd edition. Demos Medical Publishing. https://doi.org/10.4065/78.4.524.
4. Zebracki K, Vogel LC. Epidemiology of pediatric-onset spinal cord injuries in the United States. Epidemiol Spinal Cord Inj 2012;26(6):19–28.
5. DeVivo MJ, Vogel LC. Epidemiology of spinal cord injury in children and adolescents. J Spinal Cord Med 2004;27(Suppl 1):S4–10.
6. Shlobin NA, Yerkes EB, Swaroop VT, et al. Multidisciplinary spina bifida clinic: the Chicago experience. Childs Nerv Syst; 2022. https://doi.org/10.1007/S00381-022-05594-5.
7. Kaufman BA, Terbrock A, Winters N, et al. Disbanding a multidisciplinary clinic: effects on the health care of myelomeningocele patients. Pediatr Neurosurg 1994;21(1):36–44.
8. Van Speybroeck A, Beierwaltes P, Hopson B, et al. Care coordination guidelines for the care of people with spina bifida. J Pediatr Rehabil Med 2020;13(4): 499–511.
9. Davis BE, Shurtleff DB, Walker WO, et al. Acquisition of autonomy skills in adolescents with myelomeningocele. Dev Med Child Neurol 2006;48(4):253–8.
10. Garces J, Mathkour M, Scullen T, et al. First case of autonomic dysreflexia following elective lower thoracic spinal cord transection in a spina bifida adult. World Neurosurg 2017;108:988.e1–5.
11. Attia M, Engel P. Thermoregulatory set point in patients with spinal cord injuries (spinal man). Paraplegia 1983;21(4):233–48.
12. Petrofsky JS. Thermoregulatory stress during rest and exercise in heat in patients with a spinal cord injury. Eur J Appl Physiol Occup Physiol 1992;64(6):503–7.
13. Sanger TD, Delgado MR, Gaebler-Spira D, et al. Classification and definition of disorders causing hypertonia in childhood. Pediatrics 2003;111(1):e89–97.
14. Adams MM, Hicks AL. Spasticity after spinal cord injury. Spinal Cord 2005; 43(10):577–86.
15. Elbasiouny SM, Moroz D, Bakr MM, et al. Management of spasticity after spinal cord injury: current techniques and future directions. Neurorehabil Neural Repair 2010;24(1):23–33.
16. Padman R, Alexander M, Thorogood C, et al. Respiratory management of pediatric patients with spinal cord injuries: retrospective review of the duPont experience. Neurorehabil Neural Repair 2003;17(1):32–6.
17. Patel DM, Rocque BG, Hopson B, et al. Sleep-disordered breathing in patients with myelomeningocele. J Neurosurg Pediatr 2015;16(1):30–5.
18. Kim I, Hopson B, Aban I, et al. Decompression for Chiari malformation type II in individuals with myelomeningocele in the National Spina Bifida Patient Registry. J Neurosurg Pediatr 2018;22(6):652–8.
19. Merenda L, Brown JP. Bladder and bowel management for the child with spinal cord dysfunction. J Spinal Cord Med 2004;27(Suppl 1). https://doi.org/10.1080/10790268.2004.11753780.
20. Bladder management for adults with spinal cord injury: a clinical practice guideline for health-care providers. J Spinal Cord Med 2006;29(5):527–73.

21. Wallis MC, Paramsothy P, Newsome K, et al. Incidence of urinary tract infections in newborns with spina bifida: is antibiotic prophylaxis necessary? J Urol 2021; 206(1):126.

22. Merriman LS, Arlen AM, Kirsch AJ, et al. Does augmentation cystoplasty with continent reconstruction at a young age increase the risk of complications or secondary surgeries? J Pediatr Urol 2015;11(1):41.e1–5.

23. Atchley TJ, Dangle PP, Hopson BD, et al. Age and factors associated with self-clean intermittent catheterization in patients with spina bifida. J Pediatr Rehabil Med 2018;11(4):283–91.

24. McLaughlin MJ, He Y, Brunstrom-Hernandez J, et al. Pharmacogenomic variability of oral baclofen clearance and clinical response in children with cerebral palsy. Pharm Manag PM R 2018;10(3):235–43.

25. Akbar M, Abel R, Seyler TM, et al. Repeated botulinum-A toxin injections in the treatment of myelodysplastic children and patients with spinal cord injuries with neurogenic bladder dysfunction. BJU Int 2007;100(3):639–45.

26. Kennelly M, Cruz F, Herschorn S, et al. Efficacy and Safety of AbobotulinumtoxinA in Patients with Neurogenic Detrusor Overactivity Incontinence Performing Regular Clean Intermittent Catheterization: Pooled Results from Two Phase 3 Randomized Studies (CONTENT1 and CONTENT2). Eur Urol 2022;82(2). https://doi.org/10.1016/J.EURURO.2022.03.010.

27. Chulamorkodt NN, Estrada CR, Chaviano AH. Continent urinary diversion: 10-year experience of shriners hospitals for children in Chicago. J Spinal Cord Med 2004;(Suppl 1). https://doi.org/10.1080/10790268.2004.11753447.

28. Goetz LL, Hurvitz EA, Nelson VS, et al. Bowel management in children and adolescents with spinal cord injury. J Spinal Cord Med 1998;21(4):335–41.

29. Del Popolo G, Mosiello G, Pilati C, et al. Treatment of neurogenic bowel dysfunction using transanal irrigation: a multicenter Italian study. Spinal Cord 2008;46(7): 517–22.

30. Kelly MS, Wiener JS, Liu T, et al. Neurogenic bowel treatments and continence outcomes in children and adults with myelomeningocele. J Pediatr Rehabil Med 2020;13(4):685–93.

31. Brinas P, Zalay N, Philis A, et al. Use of Malone antegrade continence enemas in neurologic bowel dysfunction. J Visc Surg 2020;157(6):453–9.

32. Johns J, Krogh K, Rodriguez GM, et al. Management of neurogenic bowel dysfunction in adults after spinal cord injury. Top Spinal Cord Inj Rehabil 2021; 27(2):75–151.

33. Dearolf WW, Betz RR, Vogel LC, et al. Scoliosis in pediatric spinal cord-injured patients. J Pediatr Orthop 1990;10(2):214–8.

34. Vogel LC, Krajci KA, Anderson CJ. Adults with pediatric-onset spinal cord injury: part 2: musculoskeletal and neurological complications. J Spinal Cord Med 2002; 25(2):117–23.

35. Mehta S, Betz RR, Mulcahey MJ, et al. Effect of bracing on paralytic scoliosis secondary to spinal cord injury. J Spinal Cord Med 2004;27(Suppl 1). https://doi.org/10.1080/10790268.2004.11753448.

36. Chafetz RS, Mulcahey MJ, Betz RR, et al. Impact of prophylactic thoracolumbosacral orthosis bracing on functional activities and activities of daily living in the pediatric spinal cord injury population. J Spinal Cord Med 2007;30(Suppl 1). https://doi.org/10.1080/10790268.2007.11754598.

37. McCarthy JJ, Chafetz RS, Betz RR, et al. Incidence and degree of hip subluxation/dislocation in children with spinal cord injury. J Spinal Cord Med 2004; 27(Suppl 1). https://doi.org/10.1080/10790268.2004.11753423.

38. McCarthy JJ, Betz RR. Hip disorders in children who have spinal cord injury. Orthop Clin North Am 2006;37(2):197–202.
39. Swaroop VT, Dias LS. Strategies of hip management in myelomeningocele: to do or not to do. Hip Int 2009;19(1 SUPPL. 6). https://doi.org/10.1177/112070000901906S09.
40. Apkon SD, Fenton L, Coll JR. Bone mineral density in children with myelomeningocele. Dev Med Child Neurol 2009;51(1):63–7.
41. Moynahan M, Betz RR, Triolo RJ, et al. Characterization of the bone mineral density of children with spinal cord injury. J Spinal Cord Med 1996;19(4):249–54.
42. Vogel LC, Betz RR, Mulcahey MJ. Spinal cord injuries in children and adolescents. Handb Clin Neurol 2012;109:131–48.
43. Gour-Provençal G, Costa C. Metabolic syndrome in children with myelomeningocele and the role of physical activity: a narrative review of the literature. Top Spinal Cord Inj Rehabil 2022;28(3):15–40.
44. Almutlaq N, O'Neil J, Fuqua JS. Central precocious puberty in spina bifida children: guidelines for the care of people with spina bifida. J Pediatr Rehabil Med 2020;13(4):557–63.
45. Shang Z, Wang M, Zhang B, et al. Clinical translation of stem cell therapy for spinal cord injury still premature: results from a single-arm meta-analysis based on 62 clinical trials. BMC Med 2022;20(1):284.

Spasticity Interventions
Decision-Making and Management

Joline E. Brandenburg, MD[a,b,*], Amy E. Rabatin, MD[a,b],
Sherilyn W. Driscoll, MD[a,b]

KEYWORDS

- Spasticity • Children • Treatment • Botulinum toxin • Phenol • Complications
- Function • Baclofen

KEY POINTS

- Spasticity in children can negatively affect development, function, comfort, and sleep.
- The severity and influence of spasticity may fluctuate with age, growth, and physiological stressors.
- Not all spasticity must be treated but effective management options are available.
- Differentiating between spasticity and other motor disorders such as dystonia is important when considering treatment options.
- Spasticity management strategies can be used simultaneously and include stretching, bracing, oral and injectable medications, and neurosurgical procedures.

INTRODUCTION

Spasticity is a neurologic disorder in children that can interfere with development, function, and participation caused by a variety of processes affecting the central nervous system.[1] In the pediatric population, spasticity is most commonly associated with a diagnosis of cerebral palsy.[1,2] In fact, the majority of children with cerebral palsy have spasticity.[3] However, spasticity may also result from a myriad of other inflammatory, metabolic, infectious, congenital, neoplastic, vascular, and traumatic conditions of the brain or spine. Therefore, an understanding of the condition and management is important for the general pediatrician.

Spasticity is a form of hypertonia and is defined as an increase in muscle tone or stiffness related to an underlying abnormality of the central nervous system. It is

[a] Division of Pediatric Rehabilitation Medicine, Department of Physical Medicine and Rehabilitation, Mayo Clinic, 200 1st Street Southwest, Rochester, MN 55905, USA; [b] Department of Pediatric and Adolescent Medicine, Mayo Clinic, 200 1st Street Southwest, Rochester, MN 55905, USA
* Corresponding author. Division of Pediatric Rehabilitation Medicine, Department of Physical Medicine and Rehabilitation, Mayo Clinic, 200 1st Street Southwest, Rochester, MN 55905.
E-mail address: Brandenburg.Joline@mayo.edu

Pediatr Clin N Am 70 (2023) 483–500
https://doi.org/10.1016/j.pcl.2023.01.005
0031-3955/23/© 2023 Elsevier Inc. All rights reserved.

characterized as "velocity dependent" because the more rapidly the muscle is stretched, the more likely the muscle is to "catch."[1,4] It is often associated with an "upper motor neuron syndrome" composed of hyperreflexia, clonus, reflex overflow (ie, both legs move when checking patellar reflex on one leg), presence of a Babinski response (upgoing big toe when bottom of foot is scratched), weakness, and poor motor control.[4] The degree of spasticity may range from mild to severe (determined through validated assessments as discussed below), often varying depending on the state of the child (worse with illness, pain, emotional distress) and underlying diagnosis.[4] Spasticity must be differentiated from dystonia, the other common form of hypertonia in children, because treatments and outcomes may differ.[4] Dystonia is defined as sustained or intermittent muscle contraction, which is not dependent on velocity, resulting in abnormal movements such as posturing or twisting.[4] It is variable and may be associated with or brought on by voluntary movement. In some conditions, such as cerebral palsy, children may have spasticity, dystonia, or both.

Spasticity can affect any functional motor activity. For example, ambulatory differences include toe walking or crouch gait. Daily activities may be difficult such as reaching for a toy or achieving proper positioning or seating in a wheelchair. Scissoring of the legs or finger flexor spasticity may cause problems with perineal or hand hygiene. Skin breakdown may result. Spasticity can also cause pain. Muscle spasms may result in difficulty sleeping. However, it is also important to note that not all spasticity has negative consequences. Some children use their spasticity to maintain upright posture or stand with assistance.

The consequences of spasticity are compounded in a growing child because muscle imbalance (overactivity of one muscle compared with relatively less activity of an antagonist muscle—ie, overactive calf muscle but less-active foot dorsiflexor muscles) may result in secondary musculoskeletal complications.[5] The musculotendinous shortening seen in joint contractures causes limitations of range of motion and, thus, further functional limitations. "Lever arm dysfunction," or atypical forces placed on growing bones, may result in long bone torsion (rotational deformity) such as femoral neck anteversion (persistent inward turning of femurs bones), and tibial torsion (manifest as feet turning excessively outward or inward), scoliosis, and joint instability such as hip dysplasia with subluxation or dislocation, and foot deformities.[5]

DISCUSSION
Nature of the Problem

Disruption of central nervous system function
Regardless of the cause, mechanism, or timing, the mechanistic underpinning and drivers of spasticity are complex.[2,6–8] Spasticity is not just one disrupted pathway but rather the result of a cascade of changes that can occur with single or multiple insults to a developing central nervous system. This cascade of developmental differences can vary in location (brain versus spinal cord) or cause and timing (birth prematurity versus encephalomyelitis versus trauma) but still result in similar clinical manifestations.[2,6–8]

Spasticity can change or seem to change over time in the pediatric population. Spasticity often "evolves" as the brain and spinal cord myelinate and mature. During this developmental period, neurons and dendrites in the brain and spinal cord form and fine tune synapses and connections to establish the optimal communication needed to perform typical daily functions.[9–11] This process results in difficultly predicting the severity and location of spasticity as well as the impairment in physical function in infants and young children. In addition, the dominant type of hypertonia can change over time. For example, a child with the diagnosis of mixed-tone, spastic dystonic quadriplegic cerebral palsy may have low tone in infancy, spasticity in the preschool years and predominantly dystonia by school age.

Maldevelopment of skeletal muscle properties

Spasticity also causes maladaptive skeletal muscle changes, which are compounded by growth in children. In children with spastic cerebral palsy, muscles have increased passive stiffness with stretch[12–14] while force generation (strength) is reduced.[15,16] These functional changes to skeletal muscle relate to changes in the intrinsic properties of the muscle itself. These differences in muscle properties brought on by spasticity likely amplify the impact of spasticity on the development of joint contractures and boney rotational deformities. Unfortunately, some of these changes to muscle do not reverse or fully correct, even when spasticity is treated.[17,18] Although most of the studies done to investigate muscle properties in children with spasticity have been in children with cerebral palsy, it is likely that a similar process is occurring in children with spasticity due to different neurologic conditions.

Assessment and Evaluation

History including the functional impact of spasticity, and physical examination are key components of spasticity assessment to inform the treatment plan (**Tables 1** and **2**).

Table 1
Key history questions to assess for spasticity

Where is stiffness/spasticity appreciated?	• Upper Extremities
	  ○ Bilateral
	  ○ Unilateral
	• Lower Extremities
	  ○ Bilateral
	  ○ Unilateral
	• Trunk
	• Neck

How severe is the spasticity?	• Easy to overcome • Always present but still able to move • Always present and difficult to move • Very difficult to move or stretch
Is the spasticity getting better, worse or staying the same?	
Does the spasticity interfere with function and, if so, how?	• Diaper changes/dressing/hygiene • Reaching and other upper extremity activities • Positioning in or propelling wheelchair • Getting heel down in orthoses • Transfers, gait
Does spasticity interfere with sleep?	• Wakes with spasms • Repositioning is difficult • Stiff when first wake up
Is there pain associated with spasticity?	
Spasticity interventions currently used or tried	• Stretching—what and how often, including activities such as standing • Participation in therapies • Bracing • Oral medications • Injections • Surgeries

Table 2
Key physical examination components to assess for spasticity

Physical Examination	Examples of Abnormalities
Inspection and palpation	• Legs scissor when handled or excited • Fingers tightly fisted
Range of motion	• Difficult or unable to get ankles to a neutral position • Knees unable to be fully stretched when child supine
Strength	• Unable to sit unsupported • Unable to kick against gravity when seated or must move both legs at same time when trying to kick • Asymmetry in ability to open hand
Reflexes	• Brisk deep tendon reflexes • Reflex overflow (eg, unilateral patellar reflex elicits movement of both legs) • Clonus (rapid beating movement of ankle with brisk stretch) • Babinski response
Mobility and gait	• Bunny hop appearance to crawl • Always on toes when pulls to stand • Toe walking • One arm is flexed or does not swing the same as other arm when walking • Crouch walking
Objective spasticity assessment (not commonly performed by primary care)	• Modified Ashworth scale • Tardieu scale

The child's age, size, functional level, comfort level, neurologic status, and developmental potential should be assessed.[1]

The Modified Ashworth Scale and Tardieu Scale are rating scales used commonly in the assessment and rating of severity of spasticity by specialists (**Table 3**).[19] These scales are also used to track response to spasticity interventions. The Hypertonia

Table 3
Spasticity and dystonia scales

Type of Abnormal Tone:	Scales Commonly Used:	
Spasticity	Modified Ashworth scale • Scale from 0 to 4 (0 = No spasticity to 4 = Rigidity) • Greater the number, more severe the spasticity • Measured/reported for each muscle of interest/involvement	Modified Tardieu scale • Dynamic tone—range of movement after spastic catch • Reported as R1 (joint angle at first feel spastic catch) and R2 (joint angle at end of ROM)
Dystonia	HAT • Seven-item tool assessing passive and active movement • Used to assess and discern spasticity and dystonia	

Data from Refs.[1,4,19]

Assessment Tool (HAT) may be used to help distinguish between spasticity and dystonia.[1,4]

When to Refer?

Pediatric providers should be aware that new or worsening spasticity in a child with a static diagnosis, such as cerebral palsy or spina bifida should prompt further medical assessment because it may be a "red flag" for a new infection, illness, bowel impaction, urinary retention, skin pressure injury, occult fracture, tethered cord, syrinx, or other central nervous system process. Before referral or instituting any spasticity treatment plan changes, medical contributors to worsened spasticity should be ruled out or treated. For example, in a child with chronic constipation and worsening spasticity, ask about bowel habits (consistency, frequency, amount), appetite, abdominal pain, and consider ordering an abdominal radiograph to evaluate stool burden.

Referral to a pediatric physiatrist (physical medicine and rehabilitation physician) or pediatric neurologist is appropriate when assistance is needed with spasticity diagnosis, spasticity management, worsening of spasticity, or change in function. Pediatric physiatrists are uniquely positioned to holistically assess not only the presence of spasticity but also the impact on of spasticity on function, developmental skill acquisition, cares/positioning, pain, sleep, and musculoskeletal deformity because this is a core component of their advanced training. Early and appropriate management of spasticity will help optimize development and function and minimize complications. Differentiating between the various forms of hypertonia as well as making the distinction between severe spasticity and contracture is critical to providing appropriate treatment. The decisions regarding whether and how much to treat are important because overtreating spasticity can also result in functional decline if spasticity is used in standing or walking or for activities of daily living. Thus, it is critical to refer to a provider, such as a pediatric physiatrist, who can assess spasticity and identify when to intervene in spasticity management along with discussing a multifaceted spasticity management approach.

Therapeutic Options

Regardless of cause, child's age, or when spasticity symptoms begin, treatment paradigms are similar. Once it is decided that the child's spasticity needs intervention, a multifaceted approach to management may be used, akin to putting pieces of a spasticity puzzle together (**Figs. 1** and **2**). However, unlike a traditional puzzle, not all spasticity puzzle pieces may be used. Puzzle pieces may also be put together in differing ways to address the needs of the individual child during their lifetime. Traditionally, interventions that are least invasive and have the lowest risk of adverse events are initiated first and serve as the base or center piece (ie, stretching, see **Fig. 1**) with a gradual addition or transition of interventions depending on the child's response and severity of spasticity. The approach to spasticity management may also vary depending on whether the spasticity that needs intervention is focal (a single muscle or muscle group) or diffuse and affecting multiple areas.[20–22] Child's age, medical comorbidities, ability of family to predictably attend medical appointments, and proximity to a tertiary care center may also influence the selection of spasticity interventions. A pediatric physiatrist is well positioned to guide the determination of when and which spasticity interventions to use, dosing, and monitoring for adverse effects.

Stretching

The spasticity intervention that is least invasive and has the lowest risk of adverse effects is a stretching program. Stretching programs can vary in frequency, duration

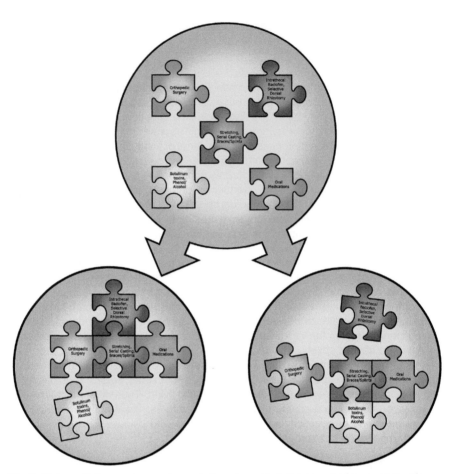

Fig. 1. The spasticity management puzzle has pieces that can arranged in a variety of ways. For each child, the puzzle may be arranged a little differently with pieces added, subtracted, or never used throughout the course of the child's lifetime. (*Courtesy of* Ms Natalie Peterson.)

for holding the stretch, and muscles stretched. A metanalysis of stretching as a therapeutic intervention for children with cerebral palsy found mixed results.[23] Stretching, even for prolonged periods or multiple times a day may not be sufficient to overcome the frequent to constant flexion positioning that occurs in children with spasticity.[23,24] Stretching programs also tend to be time intensive for families. For some, prolonged stretch during sleep with positioning orthoses may be attempted, especially for hands/wrists (finger flexors/wrist flexors), ankle (gastrocnemius), and knee (hamstrings), although evidence to support their benefit is weak.[25] Unfortunately, these nighttime positioning devices can be uncomfortable and may disrupt sleep for both the child and the family. Stretching can also occur during other activities, such as a standing program while doing schoolwork or simply transitioning from wheelchair to floor for activities in a prone position.[20–22,24]

Systemic medications
Oral medications have a greater risk of side effects than stretching but have a greater effect on spasticity reduction. Oral medications should be considered when spasticity

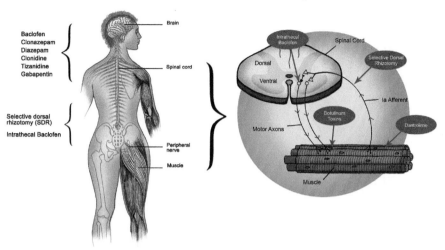

**Common Spasticity Interventions
for Individuals with Cerebral Palsy**

Fig. 2. Body diagram representation of areas of action for varying spasticity reducing interventions. For many children with spasticity, multiple interventions may be simultaneously used in a stepwise fashion to harness the varying sites and mechanisms of action of spasticity interventions. (*Courtesy of* Ms Natalie Peterson.)

affects multiple limbs, impedes function, impairs performance of cares and positioning, and/or is thought to be contributing to pain or sleep difficulties. Medications for spasticity reduction vary based on mechanism of action, dosing, administration, adverse effects, and Food and Drug Administration (FDA) approval for use in children for spasticity reduction (**Table 4**).[20–22,25–28] Although baclofen and diazepam have the strongest evidence supporting their use for spasticity management in children with cerebral palsy,[25] the choice of medication to use for spasticity management depends on a number of variables including age and comorbidities (see **Table 4**). For instance, for a 2-year-old child with quadriplegic cerebral palsy (CP), intractable epilepsy, and constipation, a medication in the benzodiazepine class or gabapentin may be considered first to avoid exacerbating other comorbidities.[20,29] For some children, a combination of medications may be needed due to having both spasticity and a dyskinetic movement disorder. In this case, a stepwise approach of titrating a medication to maximum dosing or intolerable side effect is recommended before initiating another medication. For example, in a 15-year-old child with severe spasticity and dyskinetic movement disorder due to an anoxic brain injury who is maximized on baclofen, gabapentin, and diazepam but still has hypertonia, one may reach for clonidine or dantrolene as a next medication. If low blood pressure is an issue, then dantrolene may be the better choice.[20] For infants or very young children with severe hypertonia (often spasticity and dyskinetic movement disorder), gabapentin should be considered because there is some evidence that it may help hypertonia directly but also indirectly through reducing visceral hyperalgesia and generalized neuroirritability.[29–31]

Injectable medications and compounds
For more focal spasticity reduction, botulinum neurotoxins (BoNTs), phenol, and alcohol should be considered. Of these options, BoNTs have the highest level of evidence for effectiveness in reducing spasticity.[25] However, the BoNTs do differ

Table 4
Systemic medication considerations for spasticity management in children

Medication	Dosing	Adverse Effects	Other Considerations	Mechanism of Action	FDA Approval for Spasticity in Children
Baclofen	• Maximum 40 mg/d if aged younger than 8 y • Maximum 60 mg/d if aged older than 8 y • For suspected ITB withdrawal give 10–20 mg q4 h	• Sedation • Seizures • Constipation • Hypotonia • Withdrawal can be life-threatening if abruptly stopped (Black Box Warning)	• No IV formulation • Recent patent of compounded liquids (Ozobax and Fleqsuvy) is costly and may not be covered by insurance • Dissolvable granules now available (Lyvispah) • Compounded formulations may precipitate, must shake vigorously every time • Pharmacokinetics make 4× per day dosing ideal, though most prescribe 3× per day for family convenience	Gamma aminobutyric acid type B (GABA$_B$) receptor agonist	• Tablets, granules, and oral solution approved for children aged ≥12 y • Intrathecal approved for children aged ≥4 y
Clonazepam	• No dosing listed for spasticity • Dosing for seizures as guide	• Sedation • Drooling • Withdrawal can be life-threatening if abruptly stopped • Black box warning for physical dependence, withdrawal and use with opioids	• Authors use this for spasticity interfering with sleep (dose only at bedtime) • Protein bound, so dosing can be impacted by nutritional status • Cimetidine inhibits metabolism	GABA$_A$ receptor agonist	No

	Dosing	Side effects	Notes	Mechanism	Approved
Diazepam	• 6 mo and older—1–2.5 mg orally 3–4 times daily	• Same as clonazepam	• Often used for postsurgical spasm/spasticity exacerbation • Protein bound, so dosing can be impacted by nutritional status • Cimetidine inhibits metabolism • Has highest level of evidence of all systemic meds for spasticity reduction	GABA$_A$ receptor agonist	• Approved for children aged ≥6 mo
Clonidine	• 0.02 ± 0.03 mg/kg/d, with a range of 0.0014–0.15 mg/kg/d[26]	• Sedation • Hypotension	• Oral and transdermal formulations	Alpha 2 adrenergic	No
Tizanidine	• Children aged >2 y—0.3–0.5 mg/kg/d in 4 divided doses	• Sedation • Hypotension	• Authors rarely use for spasticity	Alpha 2 adrenergic	No
Gabapentin	• Infants—5 mg/kg/d and titrate by adding either adding doses (up to 3× per day) or increasing dose • 3–11 years—10–15 mg/kg/d in 3 divided doses, up to 40 mg/kg/d for 3-y and 4-y-olds and 35 mg/kg/d up to age 11 y • >11 y—300 mg 3 times daily (may start lower), can titrate up to 3600 mg/d	• Nystagmus • Sedation	• Authors first choice for children aged <1 y and with who have profound neurologic impairment and neuroirritability • May inhibit excitatory synaptogenesis—ie, reduce excitatory synapse formation	Binds alpha 2 delta 1 ($\alpha2\delta$-1) receptors (Calcium channels)	No

(continued on next page)

Table 4
(continued)

Medication	Dosing	Adverse Effects	Other Considerations	Mechanism of Action	FDA Approval for Spasticity in Children
Dantrolene	• 0.5 mg/kg once daily for 7 d, then 0.5 mg/kg 3 times a day for 7 d, then 1 mg/kg 3 times a day for 7 d, then 2 mg/kg 3 times a day • Max 100 mg 4× per day or 12 mg/kg	• Black box warning for liver failure (not reported in children)	• Authors check LFTs before starting, during titration, and every 6 mo–1 y thereafter • Caution with other medications metabolized by liver • Authors have had to limit dosing due to increased drooling/swallowing difficulties (likely due to weakness) • Does not affect cardiac or smooth muscle • Compounded formulation can be difficult to get	Decreases calcium availability at the sarcoplasmic reticulum in the muscle	• Approved for children aged ≥ 5 y

Abbreviation: ITB, intrathecal baclofen.
Data from Refs.[20–22,25–31]

with regard to dosing, formulation, mechanism of action, and even effectiveness (**Table 5**).[32,33] BoNT is a highly purified naturally occurring substance produced by *Clostridium botulinum.* There are 7 BoNT serotypes (A–G), although few are used medically and only serotype A and B are used for spasticity management. All BoNTs are administered through injection into the targeted muscle and act by inhibiting the release of acetylcholine at the neuromuscular junction, thus interrupting the communication from the nerve to the muscle and interfering with muscle contraction. All BoNTs have the potential for similar adverse effects (see **Table 5**), although more reports of dry mouth and double vision have occurred with rimabotulinum toxin B.[32,33] BoNT injections should be performed by providers trained in dosing, medication reconstitution, and adverse effects in children. Providers must also have excellent musculoskeletal anatomy knowledge for localization of the injections. Use of electrical stimulation and ultrasound guidance increase the accuracy of muscle localization for injection.[34] Injections can be performed with the child awake and receiving topical anesthesia or distraction techniques or can be performed with varying levels of sedation. The choice in this approach should be discussed with family and may change over time. Injections should not be performed more frequently than every 12 weeks due to the mechanism of action of BoNTs and to reduce the potential for developing antibodies, which has occurred with frequent, low-dose injections.[35] Most providers also recommend that BoNTs should not be administered within 2 weeks of any vaccination or between vaccinations when administering the original series of coronavirus disease 2019 vaccinations. This recommendation is due to a theoretical risk of developing antibodies to BoNTs, although studies have not evaluated this risk.

Phenol and alcohol injections are less well studied in children with spasticity but have been used much longer than BoNTs.[21,25] Both phenol and alcohol should be injected as close to the nerve of interest as possible because they act by denaturing the myelin sheath, which then results in denervation.[36] However, this mechanism not only affects the myelin sheath of the nerve but also causes fibrosis of all tissues it is exposed to, including muscle. The spasticity reducing effect can last up to 6 months. Phenol and alcohol are frequently used in combination with BoNTs, although usually targeting differing areas. Because most children with spasticity have preserved sensation, phenol and alcohol injections should be reserved for nerves that are primarily motor (eg, obturator or musculocutaneous nerves) to reduce the risk of significant neuropathic pain. Because these injections are painful, require very precise needle placement, and often take a longer period to do than BoNT injections, anesthesia is commonly used. Adverse effects of phenol and alcohol injections include neuropathic pain, fibrosis, intoxication (high concentration alcohol), cardiac dysrhythmia, and catastrophic limb loss due to vascular injection (not reported in children; see **Table 5**).[36,37] If neuropathic pain occurs after an injection, repeating the injection as soon as possible for more complete neurolysis or initiation of gabapentin can be done. Over time, both BoNT and phenol/alcohol can lose effectiveness. This is likely due to chronic denervation and changes at the level of the muscle with repeat injections. Adjusting dosing and dilution of BoNT can be helpful if effectiveness is decreasing. Occasionally switching to another BoNT can help.[33] Waiting to start injections until spasticity is causing significant problems, spreading out time between injections as much as possible, and for those getting injections in multiple limbs, using BoNT/phenol/alcohol in combination with oral medications can all be used to prolong optimal effectiveness.

Surgical interventions
The most prolonged effective spasticity management options involve surgical interventions. In children with spasticity interfering with gait, function, or cares, a selective

Table 5
Injectable spasticity management options for focal spasticity interventions

Medication/Compound	Dosing	Adverse Effects	Other Considerations	Mechanism of Action	FDA Approval for Spasticity in Children
Onabotulinum toxin A (Botox)	• 8 u/kg or 300 u total for lower limbs • Total body dosing 10 u/kg or 340 u	• Dry mouth • Double vision • Spread to other muscles • Weakness • Swallowing difficulties • Respiratory difficulties	• Most providers will go up to 400 u in children, depending on child's weight and muscles targeted • Maximum of 300 u should be considered in medically fragile or children with CP who are nonambulatory	Blocks presynaptic release of Ach into the NMJ	Children aged ≥2 y for upper and lower limb spasticity
Abobotulinum toxin A (Dysport)	• Total body dosing 30 u/kg or 1000 u	• Dry mouth • Double vision • Spread to other muscles • Weakness • Swallowing difficulties • Respiratory difficulties	• May have longer duration of action than other toxins	Blocks presynaptic release of Ach into the NMJ	Children aged ≥2 y for upper and lower limb spasticity
Incobotulinum toxin A (Xeomin)	• Maximum 8 u/kg, 200 u per single limb, or 400 u total dosing	• Dry mouth • Double vision • Spread to other muscles • Weakness • Swallowing difficulties • Respiratory difficulties	• Lower protein concentration may reduce development of antibodies, though all toxins now have much lower protein than original during original marketing	Blocks presynaptic release of Ach into the NMJ	Children aged ≥2 y for upper limb spasticity

Agent	Dosing	Adverse effects	Special considerations	Mechanism of action	Approved for children with CP
Rimabotulinum toxin B (Myobloc)	• Not clear for children • 70–660 u/kg or 3000–22,000 u • Maximum 22,000 u	• Dry mouth • Double vision • Spread to other muscles • Weakness • Swallowing difficulties • Respiratory difficulties		Blocks presynaptic release of Ach into the NMJ	No
Alcohol	• Typically 40%–50% concentration	• Limb-threatening vascular sclerosis if injected into blood vessel • Paresthesia • Muscle fibrosis	• May shows signs of intoxication if use high concentration (75%–100%)	Denatures the myelin sheath of the peripheral nerve and may have direct neuronal degeneration resulting in the degradation of the nerve	No
Phenol	• 3%–7% concentration • Recommended pediatric dosing of <30 mg/kg • 5% phenol = 50 mg/mL • 7% phenol = 70 mg/mL	• Limb-threatening vascular sclerosis if injected into blood vessel • Paresthesia • Cardiac dysrhythmia • Muscle fibrosis	• Highly toxic, must be prepared in fume hood to appropriate percentage	Denatures the myelin sheath of the peripheral nerve and may have direct neuronal degeneration, which results in the degradation of the nerve	No

Abbreviations: Ach, acetylcholine; CP, cerebral palsy; NMJ, neuromuscular junction; u, units.
Data from Refs.[21,25,27,32,33,36,37]

dorsal rhizotomy (SDR) may be indicated. SDR is a neurosurgical procedure in which sensory nerve roots are divided into rootlets, selectively stimulated, and up to 50% to 70% of rootlets sectioned.[38,39] Traditionally, this has been reserved for children with spastic diplegic cerebral palsy, who are ambulatory, between ages 4 and 7 years, and without extensive orthopedic surgical interventions.[39] However, this can also be helpful for children with hemiplegic or quadriplegic cerebral palsy, and potentially those with other conditions in which spasticity interferes with function.[40] This procedure is not intended to change their level of function (ie, if they use a walker before surgery, it is likely they will need to use a walker even after full recovery). Palliative rhizotomy consists of a SDR followed by a ventral rhizotomy (motor nerves).[41] This procedure is reserved for nonambulatory children with severe cerebral palsy or a similar disorder and who have severe spasticity and/or dystonia.

In children with very severe spasticity affecting all limbs, those who also have significant dystonia or other dyskinetic movement disorder, or those with more degenerative or rapidly progressing spastic condition, intrathecal baclofen (ITB) pump could be considered. ITB is a system that involves implantation of a pump device subcutaneously in the abdominal wall that is approximately the diameter of a hockey puck and holds compounded baclofen. A catheter is tunneled from the pump to the spinal column with the catheter piercing the dura to deliver the baclofen to the cerebrospinal fluid in the thoracic or lumbar levels, although some have threaded the catheters higher for children with dystonic and dyskinetic movement disorders.[42] ITB typically is most effective for managing tone in lower extremities.[42] Although this can be quite helpful, adverse effects can be substantial. For children, the risk of pump infection is greater than adults. Withdrawal due to abrupt disruption of baclofen delivery, most commonly due to catheter malfunction, can be life-threatening if not recognized and treated. Withdrawal symptoms can include irritability, neuropathic itching, and increased spasticity. The first line of treatment is administration of oral baclofen, often at doses of 10 to 20 mg q4 hours depending on child's size. If withdrawal from baclofen is suspected, this should be started immediately while trying to identify the reason for the child's symptoms or transferring child to an institution that can both evaluate the pump and catheter and intervene surgically, if needed.

Combination therapy

For many children with spasticity, a combination of interventions may be needed (**Fig. 2**). When a combination of interventions is used, greater complexity develops in the treatment plan. The complexities of scaling spasticity interventions, monitoring changes in spasticity, and balancing adverse effects is well within the expertise of pediatric physiatrists. A common combination of spasticity management interventions is daily lower extremity stretching with the inclusion of a standing program with daily wear of ankle foot orthoses, oral medications, and injectable BoNTs (see **Fig. 1**). Children will typically have tried multiple medications before more invasive interventions such as SDR and ITB. Not all families elect to pursue surgical interventions for spasticity reduction. It is important that families have the opportunity for consultation with a physician with expertise in spasticity management, such as a pediatric physiatrist, to discuss all options that may be considered for their child along with goals of management. Furthermore, studies of alternative therapies such as cannabis, stem cell therapy, and hyperbaric oxygen for spasticity in children are of limited or low quality and currently insufficient to support their use.[43–45]

Rarely does an intervention eliminate spasticity. Thus, some children may benefit from injectable BoNTs or oral medications even after SDR or ITB. Importantly, none of the spasticity reducing interventions cures the child of the disorder that resulted in spasticity.

SUMMARY

Spasticity is a complex disorder that can be caused by a variety of processes affecting the central nervous system. The impact of spasticity on function, comfort, positioning, contracture, and limb deformity may change as the child grows and the central nervous system matures. There are multiple potential interventions that can be tried for spasticity reduction. Timing of initiation of interventions and which interventions to use depends on multiple factors intrinsic and extrinsic to the patient. Early referral to a physician with special training in this area, such as a pediatric rehabilitation medicine physician, is important to facilitate appropriate interventions in a timely manner. Regardless of cause, none of the spasticity reducing interventions will cure the underlying disorder.

CLINICS CARE POINTS

- Pediatricians should refer children with spasticity to a pediatric rehabilitaiton physician as soon as possible to facilitate appropirate interventions.
- As the impact of spasticity on a child's function, comfort, and limb range of motion may change as a child grows, and should be reassessed when concerns arise.
- Children with spasticity may have differing interventions depending on severity of spasticity, limbs involved, and goals of child and family.

DECLARATION OF INTERESTS

The authors declare no competing interests.

ACKNOWLEDGMENTS

The authors would like to thank Ms Natalie Peterson for her expertise in drafting the figures.

REFERENCES

1. Gormley ME Jr, Deshpande S. Hypertonia. In: Murphy KP, McMahon MA, Hourtrow AJ, editors. Pediatric rehabilitation. 6th edition. New York: Springer Publishing Company; 2020. p. 100–23.
2. Brandenburg JE, Fogarty MJ, Sieck GC. A critical evaluation of current concepts in cerebral palsy. Physiology 2019;34(3):216–29.
3. Yeargin-Allsopp M, Van Naarden Braun K, Doernberg NS, et al. Prevalence of cerebral palsy in 8-year-old children in three areas of the United States in 2002: a multisite collaboration. Pediatrics 2008;121(3):547–54.
4. Sanger TD, Delgado MR, Gaebler-Spira D, et al. Task force on childhood motor D. Classification and definition of disorders causing hypertonia in childhood. Pediatrics 2003;111(1):e89–97.
5. Driscoll SW, Skinner J. Musculoskeletal complications of neuromuscular disease in children. Phys Med Rehabil Clin N Am 2008;19(1):163–94, viii.
6. Bar-On L, Molenaers G, Aertbelien E, et al. Spasticity and its contribution to hypertonia in cerebral palsy. BioMed Res Int 2015;2015:317047.
7. Enslin JMN, Rohlwink UK, Figaji A. Management of spasticity after traumatic brain injury in children. Front Neurol 2020;11:126.

8. Mukherjee A, Chakravarty A. Spasticity mechanisms - for the clinician. Front Neurol 2010;1:149.

9. Brandenburg J, Fogarty M, Sieck G. Evaluation of diaphragm neuromuscular transmission and fatigue in a mouse model of cerebral palsy: TB-SP09. Dev Med Child Neurol 2019;61:140.

10. Kanning KC, Kaplan A, Henderson CE. Motor neuron diversity in development and disease. Annu Rev Neurosci 2010;33:409–40.

11. Mantilla CB, Brandenburg JE, Fogarty MJ, et al. Functional development of respiratory muscles. In: Polin R, Abman SH, Rowitch D, et al, editors. Fetal and neonatal physiology. Vol 1. 6th ed. Elsevier; 2021. p. 652.

12. Alhusaini AA, Dean CM, Crosbie J, et al. Evaluation of spasticity in children with cerebral palsy using Ashworth and Tardieu Scales compared with laboratory measures. J Child Neurol 2010;25(10):1242–7.

13. Brandenburg JE, Eby SF, Song P, et al. Quantifying passive muscle stiffness in children with and without cerebral palsy using ultrasound shear wave elastography. Dev Med Child Neurol 2016;58(12):1288–94.

14. Brandenburg JE, Eby SF, Song P, et al. Ultrasound elastography: the new frontier in direct measurement of muscle stiffness. Arch Phys Med Rehabil 2014;95(11):2207–19.

15. Damiano DL, Quinlivan J, Owen BF, et al. Spasticity versus strength in cerebral palsy: relationships among involuntary resistance, voluntary torque, and motor function. Eur J Neurol 2001;8(Suppl 5):40–9.

16. Wiley ME, Damiano DL. Lower-extremity strength profiles in spastic cerebral palsy. Dev Med Child Neurol 1998;40(2):100–7.

17. Brandenburg JE, Eby SF, Song P, et al. Quantifying effect of onabotulinum toxin a on passive muscle stiffness in children with cerebral palsy using ultrasound shear wave elastography. Am J Phys Med Rehabil 2018;97(7):500–6.

18. Tedroff K, Hagglund G, Miller F. Long-term effects of selective dorsal rhizotomy in children with cerebral palsy: a systematic review. Dev Med Child Neurol 2020;62(5):554–62.

19. National Institute of Neurological Disorders and Stroke Common Data Elements. Cerebral Palsy Common Data Elements. 2016. Available at: https://www.commondataelements.ninds.nih.gov/cerebral%20palsy. Accessed August 22, 2022.

20. Krach LE. Pharmacotherapy of spasticity: oral medications and intrathecal baclofen. J Child Neurol 2001;16(1):31–6.

21. Quality Standards Subcommittee of the American Academy of N, the Practice Committee of the Child Neurology S, Delgado MR, et al. Practice parameter: pharmacologic treatment of spasticity in children and adolescents with cerebral palsy (an evidence-based review): report of the Quality Standards Subcommittee of the American Academy of Neurology and the Practice Committee of the Child Neurology Society. Neurology 2010;74(4):336–43.

22. Tilton AH. Management of spasticity in children with cerebral palsy. Semin Pediatr Neurol 2004;11(1):58–65.

23. Eldridge FH, Lavin N. How effective is stretching in maintaining range of movement for children with cerebral palsy? A critical review. Int J Ther Rehabil 2016;23:386–95.

24. Kalkman BM, Bar-On L, O'Brien TD, et al. Stretching interventions in children with cerebral palsy: why are they ineffective in improving muscle function and how can we better their outcome? Front Physiol 2020;11:131.

25. Novak I, Morgan C, Fahey M, et al. State of the evidence traffic lights 2019: systematic review of interventions for preventing and treating children with cerebral palsy. Curr Neurol Neurosci Rep 2020;20(2):3.

26. Lubsch L, Habersang R, Haase M, et al. Oral baclofen and clonidine for treatment of spasticity in children. J Child Neurol 2006;21(12):1090–2.

27. Micromedex (electronic version). IBM Watson Health. Greenwood Village. Available at: www.micromedexsolutions.com. Accessed July 14, 2022.

28. Eroglu C, Allen NJ, Susman MW, et al. Gabapentin receptor alpha2delta-1 is a neuronal thrombospondin receptor responsible for excitatory CNS synaptogenesis. Cell 2009;139(2):380–92.

29. Hauer JM, Wical BS, Charnas L. Gabapentin successfully manages chronic unexplained irritability in children with severe neurologic impairment. Pediatrics 2007;119(2):e519–22.

30. Hauer JM, Solodiuk JC. Gabapentin for management of recurrent pain in 22 nonverbal children with severe neurological impairment: a retrospective analysis. J Palliat Med 2015;18(5):453–6.

31. Sacha GL, Foreman MG, Kyllonen K, et al. The use of gabapentin for pain and agitation in neonates and infants in a neonatal ICU. J Pediatr Pharmacol Ther 2017;22(3):207–11.

32. Brandenburg JE, Krach LE, Gormley ME Jr. Use of rimabotulinum toxin for focal hypertonicity management in children with cerebral palsy with nonresponse to onabotulinum toxin. Am J Phys Med Rehabil 2013;92(10):898–904.

33. Vova JA, Green MM, Brandenburg JE, et al. Brandenburg J.E., et al., A consensus statement on the use of botulinum toxin in pediatric patients. P & M (Philos Med) R 2021;14(9):1116–42.

34. Alter KE, Karp BI. Ultrasound, electromyography, electrical stimulation; techniques aiding more effective botulinum toxin therapy. In: Jabbari B, editor. Botulinum toxin treatment in clinical medicine: a disease-oriented approach. Cham: Springer International Publishing; 2018. p. 259–91.

35. Bellows S, Jankovic J. Immunogenicity associated with botulinum toxin treatment. Toxins 2019;11(9).

36. Zafonte RD, Munin MC. Phenol and alcohol blocks for the treatment of spasticity. Phys Med Rehabil Clin N Am 2001;12(4):817–32, vii.

37. Morrison JE Jr, Matthews D, Washington R, et al. Phenol motor point blocks in children: plasma concentrations and cardiac dysrhythmias. Anesthesiology 1991;75(2):359–62.

38. Grunt S, Fieggen AG, Vermeulen RJ, et al. Selection criteria for selective dorsal rhizotomy in children with spastic cerebral palsy: a systematic review of the literature. Dev Med Child Neurol 2014;56(4):302–12.

39. McLaughlin J, Bjornson K, Temkin N, et al. Selective dorsal rhizotomy: meta-analysis of three randomized controlled trials. Dev Med Child Neurol 2002; 44(1):17–25.

40. Abbott R. The selective dorsal rhizotomy technique for spasticity in 2020: a review. Child's Nerv Syst 2020;36(9):1895–905.

41. Ahluwalia R, Bass P, Flynn L, et al. Conus-level combined dorsal and ventral lumbar rhizotomy for treatment of mixed hypertonia: technical note and complications. J Neurosurg Pediatr 2021;27(1):102–7.

42. Gober J, Seymour M, Miao H, et al. Management of severe spasticity with and without dystonia with intrathecal baclofen in the pediatric population: a cross-sectional study. World Journal of Pediatric Surgery 2022;5(3):e000407.

43. McDonagh MS, Morgan D, Carson S, et al. Systematic review of hyperbaric oxygen therapy for cerebral palsy: the state of the evidence. Dev Med Child Neurol 2007;49(12):942–7.
44. Sun JM, Kurtzberg J. Stem cell therapies in cerebral palsy and autism spectrum disorder. Dev Med Child Neurol 2021;63(5):503–10.
45. Wong SS, Wilens TE. Medical cannabinoids in children and adolescents: a systematic review. Pediatrics 2017;140(5):e20171818.

Functional Impairment in Pediatric Cancer Survivorship

David W. Pruitt, MD[a],*, Matthew T. Haas, MD[b],
Priya D. Bolikal, MD[a]

KEYWORDS

- Pediatric cancer • Survivorship • Rehabilitation medicine

KEY POINTS

- Interval assessments of functional deficits, activity limitations, and participation restrictions are essential in optimizing the functional recovery and reintegration of children and adolescent survivors of cancer.
- Survivors of pediatric cancer diagnoses may show medical and/or functional impairments related to their initial cancer and immediate effects of its treatment, chronic effects of cancer therapy, or even late effects that may be identified or diagnosed years after treatment has concluded.
- Surveillance of many of the comorbidities associated with cancer survivorship is directly related to function and should involve the expertise of a pediatric rehabilitation physician (physiatrist) in the evaluation, assessment, and treatment recommendations.
- Integration of functional expertise including allied health professionals, psychology and behavioral medicine specialists, school interventionalists, and social workers is beneficial in optimizing overall functioning in survivors of pediatric cancers.

INTRODUCTION

Cancers that occur among those aged 0 to 17 years reflect a heterogenous group of diseases with a classification and categorization that is continually evolving with the emergence of new knowledge relating to the molecular, pathologic, and prognostic characteristics of these diverse malignancies.[1] The National Cancer Institute's Surveillance, Epidemiology, and End Results (SEER) Program represents the primary source for population-based data on cancer incidence in the United States.[2] Leukemias,

[a] Clinical Pediatrics and Clinical Neurology & Rehabilitation Medicine, University of Cincinnati College of Medicine, Cincinnati Children's Hospital Medical Center, 3333 Burnet Avenue, ML#4009, Cincinnati, OH 45229, USA; [b] Physical Medicine and Rehabilitation, Northwestern University Feinberg School of Medicine, Shirley Ryan AbilityLab, 355 East Erie Street, 14th Floor, Chicago, IL 60611, USA
* Corresponding author.
E-mail address: david.pruitt@cchmc.org

Pediatr Clin N Am 70 (2023) 501–515
https://doi.org/10.1016/j.pcl.2023.01.002
0031-3955/23/© 2023 Elsevier Inc. All rights reserved.

lymphomas and central nervous system (CNS) tumors combined account for 70% of the cancer cases in this age range.[1] Since the late 1960s and early 1970s, the survival rate among children diagnosed with cancer has steadily improved, and there has been a corresponding decline in the cancer-specific death rate in this population.[3] The 5-year survival rate for individuals under the age of 18 who were diagnosed with cancer between 2010 and 2016 is 85.4%.[1]

In recent years, improved understanding of the genetics and molecular biology of many pediatric cancers has led to the development of multiple new agents that offer the promise of more effective and less toxic treatment.[4] These include agents that target various cell surface antigens and engage the adaptive immune system, as well as those that interfere with key signaling pathways involved in tumor development and growth.[5] Nevertheless, targeted agents, like conventional chemotherapy, radio-therapy, and surgery, may have off-target effects and deserve long-term follow-up of their safety and efficacy.

Many survivors will experience treatment-related medical, cognitive, and psychoso-cial impairments that interfere with both the normal developmental trajectory of child-hood and the expected level of participation in regular activities. Survivors also risk the development of numerous late effects, or effects that present months or years after diagnosis and often after treatment has concluded, that compound their functional challenges. One study showed that 24.5% of pediatric cancer survivors rate both their physical and mental health-related quality of life as poor compared with 10.1% of the general population.[6] Surveillance of activity limitations and participation restrictions is critical in facilitating the inclusion of pediatric cancer survivors into their environments and assuring that optimization of their medical and psychological function can be pur-sued to prevent the progression or worsening of functional impairment.

GUIDELINES

Nearly two decades ago, the Institute of Medicine, now recognized as the National Academy of Medicine, recognized the need for a lifelong surveillance plan for child-hood cancer survivors that identifies risk based on therapeutic exposures, genetic predisposition, health-related behaviors, and comorbid health conditions for cancer survivors across the spectrum of ages.[7] Findings from a recent survey, providing the current state of survivorship care in 18 countries across 5 continents, indicated that a large proportion of pediatric-age survivors were seen by a physician familiar with late effects, whereas far fewer survivors had access to an expert after the transi-tion to adulthood, stressing that long-term follow-up is still only available for a small proportion of children diagnosed with cancer.[8–10] In efforts to improve longitudinal survivorship care, the Children's Oncology Group (COG) developed risk-based, expo-sure-related guidelines, the Long-Term Follow-Up Guidelines for Survivors of Child-hood, Adolescent, and Young Adult Cancers (LTFUG), for follow-up care of patients who have completed treatment of pediatric malignancies.[11] These guidelines can be downloaded from www.survivorshipguidelines.org. Many of the survivorship issues outlined in these guidelines are directly related to function and should involve the expertise of a physiatrist in the evaluation, assessment, and treatment recommendations.

APPROACH

Foundational to a rehabilitation medicine, or physiatric, approach is the functional assessment and history. The World Health Organization's (WHO) International Classi-fication of Functioning, Disability, and Health (ICF) offers a structured framework for describing and studying the impact of various health conditions on key domains: body structures and functions; activity limitations; and participation restrictions[12] (**Fig. 1**). Body structures are the anatomical parts of the body such as limbs or organs, and body functions include physiological and psychological functions; significant loss or deviation of either body structure or function is referred to as an impairment (eg, reduced range of motion or focal weakness). Activity limitations describe difficulties in executing an action, including activities of daily living as well as motor, cognitive and communication tasks. Lastly, participation restrictions refer to problems related to involvement in major life areas including work, school, home, community, and recreation.

In addition to understanding the primary cancer type and location, physiatrists must also consider several other factors in their assessments of pediatric cancer survivors. First, knowledge of the overall oncologic care plan helps inform providers of potential late effects (**Table 1**) that may persist or develop years after cancer diagnosis and treatment.[11] Second, effective cancer rehabilitation requires understanding where the patient is on the continuum of cancer survivorship. The most widely used classification system for cancer rehabilitation is the Dietz model, which describes rehabilitative interventions through four domains: preventative, restorative, supportive, and palliative[13] (**Table 2**). Depending on individual health conditions and functional impairments, a tailored rehabilitation plan may incorporate different services representing multiple cancer rehabilitation categories. For example, an adolescent with osteosarcoma requiring transfemoral amputation may benefit from lower extremity prosthesis and physical therapy to promote ambulation and school reintegration (restorative), occupational therapy for focused desensitization of phantom limb pain (supportive), and recommendations on physical activity and recreation to encourage general health and wellness into adulthood (preventative).

Treatment of functional impairments in pediatric cancer survivors involves individualized care plans that address the various factors contributing to the impairments as

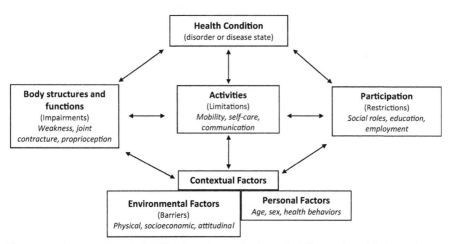

Fig. 1. WHO International Classification of Functioning, Disability and Health (ICF). The ICF conceptualizes a person's level of functioning as a dynamic interaction between her, his or their health conditions, environmental factors, and personal factors. It is a biopsychosocial model of disability, based on an integration of the social and medical models of disability and is both multidimensional and interactive. (*Adapted from*: World Health Organization 2001. The International Classification of Functioning, Disability, and Health (ICF). Geneva: WHO; with permission.)

Table 1
Late effects of pediatric and adolescent cancer survivors addressed by pediatric physiatrist

Late or Chronic Effect	Cancer Types and Risk Factors Associated with Condition in Survivorship	Recommended Screening	Physiatric Intervention
Neurologic			
Neurologic motor deficits (hemiparesis, paraplegia, tetraplegia, ataxia, spasticity, apraxia, etc.)	CNS tumors: longitudinal impairment related to initial tumor encroachment, neurosurgical intervention, cranial irradiation	Annual neurologic examination; standardized motor assessments	Descriptive prescription for physical therapy and/or occupational therapy to address specified motor impairment(s); orthotic prescription; durable medical equipment evaluation/prescription
Chemotherapy-induced peripheral neuropathy	Cancers requiring treatment with neurotoxic chemotherapies (vinka alkaloids, taxanes, platinums)	Annual examination of motor function and sensory function including light touch and proprioception	Medication management for symptomatic relief; orthotic evaluation/prescription and reassessment
Leukoencephalopathy	Transient white matter anomalies that may follow radiotherapy and high-dose chemotherapy for medulloblastoma/PNET; CNS prophylaxis for ALL	Annual neurologic examination	Neuroimaging with brain MRI; descriptive prescription for physical therapy, occupational therapy and/or speech and language pathology to address specified impairment(s); Orthotic prescription; durable medical equipment evaluation/prescription; psychology/psychiatry consultation for potential long-term neurobehavioral issues

	Risk factors	Surveillance	Management
Cerebrovascular complications	CNS irradiation; suprasellar irradiation; circle of Willis in radiation field	Annual neurologic examination; standardized motor assessments	Preventative medicine recommendations to reduce CVA risk (hypertension, diabetes, and dyslipidemia); Emergent neuroimaging in the case of suspected CVA; Neurosurgical consultation; descriptive prescription for physical therapy, occupational therapy and/or speech and language pathology to address specified impairment(s); orthotic prescription; durable medical equipment evaluation/prescription
Neurocognitive			
Intellectual ability	CNS tumors treated at earlier age, most notably in those treated with CSI	• Annual assessment of educational and/or vocational progress • Neuropsychological testing at entry into long-term follow-up, then periodically as clinically indicated • Self- or parent-reported questionnaires	• Acquisition of educational resources to provide appropriate setting and accommodations • Medication recommendation (eg, stimulants) • Referral to community-based disability and vocational services
Processing speed	Cancers treated with CNS irradiation and resultant damage to white matter; chemotherapy; history of PFS		
Attention and working memory	Cancers treated with CNS irradiation and resultant damage to white matter; chemotherapy; history of PFS; chemotherapy		
Executive functioning	Particularly those with ALL or brain tumor; surgical resection alone, chemotherapy alone; radiation		
Memory deficits (long-term declarative or explicit memory)	Tumor location or treatment involves neuroanatomical structures involved in memory (eg, midline brain tumors) secondary neurologic complications (seizures or HCP)		

(continued on next page)

Table 1
(continued)

Late or Chronic Effect	Cancer Types and Risk Factors Associated with Condition in Survivorship	Recommended Screening	Physiatric Intervention
Focal cognitive deficits	CNS tumors with focal surgical or radiation treatment to left cerebral hemisphere (language and communication abilities) or right cerebral hemisphere (visual-spatial abilities)		
Cerebellar cognitive affective syndrome (posterior fossa syndrome)	Surgical intervention for posterior fossa CNS tumors		
Adaptive functioning	Neurologic complications, cognitive dysfunction, psychological factors, parenting factors, general family functioning		
Musculoskeletal			
Amputation	Longitudinal issues subsequent to amputation of a limb including activity and participation restrictions, pain, residual limb integrity, energy expenditure	Annual examination of both residual and contralateral limb in terms of proximal joint stability (ie, overuse), range of motion, appearance of residual limb, skin; functional history to assess activity limitations and participation restrictions; prosthetic evaluation	Prosthetic troubleshooting and prescription; Descriptive Prescription for physical therapy and/or occupational therapy to address specified motor impairment(s); Durable medical equipment evaluation/prescription
Limb-sparing surgery	Children at younger age at surgery and musculoskeletal immaturity; radiation to extremity; use of biologic material (allograft or autograft) for reconstruction; obesity, infection, peripheral neuropathy	Annual examination of affected and contralateral limb in terms of neurologic symmetry with strength and sensation; functional history to assess activity limitations and participation restrictions	Descriptive prescription for physical therapy and/or occupational therapy to address specified motor impairment(s); Durable medical equipment evaluation/prescription

Osteonecrosis	Cancer survivors with a history of prolonged steroid treatment course; history of irradiation to site	Annual examination of musculoskeletal range of motion, strength, and gait; joint pain assessment; functional history to assess activity limitations and participation restrictions	Radiological imaging; NSAID for pain relief; orthopedic surgery referral; Descriptive prescription for physical therapy and/or occupational therapy to address specified motor impairment(s) including potential weight-bearing restrictions
Reduced bone mineral density, osteopenia, and osteoporosis	Cancer survivors with a history of prolonged steroid treatment course, impaired mobility	Annual evaluation of vitamin D and calcium; DEXA	Vitamin D supplementation; optimization of weight-bearing opportunities; bisphosphonate treatment
Joint contractures	Hematopoietic cell transplant patients with any history of GVHD	Annual musculoskeletal examination; NIH joint/fascia scale or photographic range of motion scale	Descriptive prescription for physical therapy and/or occupational therapy to address specified motor impairment(s); durable medical equipment evaluation/prescription

Long-term follow-up guidelines for survivors of childhood, adolescent, and young adult cancers, version 5.0. Children's Oncology Group, 2018. (Accessed September 1, 2022, at www.survivorshipguidelines.org.)

National Academies of Sciences Engineering and Medicine. Childhood cancer and functional impacts across the care continuum. 2021; Washington, D.C.: The National Academies Press.

Abbreviations: ALL, acute lymphoblastic anemia; CNS, central nervous system; CSI, craniospinal irradiation; CVA, cerebrovascular accident; GVHD, graft versus host disease; HCP, hydrocephalus; MRI, magnetic resonance imaging; PFS, posterior fossa syndrome; PNET, primitive neuro-ectodermal tumors.

Table 2			
Dietz classification for cancer rehabilitation[a]			
Preventative	**Restorative**	**Supportive**	**Palliative**
• Prehabilitation or prospective surveillance • Early intervention and education to lessen, delay or avoid cancer- or treatment-related complications	• Return prior level of function (physical, social, psychological, vocational) without substantial residual deficits	• Re-establish or maintain maximal functional independence with accommodations and adaptations	• Maximize patient comfort and quality life • Education and equipment to reduce caregiver burden

[a] Dietz JH. Rehabilitation Oncology. Somerset, NJ: John Wiley & Sons; 1981.

well as the treatment goals unique to each patient. For example, reduced mobility may be related to musculoskeletal abnormalities resulting from surgical interventions, weakness related to neuropathy or focal CNS lesions, and/or reduced cardiac or pulmonary functioning from general deconditioning, chemotherapy exposures or radiation. Addressing the various contributors with appropriate equipment or bracing, physical or occupational therapy, and promoting improved cardiovascular endurance are all important in treating the patient's mobility issues.

Based on individualized rehabilitation needs, a physiatrist can provide referrals to specialized services along with detailed prescriptions outlining specific functional deficits and therapeutic interventions (**Fig. 2**). The patient's overall functional status dictates the most appropriate setting and intensity of rehabilitation services. Inpatient rehabilitation should be considered if a patient has functional deficits requiring two or more therapy disciplines (physical therapy, occupational therapy, and/or speech therapy); can tolerate and will benefit from three or more hours of therapy per day; and needs close medical supervision and access to 24-hour nursing care. If any of the inpatient criteria are not met, patients will most likely be referred to outpatient rehabilitation. For patients with significant barriers to accessing or high risk for complications with community-based services, home-based rehabilitation may be considered.

EVALUATION

The LTFUG are designed for the assessment of potential chronic and late effects based on exposures, but there are no specific recommendations within the guidelines that direct which pediatric subspecialist should be integrated within the survivorship team to evaluate for each of the numerous late effects. In many cases, the cause of functional impairment is multifactorial and consideration of the interplay of a number of contributing conditions must ensue. For example, a recent study identified that survivors are at increased risk for exercise intolerance for many reasons (cardiac, pulmonary, neuropathic, and muscular impairments, among others).[14] Based on these findings, survivors will need interventions tailored to their specific deficits to improve their exercise intolerance.[4] **Table 1** highlights several late effects that impact functional independence.

The pediatric rehabilitation physician is uniquely poised to address several chronic and late effects in survivors of pediatric cancers based on their training and clinical approach that focuses on function and quality of life. Although pediatric physiatrists have a role in managing many of the late effects included in the LTFUG, this paper focuses on neurologic and musculoskeletal impairments.

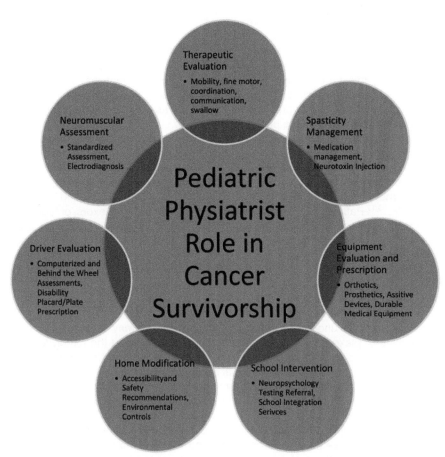

Fig. 2. Pediatric physiatry role in pediatric cancer survivorship. The pediatric physiatrist has a multidimensional role in working with survivors of childhood cancer, including both longitudinal neuromuscular assessments and an individualized functional needs assessment of the survivor and their caregiver(s).

Weakness

Focal or generalized weakness can occur as a result of tumor invasion or as a result of exposure to a variety of cancer treatments. Physiatric evaluation of patients with weakness begins with a thorough medical and functional history and neurologic examination. In patients with focal weakness, it is important to determine if the weakness is caused by a CNS, peripheral nerve, or muscular issue, as the presumed cause of the impairment will inform diagnostic evaluation and treatment. A thorough neurologic and musculoskeletal examination including strength, muscle tone, sensation, and reflexes is critical in determining where along the neuroaxis the weakness originates and how to best manage it.

In patients with a history of CNS tumors, physical examination may reveal spasticity or other forms of hypertonia, as well as hyperreflexia in the affected limbs. Evolution of these findings may warrant further workup with neuroimaging depending on the timeline of neurologic changes, cancer treatment history, as well as the patient's clinical presentation. For example, a child with a history of a brain tumor who has undergone cranial irradiation and is in remission may present with new weakness and upper motor neuron signs several months or years after completing treatment. This patient may require further neuroimaging to assess for presence of radiation necrosis or potential tumor recurrence.[15] Weakness that originates from the CNS may also be associated with spasticity that further limits patient function, and treatment may require focal spasticity management including neurotoxin injections or systemic medications for spasticity. In addition, evaluations for equipment such as orthotics, walkers, or wheelchairs can be performed by the pediatric physiatrist.

Weakness related to peripheral nerve injury may be accompanied by sensory impairments and dampened or absent reflexes. This is seen commonly in patients who develop chemotherapy-induced peripheral neuropathy after exposure to neurotoxic chemotherapeutic agents. This type of peripheral neuropathy often presents with distal symmetric motor and sensory impairments and may be accompanied by neuropathic pain.[16,17] Patients may exhibit weakness in their ankle dorsiflexors, or foot drop, that impairs gait and can increase the risk of falls.[17] Gait analysis by a physiatrist is key as there are numerous factors that lead to gait abnormalities. Potential interventions for gait abnormalities vary depending on the etiology and type of gait abnormality. Use of an ankle foot orthoses (AFO) is often recommended in cases of foot drop to improve patients' gait patterns and prevent contractures, but the specificity of the componentry and design of the AFO is critical in optimizing gait mechanics, and it is knowledge that a pediatric physiatrist can best offer for survivors.[17]

Patients who have undergone treatments for solid tumors may present with mononeuropathies or plexopathies related to direct nerve injury from the tumor, surgical intervention, or radiation therapy.[18] The pattern of weakness and sensory changes may represent a myotomal and dermatomal distribution or a peripheral nerve distribution. A thorough physical examination can very often differentiate this. If needed, further evaluation with electromyography and nerve conduction studies (EMG/NCS) can localize the nerve injury and provide prognostic recovery potential. In addition, information obtained from EMG/NCS can be used to determine if the patient is a candidate for potential nerve transfer surgery, and if so, is critical for surgical planning.

Patients with myopathies also present with weakness, and evaluation for this also begins with a functional and neurologic examination. Physical examination may reveal dampened reflexes but will not show sensory impairments as in neuropathies. The pattern of weakness is often telling as well. For example, patients with chemotherapy-induced peripheral neuropathies will display distal symmetric weakness; whereas patients with steroid myopathy display proximal muscle weakness and may have difficulty with tasks like standing up from a seated position, climbing stairs, or reaching overhead.[17] EMG/NCS can also help differentiate neuropathic versus myopathic weakness.

Neurocognitive Impairments

Neurocognitive impairments may occur in patients with exposures to antimetabolites, cranial irradiation, or neurosurgical procedures.[1,17] Neuropsychological evaluation should occur at the initiation of long-term follow-up and may need to be repeated as clinically indicated.[11] In addition, annual follow-up visits should include a review of educational or vocational progress and goals, which are key components of the physiatric evaluation. A multi-disciplinary team including a physiatrist and school intervention specialist can assist patients and families in using neuropsychological testing results to help optimize the patient's school environment to best support their learning. This may include the implementation of an Individualized Education Program (IEP) or 504 plan. As survivors of pediatric cancers enter their teenage years, consultation with a vocational rehabilitation specialist can help with career and educational planning for after high school and help identify employment opportunities that suit a patient's strengths and interests.[17]

Pain

Acute and chronic pain may occur in survivors of pediatric cancers. Cancer-related pain is often under-recognized and undertreated, particularly among pediatric patients.[19,20] A multidisciplinary approach to managing chronic pain including psychological support to assist with coping strategies and optimizing function despite pain is critical in maximizing quality of life. Still, a satisfactory evaluation of physiological pain generators is critical in optimizing the medical management of pain in the survivorship population.

The primary role of the pediatric physiatrist in the evaluation of pain in a cancer survivorship setting is to assess for biomechanical and other causes of pain and implement a treatment plan that minimizes pain and maximizes patient function. Key information gathered from the pain history including the location, onset, and character of the pain as well as exacerbating and relieving factors can help better understand the etiology. In addition, knowledge of the patient's cancer treatment history helps determine their risk of various types of pain.

Patients with a history of exposure to neurotoxic chemotherapeutic agents are at risk for neuropathic pain which is often described as a "burning" or "electric shock" sensation.[17,20] These patients may also present with other signs of nerve injury including weakness and impaired sensation. Pain is typically located distally and may be in a stocking and glove distribution. Neuropathic pain may also present in a dermatomal distribution in the case of an acute radiculopathy.

Patients with joint pain require further assessment to determine if their pain is related to arthritic changes, acute fracture, or avascular necrosis (AVN). Patients who have had exposure to steroids during their treatment course and patients have mobility limitations are at increased risk of osteopenia and osteoporosis and have an increased risk of fractures. In addition, exposure to steroid therapy or radiation increases the risk of AVN.[1,21,22] If fracture or AVN are present, consultation with an orthopedic specialist is necessary to determine weight-bearing restrictions and if surgical intervention is warranted. If the joint pain is not related to any of these conditions, further musculoskeletal examination can be performed by the physiatrist to determine the pain generator and inform further nonsurgical treatment.

Amputations

Although many patients with long bone sarcomas will be recommended for or elect limb-sparing surgeries, several patients will undergo limb amputation for definitive surgical treatment. Amputation remains a viable option for the treatment of cancer or after failed limb-salvage procedures.[1] In a recent retrospective study analyzing data from the National Cancer Database from 2004 to 2015, 19% of patients less than 20 years of age with a diagnosis of high-grade osteosarcoma underwent amputation instead of limb salvage.[23] The major indications for amputation are extremely small skeletal size (small medullary canal of the bone, so that a durable prosthesis could not be made to fit), progression on chemotherapy, and tumor encompassing the blood vessels and nerves of the limb.[1] If limb salvage is not feasible with adequate margins, amputation must be considered.[24]

Patients who have undergone amputation as part of their cancer treatments benefit from evaluation by physiatrists throughout their lifespan, though the role remains critical during survivorship. Patients who have undergone amputations require longitudinal assessments of their prosthetic devices for fit and functionality. Skin assessment is necessary to ensure skin integrity and prevent wounds. In addition pediatric amputees are at risk for bony overgrowth at the distal site of amputation, so monitoring for this is important as well.[1,17] The result of an ill-fitting prosthesis may involve skin breakdown or gait abnormalities. Gait assessment by the pediatric physiatrist can identify if a device is loose or is causing a leg length discrepancy, for example, and can guide the prosthetist on what adjustments would be most beneficial. The physiatrist will also evaluate for pain in these patients, as they are at risk for musculoskeletal pain from altered gait mechanics, pain at the site of their amputation, and phantom pain, or neuropathic pain that is present in the portion of the limb that has been amputated.[25] Treatments for these types of pain may involve a combination of prosthetic adjustments, physical or occupational therapy, and pharmacologic intervention.[25]

DISCUSSION

Despite a plethora of publications describing models of survivorship care, evaluating the use of cancer treatment summaries and survivorship care plans, and promoting risk-based health surveillance recommendations,[26,27] studies are lacking that show how these resources can be feasibly and effectively implemented in oncology and primary care settings to facilitate care coordination, reduce duplication of services, and improve survivorship outcomes.[4] Owing to the numerous late effects that must be monitored for in each childhood cancer diagnosis, it is challenging to assure each potential focus area receives adequate and essential evaluation at regular intervals. Multidisciplinary childhood cancer survivorship clinics are ideal opportunities to assure that each of the currently recognized late effects, as outlined by COG, are adequately addressed, and evaluated, but also that potential effects from new agents and techniques can also be identified and offered potential therapeutic interventions (**Fig. 3**). Even if a multidisciplinary setting is not offered for survivors, referrals for

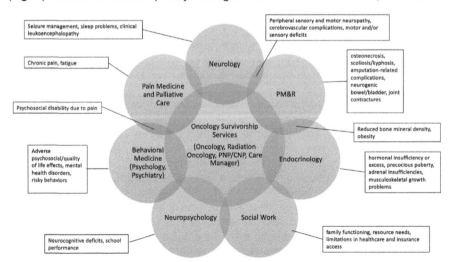

Fig. 3. Membership within a comprehensive survivorship clinic and roles of specialty services. Many pediatric specialties contribute to the ongoing care of survivors within a multidisciplinary clinic setting. In addition to the systems-based care provided by the oncology team of providers, many pediatric specialties provide both unique and collaborative care for many of the common chronic and late effects of pediatric cancer and its treatments.

pediatric physiatric services throughout both the acute setting and into survivorship can provide exceptional insight and recommendations to the oncology care team.

SUMMARY

Adult survivors of pediatric cancers have higher reports of physical impairments and activity limitations than the general population.[28] Inclusion of a pediatric physiatrist in the childhood cancer survivorship team is critical in addressing the areas of physical functioning and activity that may be impaired as a result of pediatric cancers and their treatments. The role of the physiatrist is broad but follows the ICF model in assessing the impact of health conditions as well as personal and environmental factors on body functioning, activities, and participation in school, work, and leisure. Pediatric physiatrists are an essential component, not only in evaluating many of the musculoskeletal and neurologic deficits that impact many survivors, but more importantly in guiding the transition of the survivor safely and effectively from activity limitations and participation restrictions.

CLINICS CARE POINTS

- Utilization of the Long-Term Follow-Up Guidelines for Survivors of Childhood, Adolescent, and Young Adult Cancers (LTFUG) from the Children's Oncology Group provides a risk-based, exposure-related guide for the longitudinal management of childhood cancer survivors (www.survivorshipguidelines.org)

- Pediatric physiatrists provide evaluations and interventions to manage functional deficits resulting from late or chronic effects related to impacts upon neurologic and musculoskeletal body systems.

- The pediatric physiatrist role in cancer survivorship is multidimensional including roles in neuromuscular assessment and spasticity management, therapeutic evaluation, equipment evaluation and prescription as well as school intervention.

- Optimizing school reintegration in cancer survivors is optimized by involvement of a multidisciplinary team including pediatric physiatry, neuropsychology and school intervention specialists.

DISCLOSURE

The authors have nothing to disclose.

REFERENCES

1. National Academies of Sciences Engineering and Medicine. Childhood cancer and functional impacts across the care continuum. Washington, D.C.: The National Academies Press; 2021.
2. Howlader N, Noone AM, Krapcho M, et al. SEER cancer statistics review, 1975-2016, National Cancer Institute. Bethesda (MD): National Cancer Institute; 2019.
3. Smith MA, Altekruse SF, Adamson PC, et al. Declining childhood and adolescent cancer mortality. Cancer 2014;120:2497–506.
4. Dixon SB, Chow EJ, Hjorth L, et al. The future of childhood cancer survivorship: challenges and opportunities for continued progress. Pediatr Clin North Am 2020;67:1237–51.
5. Chow EJ, Antal Z, Constine LS, et al. New agents, emerging late effects, and the development of precision survivorship. J Clin Oncol 2018;36:2231–40.

6. Weaver KE, Forsythe LP, Reeve BB, et al. Mental and physical health-related quality of life among U.S. cancer survivors: population estimates from the 2010 National Health Interview Survey. Cancer Epidemiol Biomarkers Prev 2012;21: 2108–17.

7. National Cancer Policy Board (U.S., Hewitt ME, Weiner SL, Simone JV. Childhood cancer survivorship : improving care and quality of life. Washington, D.C.: National Academies Press; 2003.

8. Norsker FN, Pedersen C, Armstrong GT, et al. Late effects in childhood cancer survivors: early studies, survivor cohorts, and significant contributions to the field of late effects. Pediatr Clin North Am 2020;67:1033–49.

9. Tonorezos ES, Barnea D, Cohn RJ, et al. Models of care for survivors of childhood cancer from across the globe: advancing survivorship care in the next decade. J Clin Oncol 2018;36:2223–30.

10. Winther JF, Kremer L. Long-term follow-up care needed for children surviving cancer: still a long way to go. Lancet Oncol 2018;19:1546–8.

11. Long-term follow-up guidelines for survivors of childhood, adolescent, and young adult cancers, version 5.0. Children's Oncology Group; 2018. Available at: www. survivorshipguidelines.org. Accessed September 1, 2022.

12. The International Classification of Functioning, Disability and Health (ICF). 2001. 2022. Available at: http://www.who.int/classifications/icf/en/.

13. Dietz JH. Rehabilitation oncology. Somerset, NJ: John Wiley & Sons; 1981.

14. Ness KK, Plana JC, Joshi VM, et al. Exercise intolerance, mortality, and organ system impairment in adult survivors of childhood cancer. J Clin Oncol 2020; 38:29–42.

15. Miyatake S, Nonoguchi N, Furuse M, et al. Pathophysiology, diagnosis, and treatment of radiation necrosis in the brain. Neurol Med -Chir 2015;55:50–9.

16. Zajaczkowska R, Kocot-Kepska M, Leppert W, et al. Mechanisms of chemotherapy-induced peripheral neuropathy. Int J Mol Sci 2019;20.

17. Pruitt D, Bolger A, Bolikal P. Cancer. In: Murphy K, McMahon M, Houtrow A, editors. Pediatric rehabilitation principles and practice. 6th ed. New York, NY: Springer Publishing Company, LLC; 2021. p. 562–90.

18. Falah M, Schiff D, Burns TM. Neuromuscular complications of cancer diagnosis and treatment. J Support Oncol 2005;3:271–82.

19. Revivo G, Amstutz D, Haas M. Chronic pain. In: Murphy K, McMahon M, Houtrow A, editors. Pediatric rehabilitation principles and practice. 6th ed. New York, NY: Springer Publishing Company, LLC; 2021. p. 163–86.

20. Krane E, Wiener L, Kao R. Pain and symptom management. In: Blsney S, Adamson P, Helman L, editors. Pizzo and poplack's pediatric oncology. Philadelphia: Wolters Kluwer; 2021. p. 1028–66.

21. Burger B, Beier R, Zimmermann M, et al. Osteonecrosis: a treatment related toxicity in childhood acute lymphoblastic leukemia (ALL)–experiences from trial ALL-BFM 95. Pediatr Blood Cancer 2005;44:220–5.

22. Niinimaki T, Harila-Saari A, Niinimaki R. The diagnosis and classification of osteonecrosis in patients with childhood leukemia. Pediatr Blood Cancer 2015;62: 198–203.

23. Evans DR, Lazarides AL, Visgauss JD, et al. Limb salvage versus amputation in patients with osteosarcoma of the extremities: an update in the modern era using the National Cancer Database. BMC Cancer 2020;20:995.

24. Hawkins DS, Brennan BM, Bolling T, et al. Ewing sarcoma. In: Pizzo P, Poplack DG, editors. Principles and practice of pediatric oncology. Philadelphia: Wolters, Kluwer; 2016. p. 855–76.

25. Stover G, Prahlow N. Residual limb pain: An evidence-based review. NeuroRehabilitation 2020;47:315–25.
26. Kadan-Lottick NS, Ross WL, Mitchell HR, et al. Randomized trial of the impact of empowering childhood cancer survivors with survivorship care plans. J Natl Cancer Inst 2018;110:1352–9.
27. Landier W, Chen Y, Namdar G, et al. Impact of tailored education on awareness of personal risk for therapy-related complications among childhood cancer survivors. J Clin Oncol 2015;33:3887–93.
28. Hudson MM, Mertens AC, Yasui Y, et al. Health status of adult long-term survivors of childhood cancer: a report from the Childhood Cancer Survivor Study. JAMA 2003;290:1583–92.

20. ...

21. ...

Promoting Recovery Following Birth Brachial Plexus Palsy

Marisa Osorio, DO[a],*, Sarah Lewis, DPT[b], Raymond W. Tse, MD[c,d]

KEYWORDS

• Brachial plexus • Birth • Management • Rehabilitation

KEY POINTS

• Twenty to thirty percent of children with birth brachial plexus palsy will have residual deficits.
• If an infant with neonatal brachial plexus palsy has not recovered fully within the first 4 weeks of life, they should be referred to a specialty clinic.
• Musculoskeletal abnormalities are common and require treatment to optimize function.
• Rehabilitation management spans infancy through adolescence, addressing pain, function, and vocational/avocational concerns.

EPIDEMIOLOGY

The incidence of neonatal brachial plexus palsy (NBPP) is 1.74 per 1000 live births, with recent data suggesting that the incidence has been decreasing over time likely owing to awareness of risk factors and strategies to reduce injury.[1] Risk factors associated with NBPP in order of frequency are shoulder dystocia, macrosomia, maternal gestational diabetes, breech presentation, and instrumented delivery.[1] Previous delivery with shoulder dystocia with or without resultant NBPP is an additional risk factor.[2] With shoulder dystocia, various maneuvers are applied to release the shoulder and deliver the infant. Traction on the shoulder girdle preferentially produces tension on the upper regions of the brachial plexus with progression into the middle and lower regions in more severe injuries.

[a] Department of Rehabilitation Medicine, University of Washington, Seattle Children's Hospital, Rehabilitation Medicine, 4800 Sand Point Way Northeast, OB 8.410, Seattle, WA 98105, USA; [b] Rehabilitation Medicine, Seattle Children's Hospital, 4800 Sand Point Way Northeast, OB 8.410, Seattle, WA 98105, USA; [c] Division of Plastic Surgery, Department of Surgery, University of Washington, 4800 Sand Point Way Northeast, OB9.527, Seattle, WA 98105, USA; [d] Division of Craniofacial and Plastic Surgery, Department of Surgery, Seattle Children's Hospital, 4800 Sand Point Way Northeast, OB9.527, Seattle, WA 98105, USA
* Corresponding author. 4800 Sand Point Way NE, OB 8.410, Seattle, WA 98105.
E-mail address: Marisa.Osorio@seattlechildrens.org

Pediatr Clin N Am 70 (2023) 517–529
https://doi.org/10.1016/j.pcl.2023.01.016
0031-3955/23/© 2023 Elsevier Inc. All rights reserved.

PRESENTATION

When only the upper trunk is involved, the motor deficits result in an "Erb posture" with the arm adducted, shoulder internally rotated, elbow extended, and forearm pronated (**Fig. 1**). When both the upper and the middle trunks are involved, there can be additional deficits in elbow extension and wrist extension. Patients may assume an "extended Erb" posture manifesting with a similar pattern but with wrist flexion (**Fig. 2**). The additional deficits of C8 and T1 roots manifest as impairments in hand function and a flaccid limb. A Horner syndrome (ipsilateral facial anhidrosis, ptosis, and miosis) can occur if the T1 root is injured proximal to its contribution to the sympathetic chain that ascends to the face (**Fig. 3**).

NATURAL HISTORY

Although the pattern of involvement and site of injury can be estimated by the postures and motor deficits at initial presentation, the degree of nerve injury at each level is more difficult to assess, and the amount of recovery is variable. The Narakas Classification is used to predict outcomes based on the number of nerve roots injured.[3] Generally, 80% of patients with Erb palsy (Narakas I, C5-6 nerve roots) have full recovery.[3] Patients with extended Erb palsy (Narakas II, C5-7 nerve roots) have a 60% chance of full recovery, and those with entire plexus involvement (Narakas III and IV, C5-T1 nerve roots) likely have avulsions and ruptures, resulting in permanent loss of function.[3,4]

ASSESSMENT, DIFFERENTIAL, AND ASSOCIATIONS

The initial assessment of an infant by a pediatrician is critical in identifying NBPP and associated or alternative conditions. In addition to the postures associated with NBPP (see **Figs. 1** and **2**), a careful neurologic examination should be conducted to identify weakness and deficits. The Moro reflex can be convenient for eliciting shoulder abduction, shoulder external rotation, and elbow flexion, and a Horner syndrome can be detected when examining eyes and pupils. A skeletal survey should also be conducted with difficult deliveries. Fractures of the clavicle and humerus can accompany brachial plexus palsy and can sometimes mimic NBPP, as infants guard against pain. If limb posturing is due to pain, the postures will resolve once the fracture is healed.

In addition to sequelae of the nerve injury, infants with NBPP may present with several associated conditions that should be taken into consideration in their overall care plan. Infants can have torticollis with preference for cervical rotation toward the

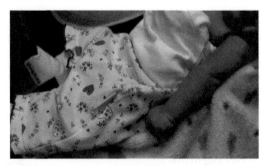

Fig. 1. Erb palsy. The typical posture at presentation.

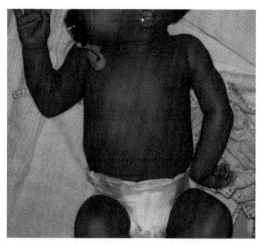

Fig. 2. Extended Erb palsy. Addition of wrist flexion due to the loss of wrist extension.

unaffected upper extremity.[5] Special attention to infant head shape and postures can identify emerging torticollis or plagiocephaly and allow for timely treatment or prevention. Diaphragm paralysis results from an associated phrenic nerve palsy and can resolve spontaneously or require surgical plication.[6,7] Although phrenic nerve palsies are typically identified in the early neonatal period, infants with NBPP can have new or worsening tachypnea or feeding difficulties after hospital discharge.[7,8] Careful examination is important for assessment of hypoxic central nervous system injury that can accompany or mimic NBPP.[9] Spinal cord injuries, Sprengel deformity, and congenital limb anomalies, such as arthrogryposis, can also mimic NBPP. Spinal cord injuries generally will involve findings in other limbs and upper motor neuron signs. Congenital anomalies can present with limited range of motion, missing skin creases, and more generalized asymmetry or dysmorphology.

MANAGEMENT OF INFANTS WITH NEONATAL BRACHIAL PLEXUS PALSY

Providers caring for newborns with brachial plexus palsy should use caution when discussing prognosis with families, as recovery is not universal. Although spontaneous resolution can occur, 20% to 30% of children have residual deficits that persist into adulthood.[4] If an infant has not recovered normal function and strength by 1 month of age or if they present at birth with a flail limb and Horner syndrome, they should be referred to a specialty clinic for timely evaluation and management.[10,11] Specialized clinics for NBPP often include a pediatric rehabilitation physician, physical and

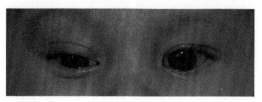

Fig. 3. Horner syndrome. Ptosis, miosis, and anhidrosis due to disruption of the sympathetic chain originating proximally from the T1 root.

occupational therapy, and surgical specialties, such as plastic surgery, neurosurgery, and orthopedic surgery. This multidisciplinary care ensures that patients receive a comprehensive approach to managing their injury and comorbidities with nonsurgical and surgical treatments. Serial evaluations of infants with measures such as the Active Movement Scale[12] help to determine the trajectory of recovery and guide diagnostic evaluations and interventions.

REHABILITATION APPROACH IN INFANTS WITH NEONATAL BRACHIAL PLEXUS PALSY

Nerve injuries can have cascading consequences in the setting of a rapidly growing and developing child. Given that muscle activity and bony relationships influence musculoskeletal growth, joint motion and morphology can become malformed in a child with NBPP. Infants with weakness lasting beyond the early neonatal period are referred for physical or occupational therapy services as standard of care.[13,14] Passive range-of-motion exercises are initiated promptly to reduce the risk of developing joint contractures. Early therapeutic management also includes caregiver education in infant positioning, motor activities, and sensory exploration. Pinning the arm against the body in infancy is no longer recommended in favor of early range of motion[13] and supportive repositioning of the limb during feeding or sleeping. Splints are also applied to mitigate contracture risk.

Glenohumeral dysplasia (**Fig. 4**) develops within the first year of life[15] and as early as 3 months of age[16] in infants with NBPP, likely owing to the significant motor imbalances about the joint and differences in muscle growth.[17,18] Dysplasia begins with glenohumeral subluxation, in which the humeral head gradually slides posteriorly out of the glenoid. Clinical signs, such as reduced passive external rotation range of motion, are used to detect glenohumeral subluxation. However, ultrasound has been shown to identify subluxation in the absence of clinical signs as early as 3 months of age (**Fig. 5**).[16,19–21] The incidence of subluxation varies in the literature from 7% to 57%,[19,22–25] likely owing to the variations in presentation and severity. These skeletal aberrations can limit long-term function, even with adequate nerve recovery, so screening for and treating these conditions early in infancy are important.

Prevention of subluxation and dysplasia through early therapy and range of motion is critical to maintaining joint motion and preserving musculoskeletal health. Stretches into shoulder external rotation are emphasized (**Fig. 6**),[22,26] as early joint mobilization does not increase the risk of subluxation and has not been reported to increase nerve injury or delay recovery.[20] The SupER splint, named for shoulder external rotation and

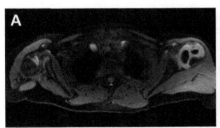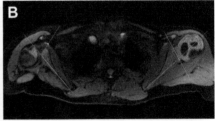

Fig. 4. Glenohumeral dysplasia. (*A*) Axial section MRI through bilateral shoulders. The patient's right limb is affected. (*B*) The humeral head is no longer aligned along the axis of the scapula. The glenoid fossa is dysplastic and has formed a pseudofossa (*red line*). This patient was 2 years old. Similar changes can be detected as early as 3 months of age.

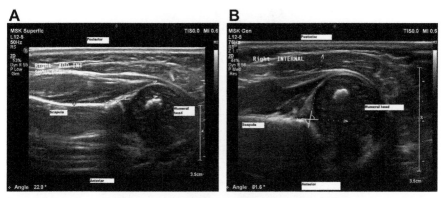

Fig. 5. Glenohumeral ultrasound. (*A*) Normal shoulder alignment. (*B*) Posterior subluxation of the humeral head.

forearm supination, has been developed to counteract prolonged posturing in shoulder internal rotation and forearm pronation (**Fig. 7**).[27] Young infants wear the splint for up to 22 hours per day. Duration of splint wear is reduced to overnight and naps when infants begin to use their arm for fine and gross motor activities, at or near 3 months of age.[28] The intent of the SupER splint is to maintain the glenohumeral joint in a reduced position while nerve recovery occurs naturally or following nerve surgery.

If these early interventions are unsuccessful in preventing subluxation, botulinum toxin injections and application of a shoulder spica cast may be used to reestablish shoulder joint alignment.[13,29,30] The botulinum toxin weakens the pull of the internal rotator muscles that displace the humeral head posteriorly. The spica cast maintains

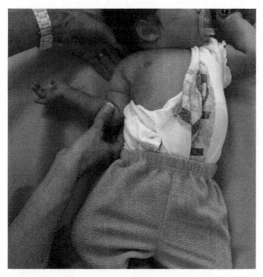

Fig. 6. Stretching to maintain passive range of external rotation. Loss of motion can lead to joint contractures and ultimately joint dysplasia. Loss/weakness of external rotation is the most common and profoundly affected motion and should be the focus of early motion. With the scapula stabilized, the shoulder is rotated externally.

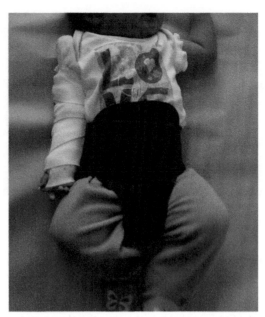

Fig. 7. Supination and external rotation (SupER) splint. Used to maintain anatomical alignment of the glenohumeral joint and prevent contracture.

the shoulder in external rotation, thereby assuring joint reduction for 4 to 6 weeks. This allows the joint to remodel and provides time for nerve recovery to external rotator muscles that balance the glenohumeral joint (**Fig. 8**).

SURGICAL TREATMENT OF NEONATAL BRACHIAL PLEXUS PALSY

The decision to proceed with surgery is not taken lightly. Approximately 10% to 30% of patients with persistent neurologic deficits from NBPP require surgery.[4] The goal of nerve reconstruction is to maximize recovery of motor and sensory functions. Given the spectrum of presentation and variations in recovery, the role of surgery continues to evolve. Although it is accepted that nerve reconstruction should happen in infancy,

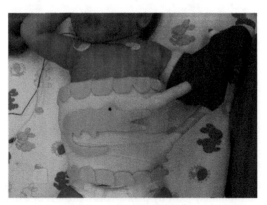

Fig. 8. Shoulder spica cast used to maintain shoulder reduction after treatment of subluxation.

Table 1
Surgical indications for reconstruction[32]

Patient Age	Findings/Persistent Deficits
1 mo	Flail/flaccid limb (no motor function, including wrist and hand) with an associated Horner syndrome (eyelid ptosis, pupil myosis, facial anhidrosis)[a]
3 mo	Limited finger extension, thumb extension, wrist extension, elbow extension, and elbow flexion (as indicated by composite Active Movement Scale score of <3.5/10)
6 mo	No elbow flexion
9 mo	Failed Cookie test (ability to bring hand to mouth while sitting with elbow at side)
>9 mo	Significant isolated deficits

[a] Horner syndrome is indicative of a proximal injury with likely avulsion of the root from spinal cord.
Data from Borschel G, Clarke H. Obstetrical brachial plexus palsy. Plast Reconstr Surg 2009;124(1 Suppl):144e-55e.

there is a lack of consensus for the timing and indications for surgery. One evidence-based algorithm was developed in Toronto (**Table 1**).[31] Surgical indications for more distal deficits are determined earlier because reinnervation requires axon regrowth, occurring at a rate of 1 mm per day, from the site of reconstruction to the location of the muscle.

Nerve reconstruction could involve exploration of the brachial plexus with excision of ruptured or neuromatous sections, followed by reconstruction using multiple cables of nerve grafts. Because of redundant sensory functions, the sural nerve is an expendable donor and can be harvested through small incisions and spliced or interposed into a defect.

In situations whereby nerve roots have been avulsed from the spinal cord, the availability of regenerating proximal axons is limited. Additional innervation can be obtained from other sources, including a portion of cranial nerve X or the intercostal nerves (**Fig. 9**).[32] The proximal innervation of donor nerves is left intact, whereas the distal end of those nerves is coapted to provide axons to distal targets, in what is known as an extraplexus nerve transfer. Through higher cortical brain plasticity, patients can relearn how to control the new pattern of motor innervation.

The same strategy of nerve transfer can also be used in incomplete palsies whereby only a portion of the brachial plexus is affected. Motor fascicles with redundant innervation from the intact portions of the brachial plexus can be used to innervate affected muscles in what is known as an intraplexus nerve transfer (see **Fig. 9**).[32]

Nerve recovery, whether natural or postsurgical, will eventually plateau, and if arm function remains limited, additional surgical treatment options are considered beyond the infant stage. Children are evaluated for musculoskeletal surgical reconstruction options to maximize their function and reduce the progression of musculoskeletal deformities.[33] Deficiencies in external rotation of the shoulder are most common, likely given the vulnerable location of its innervation that courses along the most superior aspect of the upper trunk.[34] Patients manifest with functional difficulties in overhead activities, including washing or combing hair, reaching, and throwing. Shoulder release and tendon transfer involves partial release of the shoulder ligaments and tendons to allow for greater passive external rotation and abduction range. Shoulder internal rotator muscles are then rerouted to a new point of insertion to act as shoulder external rotators and abductors.

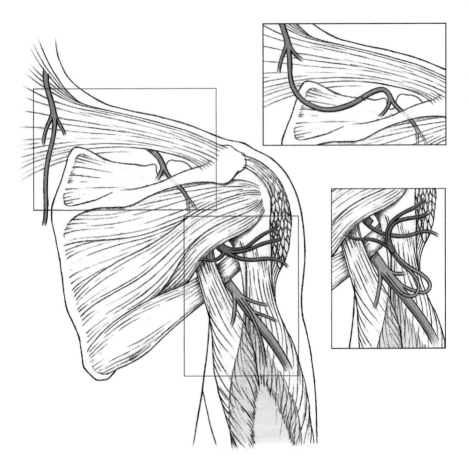

Fig. 9. Extraplexus nerve transfer using cranial nerve X coapted to suprascapular nerve and intraplexus nerve transfer using radial coapted to axillary.

Other persistent deficits can occur in a variety of circumstances, especially with more severe palsies. Lack of wrist extension or thumb abduction can be addressed via tendon transfers. Limited forearm pronation can be addressed via biceps tendon rerouting or osteotomies, and residual shoulder deficits can be improved via rotational humerus osteotomy to reorient the limb into a more functional posture. If no elbow flexion has recovered or in other select circumstances, a free functional muscle transplantation can be undertaken.

COMORBIDITIES IN THE DEVELOPING CHILD WITH NEONATAL BRACHIAL PLEXUS PALSY

Partnership with pediatricians goes beyond the infant stage and concerns for nerve recovery. Children and adolescents with NBPP may present with additional comorbid conditions that warrant multisystem screening procedures to identify problems, guide treatments, and inform referrals for specialty care. For example, language delays have been identified in children with NBPP between 24 and 36 months of age at a higher rate than reported in the general population.[35] Special attention to language development in preschool-age children may identify delays and allow for timely referral to speech and language therapy.

Central nervous system and developmental disorders have also been reported in children with NBPP, including cerebral palsy, generalized hypotonia, attention-deficit/hyperactivity disorder, and developmental coordination disorder.[36,37] Additional studies are required to establish whether children with NBPP are at increased risk for these conditions compared with other children.

Accidental or self-inflicted skin injury can occur in children with NBPP related to lack of protective sensation, dysesthesias, or psychological distress.[38] Routine integumentary examination of the affected upper extremity can reveal early signs of skin breakdown. Self-biting of the forearm, hand, fingers, or thumb occurs most frequently in young children with involvement of C5-T1 nerve roots.[39,40] Repeated skin breakdown can lead to skin infections, osteomyelitis, or distal phalanx loss.[38,39]

The underlying nerve injury and secondary musculoskeletal deformities have been identified as sources of pain with several studies reporting pain in 45% to 54% of the study populations.[41–43] In 1 study, pain occurred daily in 40% of adolescents with NBPP who underwent nerve surgery as infants.[23] Despite the frequency of pain, most children feel the limb appearance and function contribute most to the differences in quality of life compared with peers.[44,45]

As children with NBPP age, they develop secondary contractures owing to differences in limb growth and joint development, with more severe injuries resulting in more significant differences.[46] Animal studies have shown significant losses of muscle length and mass occurred with preganglionic avulsions and ruptures.[47] In studies of children with NBPP of all severities, the affected limb measured between 92% and 95% the length of the unaffected limb, and those with more severe injuries had larger differences.[48,49] Contractures contribute to the appearance of further limb shortening with internal rotation (60%) and elbow flexion (48%) contractures being the most common.[50,51]

Children and adolescents with NBPP are more frequently overweight or obese than the general US population.[52] A birth weight greater than 4000 g is associated with increased risk for obesity in children with NBPP.[52] Because macrosomia is a risk factor for NBPP,[1] close monitoring of body mass index throughout childhood and adolescence is warranted for overall health and well-being.

REHABILITATION APPROACH FOR THE DEVELOPING CHILD WITH NEONATAL BRACHIAL PLEXUS PALSY

Rehabilitation strategies target prevention of musculoskeletal deformities and improvement in overall function throughout the lifespan. Children and adolescents are referred to physical and occupational therapy for episodic treatment to address pain and functional goals. Interventions can include splinting and serial casting to treat elbow flexion contractures.[53] Kinesio taping and neuromuscular stimulation have been shown to improve range of motion, posture, and function.[54–56] Constraint therapy has also been used with improvements in function when there is developmental disregard.[57]

Rehabilitation management also emphasizes exercise and participation in recreational activities for overall well-being and maintaining healthy weight. Children can have reduced limb use and/or functional changes, as they are unable to compensate for the increased weight of the affected limb.

Ergonomic considerations are addressed for school-aged children to ensure that accommodations are implemented to support learning. For example, children often have pain in their neck, back, and shoulders because of backpack use. A second set of books at school can reduce the load carried in a backpack. Children with Erb palsy can also have subtle deficits in hand function of both affected and unaffected limbs,[58,59] and they may change hand dominance owing to the brachial plexus palsy. Accommodations can include extra time for writing or typing assignments to reduce hand fatigue. Because of contractures, many children adopt compensatory postures to position their hand for typing. These postures cause fatigue and strain in the neck and shoulder muscles, which can be mitigated with adjustable arm rests. One-handed typing programs, split keyboards, and dictation software are additional adjustments to make work more accessible.

As children reach adolescence, rehabilitation management addresses adaptations for driving when needed and provides guidance surrounding career planning and navigating accommodations in postsecondary education.

SUMMARY

Approximately 20% to 30% of children with NBPP experience permanent residual deficits from the nerve injury that can lead to musculoskeletal deformities, pain, and alterations in function.[3] Infants with persistent weakness beyond 1 month of age warrant referral to a specialty brachial plexus clinic where a multidisciplinary approach to the nonsurgical and surgical management can optimize their overall outcome and addresses the range of needs from infancy to adolescence.

CLINICS CARE POINTS

- Neonatal brachial plexus palsy causes permanent deficits in 20% to 30% of children.
- There can be secondary musculoskeletal changes, particularly at the glenohumeral joint, that can limit function even when neurologic recovery is adequate.
- If an infant with neonatal brachial plexus palsy has not recovered fully within the first 4 weeks of life or if there are concerns about injury involving the entire plexus, they should be referred to a specialty clinic.

DISCLOSURE

The authors have nothing to disclose.

COMMERCIAL/FINANCIAL CONFLICTS OF INTEREST

None.

FUNDING

None.

REFERENCES

1. van der Looven R, Le Roy L, Tanghe E, et al. Risk factors for neonatal brachial plexus palsy: a systematic review and meta-analysis. Dev Med Child Neurol 2020;62(6):673–83.
2. Donnelly V, Foran A, Murphy J, et al. Neonatal brachial plexus palsy: an unpredictable injury. Am J Obstet Gynecol 2002;187(5):1209–12.

3. Buterbaugh K, Shah A. The natural history and management of brachial plexus birth palsy. Curr Rev Musculoskelet Med 2016;9:418–26.

4. Pondaag W, Malessy M, van Dijk J, et al. Natural history of obstetric brachial plexus palsy: a systematic review. Dev Med Child Neurol 2004;46:138–44.

5. Hervey-Jumper S, Justice D, Vanaman M, et al. Torticollis associated with neonatal brachial plexus palsy. Pediatr Neurol 2011;45:305–10.

6. Yoshida K, Kawabata H. The prognostic value of concurrent phrenic nerve palsy in newborn babies with neonatal brachial plexus palsy. J Hand Surg Am 2015;40:1166–9.

7. Rizeq Y, Many B, Vacek J, et al. Diaphragmatic paralysis after phrenic nerve injury in newborns. J Pediatr Surg 2020;55(2):240–4.

8. Héritier O, Vasseur Maurer S, Reinberg O, et al. Respiratory distress in a one-month-old child suffering brachial plexus palsy. J Paediatr Child Health 2013;49(1):E90–2.

9. Chen H, Blackwell S, Yang L, et al. Neonatal brachial plexus palsy: associated birth injury outcomes, hospital length of stay and costs. J Matern Fetal Neonatal Med 2022;35(25):5736–44.

10. Schmieg S, Nguyen J, Pehnke M. Team approach: management of brachial plexus birth injury. JBJS Rev 2020;8(7):e1900200.

11. Malessy M, Pondaag W. Nerve surgery for neonatal brachial plexus palsy. J Pediatr Rehabil Med 2011;4(2):141–8.

12. Curtis C, Stephens D, Clarke H, et al. The Active Movement Scale: an evaluative tool for infants with obstetrical brachial plexus palsy. J Hand Surg Am 2002;27(3):470–8.

13. Duijnisveld B, van Wijlen Hempel M, Hogendoorn S, et al. Botulinum toxin injection for internal rotation contractures in brachial plexus birth palsy. A minimum 5-year prospective observational study. J Pediatr Orthop 2017;37(3):e209–15.

14. Smith B, Daunter A, Yang L, et al. An update on the management of neonatal brachial plexus palsy-replacing old paradigms: a review. JAMA Pediatr 2018;172(6):585–91.

15. Gharbaoui I, Gogola G, Aaron D, et al. Perspectives on glenohumeral joint contractures and shoulder dysfunction in children with perinatal brachial plexus palsy. J Hand Ther 2015;28(2):176–83.

16. Iorio M, Menashe S, Iyer R, et al. Glenohumeral dysplasia following neonatal brachial plexus palsy: presentation and predictive features during infancy. J Hand Surg Am 2015;40(12):2345–23451.e1.

17. Crouch D, Hutchinson I, Plate J, et al. Biomechanical basis of shoulder osseous deformity and contracture in a rat model of brachial plexus birth palsy. J Bone Joint Surg Am 2015;97(15):1264–71.

18. Cheng W, Cornwall R, Crouch D, et al. Contributions of muscle imbalance and impaired growth to postural and osseous shoulder deformity following brachial plexus birth palsy: a computational simulation analysis. J Hand Surg 2015;40(6):1170–6.

19. Pöyhiä TH, Lamminen AE, Peltonen JI, et al. Brachial plexus birth injury: US screening for glenohumeral joint instability. Radiology 2010;254(1):253–60.

20. Justice D, Rasmussen L, Di Pietro M, et al. Prevalence of posterior shoulder subluxation in children with neonatal brachial plexus palsy after early full passive range of motion exercises. PMR 2015;7(12):1235–42.

21. Menashe S, Ngo A, Osorio M, et al. Ultrasound assessment of glenohumeral dysplasia in infants. Pediatr Radiol 2022;52(9):1648–57.

22. Bauer A, Lucas J, Heyrani N, et al. Ultrasound screening for posterior shoulder dislocation in infants with persistent brachial plexus birth palsy. J Bone Joint Surg Am 2017;99:778–83.

23. van der Sluijs J, van Ouwerkerk W, de Gast A, et al. Deformities of the shoulder in infants younger than 12 months with an obstetric lesion of the brachial plexus. J Bone Joint Surg Br 2001;83(4):551–5.

24. Moukoko D, Ezaki M, Wilkes D, et al. Posterior shoulder dislocation in infants with neonatal brachial plexus palsy. J Bone Joint Surg Am 2004;86-A(4):787–93.

25. Dahlin L, Erichs K, Andersson C, et al. Incidence of early posterior shoulder dislocation in brachial plexus birth palsy. J Brachial Plexus Peripher Nerve Inj 2007; 2:24.

26. Kozin SH. Correlation between external rotation of the glenohumeral joint and deformity after brachial plexus birth palsy. J Pediatr Orthop 2004;24(2):189–93.

27. Durlacher K, Bellows D, Verchere C. Sup-ER orthosis: an innovative treatment for infants with birth related brachial plexus injury. J Hand Ther 2014;27(4):335–9.

28. Verchere C, Durlacher K, Bellows D, et al. An early shoulder repositioning program in birth-related brachial plexus injury: a pilot study of the Sup-ER protocol. Hand (NY) 2014;9(2):187–95.

29. Ezaki M, Malungpaishrope K, Harrison RJ, et al. Onabotulinum toxinA injection as an adjunct in the treatment of posterior shoulder subluxation in neonatal brachial plexus palsy. J Bone Joint Surg Am 2010;92(12):2171–7.

30. Greenhill D, Wissinger K, Trionfo A, et al. External rotation predicts outcomes after closed glenohumeral joint reduction with botulinum toxin type A in brachial plexus birth palsy. J Pediatr Orthop 2018;38(1):32–7.

31. Borschel G, Clarke H. Obstetrical brachial plexus palsy. Plast Reconstr Surg 2009;124(1 Suppl):144e–55e.

32. Tse R, Kozin S, Malessy M, et al. International Federation of Societies for Surgery of the Hand Committee report: the role of nerve transfers in the treatment of neonatal brachial plexus palsy. J Hand Surg Am 2015;40(6):1246–59.

33. Waters P, Smith G, Jaramillo D. Glenohumeral deformity secondary to brachial plexus birth palsy. J Bone Joint Surg Am 1998;80:668–77.

34. Siqueira M, Foroni L, Martins R, et al. Fascicular topography of the suprascapular nerve in the C5 root and upper trunk of the brachial plexus: a microanatomic study from a nerve surgeon's perspective. Neurosurgery 2010;67(2 Suppl Operative):402–6.

35. Chang K, Yang L, Driver L, et al. High prevalence of early language delay exists among toddlers with neonatal brachial plexus palsy. Pediatr Neurol 2014;51: 384–9.

36. Buitenhuis S, van Wijlen-Hempel R, Pondaag W, et al. Obstetric brachial plexus lesions and central developmental disability. Early Hum Dev 2012;88:731–4.

37. Acar G, Ekici B, Bilir F, et al. Obstetric brachial plexus palsy: 20 years' experience at a tertiary center in Turkey. Turk Arch Pediatr 2013;48(1):13–6.

38. Al-Qattan MM. Self-mutilation in children with obstetric brachial plexus palsy. J Hand Surg 1999;24(5):547–9.

39. McCann M, Waters P, Goumnerova L, et al. Self-mutilation in young children following brachial plexus birth injury. Pain 2004;110:123–9.

40. Heise C, Zaccariotto M, Martins R, et al. Self-biting behavior in patients with neonatal brachial plexus palsy. Childs Nerv Syst 2022;38(9):1773–6 [published online ahead of print, 2022 Jun 20].

41. Ho E, Curtis C, Clarke H. Pain in children following microsurgical reconstruction for obstetrical brachial plexus palsy. J Hand Surg Am 2015;40(6):1177–83.

42. de Heer C, Beckerman H, de Groot V. Explaining daily functioning in young adults with obstetric brachial plexus lesion. Disabil Rehabil 2015;37(16):1455–61.
43. Spaargaren E, Ahmed J, Van Ouwerkerk W, et al. Aspects of activities and participation of 7–8 year-old children with an obstetric brachial plexus injury. Europ J Paediatr Neurol 2011;15:345–52.
44. Squitieri L, Larson B, Change K, et al. Understanding quality of life and patient expectations among adolescents with neonatal brachial plexus palsy: a qualitative and quantitative pilot study. J Hand Surg Am 2013;38(12):2387–97.
45. Manske M, Abarca N, Letzelter J, et al. Patient-reported outcomes measurement information system scores for children with brachial plexus birth injury. J Pediatr Orthop 2021;41(3):171–6.
46. Van der Sluijs J, van der Sluijs M, van de Bunt F, et al. What influences contracture formation in lower motor neuron disorders, severity of denervation or residual muscle function? An analysis of the elbow contracture in 100 children with unilateral brachial plexus birth injury. J Child Orthop 2018;12(5):544–9.
47. Dixit N, McCormick C, Warren E, et al. Preganglionic and postganglionic brachial plexus birth injury effects on shoulder muscle growth. J Hand Surg Am 2021; 46(2):146.e1–9.
48. Bae DS, Ferretti M, Waters PM. Upper extremity size differences in brachial plexus birth palsy. Hand (N Y) 2008;3(4):297–303.
49. McDaid P, Koxin S, Thoder J, et al. Upper extremity limb-length discrepancy in brachial plexus palsy. J Pediatr Orthop 2002;22(3):364–6.
50. Hoeksma A, Ter Steeg A, DijkstraP, et al. Shoulder contracture and osseous deformity in obstetrical brachial plexus injuries. J Bone Joint Surg Am 2003; 85-A(2):316–22.
51. Ho E, Kim D, Klar K, et al. Prevalence and etiology of elbow flexion contractures in brachial plexus birth injury: a scoping review. J Pediatr Rehabil Med 2019;12(1): 75–86.
52. Singh A, Mills J, Bauer A, et al. Obesity in children with brachial plexus birth palsy. J Pediatr Orthop B 2015;24:541–5.
53. Ho ES, Zuccaro J, Klar K, et al. Effectiveness of non-surgical and surgical interventions for elbow flexion contractures in brachial plexus birth injury: A systematic review. J Pediatr Rehabil Med 2019;12(1):87–100.
54. Hassan B, Abbass M, Elshennawy S. Systematic review of the effectiveness of Kinesio taping for children with brachial plexus injury. Physiother Res Int 2020; 25(1):e1794.
55. Russo S, Rodriguez L, Kozin S, et al. Therapeutic Taping for Scapular Stabilization in Children With Brachial Plexus Birth Palsy. Am J Occup Ther 2016;70(5). 7005220030p1.
56. Elnaggar R. Shoulder function and bone mineralization in children with obstetric brachial plexus injury after neuromuscular electrical stimulation during weight-bearing exercises. Am J Phys Med Rehabil 2016;95(4):239–47.
57. Zielinski I, van Delft R, Voorman J, et al. The effects of modified constraint-induced movement therapy combined with intensive bimanual training in children with brachial plexus birth injury: a retrospective data base study. Disabil Rehabil 2021;43(16):2275–84.
58. Immerman I, Alfonso D, Ramos L, et al. Hand function in children with an upper brachial plexus birth injury: results of the nine-hole peg test. Dev Med Child Neurol 2012;54(2):166–9.
59. Matthews D. Function of the unaffected arms of children with neonatal brachial plexus injuries. Europ J Paediatr Neurol 2018;22(4):581.

Introduction to Limb Deficiency for the Pediatrician

Phoebe Scott-Wyard, DO

KEYWORDS

- Limb deficiency • Overuse syndrome • Prosthesis • Congenital limb deficiency
- Amputation

KEY POINTS

- Pediatricians often serve as the managing physician for children with a limb deficiency, particularly if there is no local Physical Medicine & Rehabilitation (PM&R) physician. It is helpful to collaborate with a team (physical/occupational therapists, prosthetists).
- Most cases of congenital limb deficiency are non-syndromic; however, the exceptions involve multiple bones, longitudinal bone deficiencies, or radial bone deficiencies. Vascular disruption sequence is frequently misdiagnosed as amniotic band syndrome.
- If a child requires surgical intervention, it is important to preserve joints, preserve length/growth plates, and consider through-joint/disarticulation amputations over trans-osseus amputations, due to the risk of painful terminal bony overgrowth.
- Not all children need to be fit with a prosthesis nor do multi-limb amputees need to have prosthetic fitting of all limbs. Consider functional goals before prosthetic prescription.
- Chronic compensatory use of residual limbs can put the child at risk for overuse injury later. Discuss environmental adaptations to prevent this (eg, avoid hopping for the unilateral lower limb amputee and avoid typing for the unilateral upper limb amputee).

INTRODUCTION

A pediatrician may not care for many children with limb differences during their career; however, due to the paucity of physicians experienced in amputee care, it is likely that the responsibility of directing the care of these children will fall to the primary care provider. This review of some of the basic tenets of amputee care is meant to be a starting point for clinicians caring for children with limb differences to improve access to knowledgeable providers for this population of patients.

Division of Pediatric Rehabilitation, Department of Orthopedics, Rady Children's Hospital, University of California – San Diego, 3020 Children's Way, MC5096, San Diego, CA 92123-4223, USA
E-mail address: pscottwyard@rchsd.org

Pediatr Clin N Am 70 (2023) 531–543
https://doi.org/10.1016/j.pcl.2023.01.011
pediatric.theclinics.com

Overall, limb deficiency continues to be rare, regardless of cause. In a recent study across seven years, the prevalence of lower limb deficiency was 38.5 cases per 100,000 children with commercial insurance in the United States. Of these cases, 84% were congenital limb deficiencies, followed by 13.5% due to trauma, and 0.5% from cancer.[1] In a 33-year review of the population database in Alberta, they found a congenital limb deficiency prevalence of 5.6/10,000 total births, or one case per 1800 births (consistent with prior studies which found a range of 1 per 1300 to 2000 live births).[2] In this review, upper limbs were more than two times more often affected than lower limbs. Five percent had chromosome abnormalities and less than one percent were due to teratogens.[3]

It is important to have an understanding of nomenclature when treating children with limb deficiency, as there is a broad spectrum of clinical presentations. For traumatic amputations, the classification used for children is the same as used adults, named for the joint or location of the body that has been amputated, for example, transtibial, transfemoral, and knee disarticulation. In the case of congenital amputations, the limb is characterized as either transverse (absence of all anatomical elements distal to a specified level of the limb as in the case of most traumatic amputations) or longitudinal (absence or hypoplasia of some anatomical elements longitudinally or along the length of a limb). Historical terminology should be avoided due to its confusing nature (eg, hemimelia or amelia).[2]

A review of the causation of congenital limb deficiency is more complex than can be delineated in this forum. Owing to the timing of limb development in the early first trimester when mothers often are unaware they are pregnant, it is often difficult to identify direct causality. In addition, it is important to note that of the more than 120 clinically defined congenital limb deficiencies, less than 40% have a known molecular origin. Most of non-syndromic, single-limb cases are sporadic, and not heritable. If there is any concern for a syndromic cause, it is highly recommended to refer for genetic consultation.[2] In children born with a congenital transverse unilateral upper limb deficiency (also known as symbrachydactyly), there are often residual digits or "nubbins," felt to be due to an attempt at regeneration after vascular disruption during development in utero.[4] This is a distinct entity when compared with amniotic band syndrome, an extremely rare phenomenon that frequently involves more than one limb, has scars that are tourniquet-like, lymphedema, and more often exhibits syndactyly of fully formed digits. It is important to recognize this difference when counseling new parents, as vascular disruption sequence is frequently misdiagnosed as amniotic band syndrome (**Figs. 1** and **2** for examples of each). Despite improvements in prenatal imaging, congenital limb deficiencies are frequently discovered at the time of birth. Prenatal ultrasound screening has a detection rate of 42% for upper limb anomalies, and three-dimensional ultrasound might increase this to 50%.[5]

Initial Examination and Diagnostic Evaluation

There are a few "red flags" to watch out for on the examination, which may require further workup. For children with radial longitudinal deficiency, the clinician may note an ipsilateral hypoplastic or absent thumb. Approximately one-third of radial ray deficiencies are syndromic, and therefore workup should include an evaluation of hematologic, cardiac, and renal systems. This may include echocardiogram, renal ultrasound, complete blood count, and Diepoxybutane Test (DEB Test) is used to screen for Fanconi Anemia (FA) chromosome breakage assay.[6]

Upper limb deficiencies tend to be more often associated with syndromes, and these can frequently have cardiac malformations, such as in the case of VACTERL association, thrombocytopenia–absent–radius (TAR) syndrome, Holt Oram syndrome, Trisomy

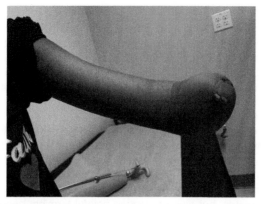

Fig. 1. Example of left below-elbow transverse congenital limb deficiency due to vascular disruption sequence, with distal residual digits.

13 and Trisomy 18.[5] Therefore, an echocardiogram would be important in evaluating a child with an upper limb abnormality, particularly radial longitudinal deficiency. Genetic consultation and chromosomal microarray should be considered in children with multiple limb involvement or longitudinal deficiency, with molecular testing of a single gene if the phenotype is clear. In the case of transverse congenital deficiency, placental pathology may be helpful to determine if amniotic banding was present.

It is often helpful to obtain radiographs of the affected and contralateral limb to determine the extent of the bony abnormality. A skeletal survey can help evaluate for skeletal dysplasia and spinal abnormalities. Any abnormalities on the neurological exam should prompt an MRI of the brain. It can also be helpful to examine the parents for any limb deformities.[2]

When examining infants and children with a congenital upper limb deficiency, it is important to observe the pectoralis muscles and chest to assess for any asymmetry. This is the hallmark feature of Poland syndrome, which can have multiple clinical implications, from severe chest/breast hypoplasia to dextrocardia.[7]

It is also recommended to evaluate the function and use of all limbs in children with multiple limb involvement, as full consideration of their functional needs must be undertaken before considering any surgical or prosthetic intervention.

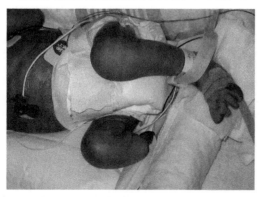

Fig. 2. Photo of infant with right transtibial congenital amputation due to amniotic band syndrome. (Photo courtesy of Sara McLaughlin, PT.)

Surgical Considerations

Families faced with surgical intervention for a child with a congenital limb deficiency often struggle with the idea of taking another part of a limb that they have already mourned as being abnormal from birth. Parents should be encouraged to keep a journal of their thoughts and feelings regarding the surgery and to take photos and even footprints/handprints, if appropriate, to help with coping. These memories can even be shared with the child later, when developmentally appropriate, to help them understand the choices that were made.

When a child is being evaluated for surgical intervention of their limb difference, there are some important considerations that must be taken into account. Firstly, preserving the length and growth plates of a residual limb will aid in improved function, and later growth modulation can be done surgically for optimal prosthetic fit. Second, through-joint disarticulation amputation is superior to trans-osseous amputation, not only preserving growth plates, but also preventing painful terminal bony overgrowth and allow for distal weight-bearing. Third, preserving joints whenever possible will not only improve function but also decrease the cost of required prosthetic componentry (eg, knee). Fourth, proximal joints should be addressed and stabilized before any distal surgical intervention, such as in the case of hip dysplasia occurring with fibular deficiency. In the case of a child with multiple limb involvement, it is beneficial to evaluate all limbs with a multidisciplinary team including occupational and physical therapists to determine the best course of treatment. For example, some children with bilateral upper limb deficiency may use their lower limbs to perform activities of daily living.[8]

In children with congenital upper limb deficiency, surgical decision-making is not straightforward. Children who have had surgery to add digits, straighten the arm, or wear a prosthesis report more improvement in perceived quality of life due to their personal coping mechanisms than due to the surgical interventions themselves.[9] Once again, it is helpful to involve a multidisciplinary team in these cases, including an occupational therapist and hand surgeon experienced in upper limb deficiency. Removal of the residual digits or nubbins of children with congenital limb deficiency is not recommended, as this can promote neuroma formation, and they can often be functional (eg, for touchscreen use).[10]

Prosthetic Management

The ideal management of children with limb deficiency is by a multidisciplinary team that includes an occupational therapist, physical therapist, social worker, prosthetist, and nurse, guided by a pediatric rehabilitation physician. Orthopedic surgeons are also involved in specific situations as noted above. The team approach allows collaboration in real time to best provide holistic care that is tailored to the individual child's needs. Pediatric rehabilitation physicians are specially trained in the care of children with complex physical disabilities, including those with limb deficiency. However, there is a paucity of pediatric rehabilitation physicians which has created an unfortunate gap in care for these children. As a primary care provider, one does not need to be an expert in prosthetic devices to prescribe the correct one. Knowledge of basic concepts and a willing, experienced prosthetist as a partner in care are the primary tools necessary. It is important to note that not all children benefit from prostheses. Children with multiple limb deficiencies may benefit from adaptive equipment and power mobility rather than several cumbersome prosthetic devices. There are continual prosthetic innovations transpiring; however, sometimes the simplest prosthetic option is the best. Children should master basic prosthetic use before addition of advanced components or controls.

For patients with upper limb deficiency, it is recommended to provide families with education regarding upper extremity prosthetic devices, with an occupational therapist and/or prosthetist, and allowing them to make an informed decision regarding prosthetic fitting due to the high rejection rate. In one international analysis of rejection, those fit before age two years (for congenital limb deficiency) or within six months of amputation (for acquired limb deficiency) were 16 times more likely to continue prosthesis use.[11] In addition, it is important to establish a daily wear pattern to promote integration into the child's body image, which can be challenging for some families.[12] The simpler the prosthetic device, the more easily it will be assimilated, for example, the "hook" terminal device is much easier for prosthetic training and function than a terminal device that looks like a hand.[13] Some of the main prosthetic types are cosmetic (meant to look like a hand or arm, able to be positioned but with minimal functional use), body-powered (worn with a harness, with functional opening or closing of a terminal device using a cable activated by shoulder movement), myoelectric or externally powered (using surface electrodes to activate a motor that causes movement in a terminal device), and activity-specific (eg, for swimming, riding a bike, or playing the violin). Previously, myoelectric prosthetic arms were heavy and expensive, rarely fit in children outside of charity centers, but commercial devices like the Hero Arm by Open Bionics have helped develop lightweight, durable options that are more accessible to children (**Fig. 3**). Regardless of type of upper limb prosthesis, training with an occupational therapist is crucial in its successful use.[13] Some children with bilateral upper limb deficiency prefer to use their limbs together in a bimanual pattern for functional tasks rather than prosthetic devices (**Fig. 4**).

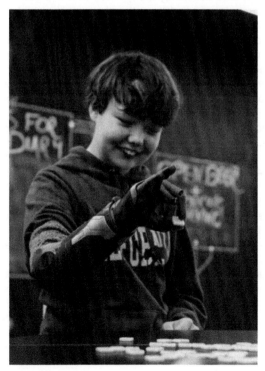

Fig. 3. Hero Arm by Open Bionics, one example of a three-dimensional printed myoelectric prosthesis. (Photo courtesy of Open Bionics.)

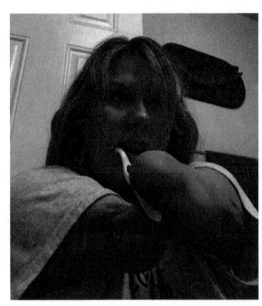

Fig. 4. Example of bimanual technique used for activities of daily living such as brushing teeth in a young adult with bilateral upper limb deficiency. (Photo courtesy of Bella Tucker.)

Children with lower limb deficiency are typically fit with prosthetic legs when pulling to stand, approximately 10 to 12 months of age. In the child with bilateral lower limb deficiency, arm span is often used to determine appropriate height in prosthetic legs. For congenital amputees, physical therapy is typically needed during early years and/or when changing components. For acquired amputees, physical therapy can be helpful with initial prosthetic fitting. Crutches or a walker should be provided for unilateral amputees or a manual wheelchair for bilateral amputees for use when prosthetic devices are broken or if they have complications from prosthetic wear.

If a child has undergone surgical revision of their congenital limb deficiency or traumatic amputation, it is important to fit with an elastic shrinker once the incision is healed to prepare the limb for prosthetic fitting. The shrinker sock helps to decrease swelling and assists with desensitization of the residual limb. After 2 to 4 weeks in a shrinker sock, the limb is ready for prosthetic fitting; if measurements are taken too early, the socket will be too big and will fall off when worn.

A prosthetic prescription should include the side and level of prosthesis (eg, right transradial upper limb prosthesis or left transfemoral lower limb prosthesis). If type of components is known, include this in the prescription. For lower limb amputees, it is important to document their potential for ambulation using Medicare's lower limb prosthesis functional classification level, or K-level, as this is often requested by insurance payors and determines if certain prosthetic components will be covered (**Fig. 5**). To initiate fitting, the prosthetist takes a mold of the residual limb, either using three-dimensional scanning or a cast. A positive model is made from the mold, over which the clear test or "check" socket is fabricated, used for initial fitting. After the check socket has been successfully fit over the residual limb and any areas of discomfort have been modified, the definitive socket is made, and the prosthetic components and alignment are added. Patients can choose the design of their socket (if desired), using fabric of their choice or possibly skin-tone to make it more cosmetic. They

K Level	Ambulation potential
0	Does not have the ability or potential to ambulate or transfer safely with or without assistance and a prosthesis does not enhance their quality of life or mobility.
1	Has the ability or potential to use a prosthesis for transfers or ambulation on level surfaces at fixed cadence. (e.g., limited and unlimited household ambulator)
2	Has the ability or potential for ambulation with the ability to traverse low level environmental barriers such as curbs, stairs, or uneven surfaces. (e.g., limited community ambulator)
3	Has the ability or potential for ambulation with variable cadence. (e.g., community ambulator who has the ability to traverse most environmental barriers and may have vocational, therapeutic, or exercise activity that demands prosthetic utilization beyond simple locomotion)
4	Has the ability or potential for prosthetic ambulation that exceeds basic ambulation skills, exhibiting high impact, stress, or energy levels. (e.g., child, active adult, or athlete)

Fig. 5. Lower limb prosthetic functional classification levels. (*Adapted from* Lower Limb Prosthetic Workgroup Consensus Document, Centers for Medicare and Medicaid Services, 2017. https://www.cms.gov/Medicare/Coverage/DeterminationProcess/downloads/LLP_Consensus_Document.pdf.)

should be evaluated every 4 to 6 months by their prosthetist for adjustments to the prosthesis for growth.

Clinical Follow-up

When evaluating a child with a limb difference in clinic, it is important to always remove any prosthetic devices to inspect the skin condition underneath, as well as to take an accurate weight. Prosthetic devices can vary widely in weight due to the componentry used, and would create an inaccurate weight measurement. However, for those with an above-knee limb difference, removal of the prosthesis may require removal of outer clothing and if the scale is in a public part of the clinic, privacy may make this challenging. In that case, it is recommended to weigh the child with the prosthesis and separately weigh the prosthesis after removal and subtract its weight.

Obesity is a well-recognized challenge in the care of children, with significant implications on both present and future health status.[14] In the amputee, obesity not only carries the same health implications, but also presents challenges in balance and prosthetic socket fit. However, it is notably difficult to establish weight standards when children are missing part or all of a limb. Uncorrected body mass index was found to underestimate body fat in unilateral lower limb amputees, and overestimate body fat in subjects with bilateral lower limb amputations.[15] Unfortunately, although skinfold thickness is a better measurement of adiposity, no reference standards exist. Furthermore, estimating fractional weight loss from each amputation using nomograms is also inaccurate. One adult study has validated the use of the Department of Defense circumference method (measuring neck, waist, hip and comparing against normalized data) for estimation of body fat percentage in people with lower limb loss.[16] This author recommends following trends of weight over time and counseling patients about physical activity and adaptive sports when appropriate.

For patients who wear a prosthesis, the encased skin can display a multitude of dermatologic problems, including fungal or bacterial infections, chronic choke syndrome, and contact dermatitis.[17] Treatment should include suspending prosthetic wear until completely healed, asking the prosthetist to evaluate prosthetic socket fit, and reviewing hygiene of prosthetic-skin interface. Prosthetic liners can be easily cleaned using soap and water, and children should be encouraged to perform this hygiene practice and regular skin checks themselves. In addition, hyperhidrosis of the residual limb is common in children with limb deficiency, due to the lack of full extremity skin area to control body temperature. There are a multitude of treatments available, without adequate efficacy and safety information for the use in children.[18] It is recommended to remove the prosthetic socket during the day and dry the residual limb if excessive sweating causes skin breakdown or problems with prosthetic socket suspension.

Children who have undergone an amputation through the diaphysis of a long bone (eg, traumatic amputations) are at risk of terminal bony overgrowth, where the distal end of the bone continues growing and creates a sharp, painful bony prominence at the end of the residual limb with skin breakdown. This requires urgent surgical consultation and consideration of stump capping or other surgical revision (**Fig. 6**).

Complaints of pain in the residual limb should be investigated for the source, as this could be due to a multitude of causes, including but not limited to neuroma or bursa formation, terminal bony overgrowth, heterotopic ossification, or in the case of a cancer survivor, tumor recurrence. Patients who have undergone traumatic amputation are at risk of neuroma formation, consisting of a ball of disorganized neural tissue that forms from transected nerves that can be extremely painful and cause pain in the residual limb and/or with prosthetic wear.[19] Recommended evaluation should include radiography to evaluate for bony cause and if negative, ultrasound or MRI to evaluated for neuroma or other soft tissue cause. Treatment includes surgical excision, and targeted muscle reinnervation (TMR), wherein the nerve is sewn to a muscle to prevent future neuroma formation.[20] Phantom pain, or pain felt in the missing limb, is uncommon in children, however, is more prevalent if they had a high preoperative

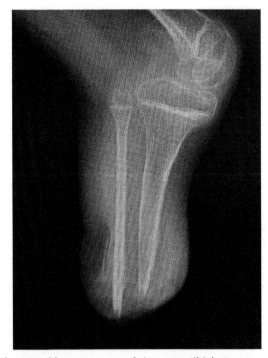

Fig. 6. Example of terminal bony overgrowth in a transtibial amputee. (Photo courtesy of Sara McLaughlin, PT.)

pain level or were treated with chemotherapy agents.[21,22] Treatments available include pharmacological agents, surgical intervention (eg, TMR), psychological (eg, biofeedback, mirror therapy), application of a transcutaneous electric nerve stimulation (TENS) unit, nerve blocks, acupuncture, and others.

Mental Health Concerns

A person's perception of their limb difference will evolve over the course of their lifetime, shifting as they contend with diverse milestones, and changing with their environment, identity, experiences, and age.[9] Studies that investigated factors affecting self-esteem in children with congenital or acquired limb deficiency found that the child's classmate, parent, teacher, and friend support network all were significant predictors of self-esteem.[23,24] In patients with an acquired amputation, there are increased levels of depression and disturbance in body image, as well as social shame postoperatively.[25] In one study comparing adults with upper limb and lower limb acquired amputations, significantly increased rates of depression and anxiety were reported in the upper limb amputees, even higher if the dominant hand was the one amputated.[26]

It is not uncommon for teenagers with upper limb deficiency who have historically not worn a prosthesis to take a sudden interest in prosthetic fitting, frequently as a result of adolescent awareness of body image and low self-esteem. In this clinician's experience, it is helpful to refer to counseling to address these issues before considering fitting, as well as establishing realistic goals of use for a prosthesis.

Although there are no studies quantifying bullying in children with limb deficiency, it has been shown that children with disabilities experience a higher rate of bullying when compared with the nondisabled population.[27,28] In addition to screening for bullying, it is recommended to encourage engagement in extracurricular activities, as this has been correlated with improved self-esteem and lower rates of bullying in children with disabilities.[29]

The importance of community is well established for people of all abilities, and there are numerous resources available to children with limb differences and their families, such as online support groups, trained peer mentors, advocacy organizations, and camps (see end of article for list of resources).

Overuse Injury

Owing to the need for alteration of typical body biomechanics in limb deficiency, patients are at heightened risk of developing overuse problems secondary to maladaptive compensatory patterns of movement. In one study of adults with unilateral acquired or congenital upper limb deficiency investigating overuse, the most frequent problem reported was carpal tunnel syndrome, followed by shoulder pain, neck pain, and elbow pain.[30] Whether the clinician is evaluating a child with a lower limb deficiency that uses crutches or a wheelchair, or a child with an upper limb difference that types/texts/writes with a single hand, it is important to screen for symptoms of carpal tunnel syndrome. It is recommended to discuss adaptations and compensatory techniques for any repetitive activities that use the non-affected side in these patients to prevent such outcomes (eg, dictation software in lieu of typing).

In the school-age child, it is recommended to get an evaluation for an individualized education plan (IEP) or 504 plan through the school district to ensure adequate physical supports are in place for their academic success (eg, elevator access, two sets of books, notes-taker, or dictation software).

The clinician should discourage prolonged hopping in the unilateral lower limb amputee, and provide crutches for home use when not wearing a prosthesis to avoid increased physiologic load on the knee and hip and risk of injury or osteoarthritis.[31]

Resources

Owing to the high cost of prosthetic devices, many patients struggle with funding options. Here is a list of some charitable organizations that can be used for assistance.

- Challenged Athlete's Foundation (www.challengedathletes.org)—provides grants for sports-related equipment and activities for people with physical disabilities.
- Jordan Thomas Foundation (www.jordanthomasfoundation.org)—provides assistance for any type of prosthesis for children (including sport or activity specific).
- Amputee Blade Runners (www.amputeebladerunners.com)—provides free running prosthetic legs.
- Limbs for Life (www.limbsforlife.org)—global nonprofit organization that provides prosthetic care for individuals who cannot otherwise afford it.
- 50 Legs (www.50legs.org)—provides support for prosthetic care for amputees.
- Jami Marseilles Warriors with Hope, Inc (www.warriorswithhope.org)—provides financial assistance to those recovering from cancer or amputation.
- Heather Abbott Foundation (www.heatherabbottfoundation.org)—helps provide customized prostheses to those who have suffered limb loss through traumatic circumstances.
- Steps of Faith (www.stepsoffaithfoundation.org)—provides assistance to uninsured or underinsured people who need prosthetic care.
- Who Says I Can't Foundation (www.whosaysicant.org)—provides support for adaptive equipment and prosthetic devices for sports.

Resources for professionals

- Association of Children's Prosthetic-Orthotic Clinics (www.acpoc.org)—multidisciplinary professional organization that connects, supports and educates those that serve children who use orthotic or prosthetic devices.
- American Congress of Rehabilitation Medicine (www.acrm.org)—interprofessional organization with the mission to improve the lives of people with disabilities.
- The Orthotics & Prosthetics Virtual Library (www.oandplibrary.org)—collection of digital resources for orthotic and prosthetic providers.

Resources for families (above sites also have family resources)

- No Limits Foundation (www.nolimitsfoundation.org)—provides camps around the United States for children with limb differences.
- Lucky Fin Project (www.luckyfinproject.org)—international organization that connects families with children with upper limb difference.
- Amputee Coalition (www.amputee-coalition.org)—national organization that provides education, support, and advocacy for people living with limb loss.

Additional reading

a. Scott-Wyard P, Yip V, Rotter DB. "Limb Deficiencies." *Pediatric Rehabilitation: Principles and Practice* (2020): 410-432.
b. Krajbich JI, Pinzur MS, Potter BK, Stevens PM, editors. *Atlas of Amputations and Limb Deficiencies*, 4th edition. American Academy of Orthopaedic Surgeons, 2016.
c. Association of Children's Prosthetic & Orthotic Clinics (ACPOC): professional organization that supports and educates those that serve children who use orthotic and prosthetic devices. www.acpoc.org,

d. No Limits Foundation life hacks videos: https://nolimits.elevate.commpartners. com/life-hacks.
e. Louer CR Jr, Scott-Wyard P, Hernandez R, Vergun AD. Principles of Amputation Surgery, Prosthetics, and Rehabilitation in Children. *J Am Acad Orthop Surg*. 2021 Apr 20. Epub ahead of print. PMID: 33878082.

CLINICS CARE POINTS

- Longitudinal deficiencies or those involving the radial aspect of the upper limb are more likely to be syndromic and require a thorough medical and genetic workup.
- Consider the functional use of all limbs before any surgery or prosthetic prescription. Always remove any prosthetic devices for a physical exam and accurate weight.
- Simple/functional prostheses are often more easily accepted by the user than technologically complex ones.
- Screen for bullying and overuse syndromes at each visit. Children with disabilities experience a higher rate of bullying when compared with the nondisabled population.

DISCLOSURE

Dr P. Scott-Wyard is a paid consultant for Hanger Clinics, Inc and is Vice-President of Association of Children's Prosthetic-Orthotic Clinics.

REFERENCES

1. McLarney M, Pezzin LE, McGinley EL, et al. The prevalence of lower limb loss in children and associated costs of prosthetic devices: a national study of commercial insurance claims. Prosthet Orthot Int 2021;45(2):115–22.
2. Wilcox WR, Coulter CP, Schmitz ML. Congenital limb deficiency disorders. Clin Perinatol 2015;42(2):281–300.
3. Bedard T, Lowry RB, Sibbald B, et al. Congenital limb deficiencies in Alberta-a review of 33 years (1980-2012) from the Alberta Congenital Anomalies Surveillance System (ACASS). Am J Med Genet 2015;167A(11):2599–609.
4. Holmes LB, Nasri HZ. Terminal transverse limb defects with "nubbins". Birth Defects Res 2021;113(13):1007–14.
5. Alrabai HM, Farr A, Bettelheim D, et al. Prenatal diagnosis of congenital upper limb differences: a current concept review. J Matern Fetal Neonatal Med 2017; 30(21):2557–63.
6. Le JT, Scott-Wyard PR. Pediatric limb differences and amputations. Phys Med Rehabil Clin N Am 2015;26(1):95–108.
7. Baldelli I, Baccarani A, Barone C, et al. Consensus based recommendations for diagnosis and medical management of Poland syndrome (sequence). Orphanet J Rare Dis 2020;15(1):201.
8. Louer CR Jr, Scott-Wyard P, Hernandez R, et al. Principles of amputation surgery, prosthetics, and rehabilitation in children. J Am Acad Orthop Surg 2021;29(14): e702–13.
9. Lightdale-Miric N, Tuberty S, Nelson D. Caring for children with congenital upper extremity differences. J Hand Surg Am 2021;46(12):1105–11.
10. Mullick S, Borschel GH. A selective approach to treatment of ulnar polydactyly: preventing painful neuroma and incomplete excision. Pediatr Dermatol 2010; 27(1):39–42.

11. Biddiss EA, Chau TT. Multivariate prediction of upper limb prosthesis acceptance or rejection. Disabil Rehabil Assist Technol 2008;3(4):181–92.

12. Engdahl SM, Meehan SK, Gates DH. Differential experiences of embodiment between body-powered and myoelectric prosthesis users. Sci Rep 2020;10(1): 15471.

13. Johnson SS, Mansfield E. Prosthetic training: upper limb. Phys Med Rehabil Clin N Am 2014;25(1):133–51.

14. Horesh A, Tsur AM, Bardugo A, et al. Adolescent and Childhood Obesity and Excess Morbidity and Mortality in Young Adulthood-a Systematic Review. Curr Obes Rep 2021;10(3):301–10.

15. Frost AP, Norman Giest T, Ruta AA, et al. Limitations of body mass index for counseling individuals with unilateral lower extremity amputation. Prosthet Orthot Int 2017;41(2):186–93.

16. George BG, Pruziner AL, Andrews AM. Circumference method estimates percent body fat in male us service members with lower limb loss. J Acad Nutr Diet 2021; 121(7):1327–34.

17. Meulenbelt HE, Geertzen JH, Dijkstra PU, et al. Skin problems in lower limb amputees: an overview by case reports. J Eur Acad Dermatol Venereol 2007;21(2): 147–55.

18. Lannan FM, Powell J, Kim GM, et al. Hyperhidrosis of the residual limb: a narrative review of the measurement and treatment of excess perspiration affecting individuals with amputation. Prosthet Orthot Int 2021;45(6):477–86.

19. Buch NS, Qerama E, Brix Finnerup N, et al. Neuromas and postamputation pain. Pain 2020;161(1):147–55.

20. Dumanian GA, Potter BK, Mioton LM, et al. Targeted muscle reinnervation treats neuroma and phantom pain in major limb amputees: a randomized clinical trial. Ann Surg 2019;270(2):238–46.

21. Krane EJ, Heller LB. The prevalence of phantom sensation and pain in pediatric amputees. J Pain Symptom Manage 1995;10:21–9.

22. Wilkins Krista La, McGrath Patrick Jb, Finley Allen Ga,c, et al. Joeld Phantom limb sensations and phantom limb pain in child and adolescent amputees. Pain 1998; 78(1):7–12.

23. Varni JW, Rubenfeld LA, Talbot D, et al. Determinants of self-esteem in children with congenital/acquired limb deficiencies. J Dev Behav Pediatr 1989; 10(1):13–6.

24. Varni JW, Setoguchi Y, Rappaport LR, et al. Effects of stress, social support, and self-esteem on depression in children with limb deficiencies. Arch Phys Med Rehabil 1991;72(13):1053–8.

25. Bennett J. Limb loss: The unspoken psychological aspect. J Vasc Nurs 2016; 34(4):128–30.

26. Desteli EE, İmren Y, Erdoğan M, et al. Comparison of upper limb amputees and lower limb amputees: a psychosocial perspective. Eur J Trauma Emerg Surg 2014;40(6):735–9.

27. Carrillo LA, Sabatini CS, Brar RK, et al. The Prevalence of Bullying Among Pediatric Orthopaedic Patients. J Pediatr Orthop 2021;41(8):463–6.

28. Pinquart M. Systematic review: bullying involvement of children with and without chronic physical illness and/or physical/sensory disability-a meta-analytic comparison with healthy/nondisabled peers. J Pediatr Psychol 2017;42(3): 245–59.

29. Haegele JA, Aigner C, Healy S. Extracurricular activities and bullying among children and adolescents with disabilities. Matern Child Health J 2020;24(3): 310–8.
30. Burger H, Vidmar G. A survey of overuse problems in patients with acquired or congenital upper limb deficiency. Prosthet Orthot Int 2016;40(4):497–502.
31. Wasser JG, Acasio JC, Hendershot BD, et al. Single-leg forward hopping exposures adversely affect knee joint health among persons with unilateral lower limb loss: a predictive model. J Biomech 2020;109:109941.

Evaluation and Treatment of the Child with Acute Back Pain

Kevin P. Murphy, MD[a],*, Cristina Sanders, DO[b],
Amy E. Rabatin, MD[c,d]

KEYWORDS

- Back pain children • Risk factors • Spondylolysis • Spondylolisthesis
- Spinal tumors • Discitis

KEY POINTS

- Over 80% of back pain in children is benign and mechanical in nature, improving by natural history or within 2 weeks of conservative care.
- Back pain in children not improving within 2 weeks of conservative care requires in-depth assessment, including complex imaging, laboratory studies, and consultative services as indicated.
- Pediatric back pain is common, associated with active and sedentary lifestyles, deconditioning, and excessive body mass index.
- Spondylolysis and spondylolisthesis comprise almost 10% of pediatric back pain alone, often caused by hyperextension activities of the lumbar spine and treated most commonly with conservative care.
- Back pain in children is associated with decreased quality of life, including increased school days missed and decreased participation in sports and self-cares.

EVALUATION AND TREATMENT OF ACUTE LOW-BACK PAIN IN CHILDREN
Introduction

Back pain in children is a relatively common occurrence. Prevalence of childhood back pain is estimated anywhere from 20% to 30%, increasing with age.[1,2] Accurate

[a] Department of Physical Medicine and Rehabilitation, Sanford Health Systems, Bismarck North Dakota and Northern Minnesota, Northland Pediatric Rehabilitation Medicine LLC, 4710 Matterhorn Circle #309, Duluth, MN 55811, USA; [b] Pediatric Rehabilitation Medicine, Monument Health Department Neurology and Rehabilitation, Monument Health System, 677 Cathedral Drive, Suite 240, Rapid City, SD 57701, USA; [c] Division of Pediatric Rehabilitation Medicine, Department of Physical Medicine and Rehabilitation, Mayo Clinic, 200 1st Street Southwest, Rochester, MN 55905, USA; [d] Department of Pediatric and Adolescent Medicine, Mayo Clinic, 200 1st Street Southwest, Rochester, MN 55905, USA
* Corresponding author.
E-mail address: kevin.murphy@sanfordhealth.org

Pediatr Clin N Am 70 (2023) 545–574
https://doi.org/10.1016/j.pcl.2023.01.013
0031-3955/23/© 2023 Elsevier Inc. All rights reserved.

estimates are difficult to obtain, as studies are limited in number and research design, making the true incidence somewhat unknown.[3] The great majority of childhood back pain is benign and mechanical in nature (**Fig. 1**).[1,2,4] Symptoms for benign mechanical back pain usually resolve within 2 to 4 weeks of conservative care, such as rest, ice, and physical therapy (PT). Symptoms are associated with activity, poor posture, and increased body mass index (BMI).[4,5] Symptoms persisting beyond 4 weeks of conservative care, in the compliant patient, serve notice for the potential of more concerning pathologic condition.[1,2,4] Additional factors that warrant a more aggressive medical evaluation, commonly known as "red flags," include the following: back pain in a child under the age of 5 years, systemic symptoms, night pain, bowel and bladder incontinence in the previously continent child, neurologic symptoms and/or deficits, morning stiffness, and peripheral joint disease (**Fig. 2**).[5] Pain awakening the child at night is distinguished from pain that keeps the child from going to sleep, the latter more common and often associated with increased activity.[1] A detailed history and examination are required in all children with back pain; especially in those under the age of 12 years. Extra caution for the possibility of underlying aggressive pathologic condition is the rule in this population, including careful follow-up to assure full resolution of symptoms.[4]

The Pediatric Rehabilitation Medicine (PRM) physician plays a leadership role in the diagnosis and treatment of the child with a painful back, of every type, including associated factors and secondary conditions. Referral to the PRM physician is appropriate for assistance when needed in back pain diagnosis, management, worsening of symptoms, or change in function. As part of this role, PRM physicians identify and assist with appropriate referrals to higher levels of care and surgical review when

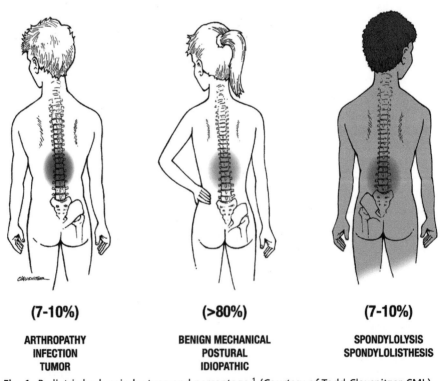

| (7-10%) | (>80%) | (7-10%) |

ARTHROPATHY	BENIGN MECHANICAL	SPONDYLOLYSIS
INFECTION	POSTURAL	SPONDYLOLISTHESIS
TUMOR	IDIOPATHIC	

Fig. 1. Pediatric back pain by type and percentage.[1] (*Courtesy of* Todd Clausnitzer CMI.)

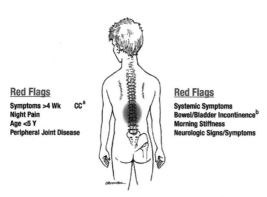

Red Flags

Symptoms >4 Wk   CC[a]
Night Pain
Age <5 Y
Peripheral Joint Disease

Red Flags

Systemic Symptoms
Bowel/Bladder Incontinence[b]
Morning Stiffness
Neurologic Signs/Symptoms

Fig. 2. Red flags for back pain in children. [a]Conservative care. [b]Previously continent child. (*Courtesy of* Todd Clausnitzer CMI.)

necessary. Early and appropriate management of back pain helps to optimize functional outcome and minimize complications.

BENIGN MECHANICAL BACK PAIN

Identification and treatment of benign back pain are imperative, as studies have associated pediatric back pain with development or continuation of back pain in adulthood.[6] Benign back pain in children and adolescents is typically mechanical or musculoskeletal in nature.[6–8] Mechanical back pain arises from stress or strain on the back, including supporting musculature. It is generally nonspecific, self-limited, and often not attributable to identifiable pathologic condition. Duration of benign back pain is typically 2 to 4 weeks, may be associated with high amounts or low amounts of physical activity, and improves with conservative treatment, including activity modification.[7–9] Mechanical back pain may be associated with poor posture, stressed thoracolumbar fascia, tight hamstrings, weak core musculature, overuse or trauma, biomechanical differences including increased or decreased flexibility, and incomplete ossification of bony components of the spine depending on age.[6,8] Pain behaviors can limit physical function, including general physical activity, self-cares, sports, and school participation.[6,9] With benign back pain, red flags on history and physical examination will be negative (see **Fig. 2**).

Risk factors for benign back pain include female sex, increasing age, growth acceleration, obesity, physical activity level (high or low levels), physical activity type such as spinal extension-based sports, previous back injury, family history of back pain, history of widespread pain, history of sleep problems, smoking exposure, and adverse psychosocial stresses.[4,5,7–10] Examples of low-level physical activity, or sedentary lifestyle, include 2 or more hours daily of screen time, computer, video games, or watching television. High-level activities include sports type (axial loading, extension based, twisting) with heightened levels of competition; continuous, frequent, stressful physical activities with minimal rest resulting in overuse and insufficient conditioning.[6] Moderate physical activity is protective against back pain.[11] Of note, scoliosis has shown no association with low-back pain specifically over longitudinal studies, however if untreated may be correlated with pain.[7,12] Evidence is mixed on back pain associated with loads, such as from a backpack. The American Academy of Pediatrics does however recommend backpacks weigh no more than 10% to 20% of the child's weight.[4,5,8] Some evidence suggests carrying a backpack on a single shoulder may contribute to back pain.[9,13]

History in benign back pain should be free of red flags (see **Fig. 2**). Mechanical symptoms, neurologic symptoms, and symptoms that would indicate systemic or inflammatory processes are important to identify.[10] **Table 1** lists key elements of a history for back pain. A flowchart is provided for evaluation and treatment of benign back pain in **Fig. 3**. A physical examination should be performed with appropriate visualization of the spine and should include musculoskeletal and neurologic assessments. The physical examination may elicit pain and demonstrate compensatory maneuvers and should be negative for neurologic deficits. **Table 2** lists key elements of a physical examination for back pain as the presenting symptom. Imaging can usually be avoided for benign back pain, per American College of Radiology guidelines. Imaging is warranted when red flags are present.[5,14] Initial imaging includes posteroanterior and lateral plain radiographs of the appropriate spinal levels. MRI, computed tomography (CT), and/or laboratory evaluation are necessary in certain instances and are often diagnoses-specific (please refer to specific conditions discussed later in this article). If concerning features are identified, laboratory evaluation may include complete

Table 1
Key history elements with examples to include in evaluation of back pain

Key History Elements	Examples
Symptom onset, duration, frequency, progression	Acute, subacute, chronic, intermittent, and/or relapsing
Trauma association	Acute macrotrauma or repetitive microtrauma
Location	Point to specific location
Characteristics	Quality, description, frequency, radiation
Pain rating/intensity	Rating 0–10, visual analogue scales
Aggravating and alleviating/palliating positions, activities, and factors	Mechanical symptoms: Sitting, standing, laying down, walking, running, bending forward or back
Physical activity	Type, amount, and frequency, including sports participation
Associated symptoms	• Joint redness, swelling; or warmth • Limb numbness, tingling, or weakness • Joint hypermobility, including any dislocation or subluxations • Stiffness in morning lasting more than 30 min • Red flags (see **Fig. 2**)
Sleep quality	Pain preventing from falling asleep or pain awakening at night
Functional impact of pain/pain behaviors	• Ability to go to school, work, play sports, and so forth • Pediatric-oriented functional disability scales
Mental health history	Depressive symptoms
Medical, social, and family history	• Medical history: Include recent illness, treatment with immunosuppressive agents • Social history: Who lives at home, school status • Family history: Pain, orthopedic-, neurologic-, rheumatologic-, and HLA-B27–related diseases
Treatment to date	• Participation in therapy (physical therapy, occupational therapy) • Medications tried/using, including oral and topical • Other conservative/nonpharmacologic interventions (ice/heat, chiropractic care, massage, acupuncture, orthotics/shoe inserts) • Pain management strategies (cognitive behavioral therapy, biofeedback, mind-body techniques)

Back Pain Evaluation Flowchart

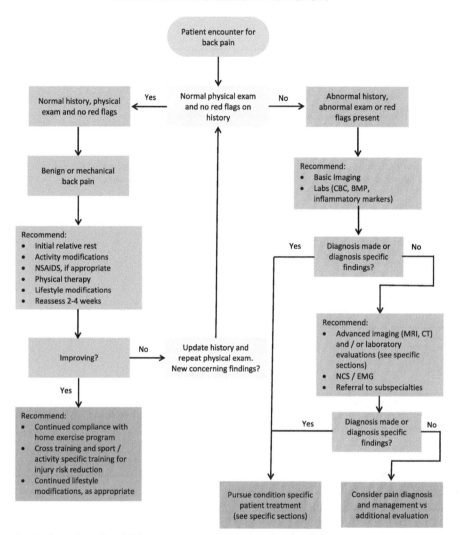

Fig. 3. Flow chart for children presenting with acute low-back pain. BMP, Basic Metabolic Panel; EMG, Electromyography; NCS, Nerve Conduction Studies.

blood count, chemistry panel, and inflammatory markers, such as erythrocyte sedimentation rate (ESR), C-reactive protein (CRP), Lyme titer, rheumatoid factor, and antinuclear antibodies.[4,5,7,8]

Treatment for benign back pain typically includes relative rest, activity modification, limited use of nonsteroidal anti-inflammatory drugs (NSAIDs), and close follow-up.[4,6,8] PT is typically recommended with stressed adherence to a prescribed home exercise program.[10] PT focus includes core strengthening and stabilization, mobility, and stretching, including hamstrings and hip flexors, biomechanics, posture assessment, and myofascial release techniques if appropriate.[8] Modalities such as superficial ice or heat may be recommended. Therapeutic ultrasound over an open growth plate or physis is

Table 2
Key physical examination elements with examples to include in evaluation of back pain

Key Physical Examination Elements	Examples
Inspection with visualization of the spine in standing and sitting positions	• Posture (excessive lordosis, postural round back, or rigid kyphosis) • Alignment (scoliosis, pelvic obliquity, scapular asymmetry) • Muscle bulk • Skin: Rashes, hair tufts
Palpation of the spine and surrounding musculature	• Areas of pain or tenderness (spinous processes, paraspinal muscles, SI joints) • Step off deformities (especially lumbar)
Range of motion of spine and extremities	• Flexion, extension, rotation, and lateral bending • Hip pathologic condition can mimic back pain • Hamstring and hip flexor tightness • Assess for hypermobility/Beighton score
Neurologic assessment	• Strength/manual muscle testing: Upper and lower extremities and core • Sensation: Dermatomes • Tone/spasticity • Deep tendon reflexes • Abdominal reflex • Babinski • Clonus • Proprioception
Gait	• Symmetry of movement • Include toe and heel walking • Foot drop • Assess for Trendelenburg • Assess for leg length discrepancy
Special tests for spine as well as hip (MacDonald, Achar, Houghton, Lamb)	• FABER (flexion, abduction, external rotation)/Patrick test • FAIR (flexion, adduction, internal rotation) • Straight leg raise • Slump test • Stork test • Thomas test

contraindicated, and its use is restricted in skeletally immature patients.[15] Remaining as physically active as possible during recovery helps to relieve soft tissue tightness and prevent weakness. Activities may include walking, swimming, and other low-impact aerobics. Bedrest should be avoided.[4] Functional progression of therapy and activity may occur as biomechanics improve and comfort levels increase. Psychological support through cognitive behavioral therapy can address any psychosocial components associated with pain often absent but not excluded with benign mechanical type.[9,10] Lifestyle modifications, including dietary changes, weight loss, and smoking cessation with reduced exposure to secondary smoke, are recommended and supported.[9,12]

Programs for prevention or injury risk reduction can include strength and conditioning education and strategy acquisition before the start of a sport season or activity. Appropriately trained coaches and trainers, adequate rest from sport and repetitive activity, as well as appropriately fitting equipment can all contribute to back pain prevention for children and adolescents.[4,8] Yoga and Pilates can help develop strength in abdominal and back muscles essential for core fitness and truncal support.[9] As in the adult population, low-impact aerobics and yoga in the pediatric population reduces back pain intensity and associated risk factors, increasing overall sense of well-being.[9] Such exercise can be very helpful in preventing injuries and disease into adulthood, including benefits to mental health and executive functions.[16] A discussion encouraging and recommending exercise should be a part of all annual medical provider encounters across the lifespan and integrated into routine family culture as possible.[4]

NOTABLE CONDITIONS WITH IDENTIFIABLE PATHOLOGIC CONDITION

Fig. 4 highlights common regions of back pain discussed by spinal and sacral segments in this section. **Table 3** highlights presentations, physical examination findings, basic evaluation, and management recommendations for notable conditions with identifiable pathologic condition causing back pain. Notable conditions highlighted in **Table 3** include spondylolysis,[17-22] spondylolisthesis, Scheuermann disease (SD),[23,24] postural round back,[25-27] radiculopathy,[28,29] slipped vertebral ring apophysis,[30] ankylosing spondylitis (AS),[31,32] and iliac apophysitis.

Spondylolysis is a unilateral or bilateral fracture of the pars interarticularis.[2] Sports commonly involved with spondylolysis include football, gymnastics, swimming, figure skating, and diving. Repetitive microtrauma is theorized to be the cause for the pars fractures.[2,4] In the setting of continued biomechanical stress, spondylolysis can progress to spondylolisthesis.[33] Spondylolisthesis is a bilateral fracture of the pars interarticularis involving anterior displacement of a vertebral body in relation to adjacent vertebrae.[2] Vertebral displacement can result in central spinal and/or peripheral neural

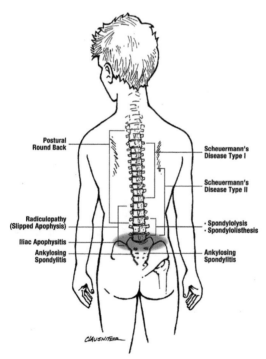

Fig. 4. Common conditions of back pain in children by spinal region. (*Courtesy of* Todd Clausnitzer CMI.)

Table 3
Notable conditions with identifiable pathologic condition

Condition	Common Presentation	Physical Examination (PE) Findings	Cause	Evaluation	Management-Prognosis
Spondylolysis	• Back pain with extension; may radiate into leg • Associated with activities involving repetitive flexion-extension of the lumbar spine[17]	• Reduced range of back motion, especially in extension • Point tenderness may be present • Positive stork test[4,5,22] • Pain with hyperextension • Pain with increased activity • Pain radiation into gluteal muscles and lower extremity	• Unilateral or bilateral fracture of the pars interarticularis secondary to repetitive microtrauma[2,4,17] • Fourth or fifth vertebrae most frequently involved • Rare to see under the age of 2 • Prevalence increases between 5 and 7 y of age approaching 7% as in the adult population[2,4]	• Plain radiographs lumbar spine (anteroposterior [AP], lateral) show defect in up to 75%, more so with bilateral involvement[18] • Lumbar spine oblique radiographs ("Scotty dog sign") not always needed[19] • MRI more sensitive, may identify prelytic lesions[20,21]	• Relative rest • PT: Initially avoid spinal extension • Activity modifications: Avoid pain-provoking activities[4] • Thoracic lumbar sacral orthosis (TLSO), soft or custom molded, in selected patients • Surgical intervention is rare[4]
Spondylolisthesis	• Back pain with extension; may radiate into leg • Associated with activities involving repetitive flexion-extension of the lumbar spine[17] • May have neurologic symptoms	• Reduced range of back motion, especially in extension • Point tenderness may be present • Positive stork test • Pain with hyperextension • Pain with increased activity • Pain radiation into gluteal muscles and lower extremity • Rare: Cauda equina syndrome	• Bilateral fracture of the pars interarticularis involving anterior displacement of a vertebral body in relation to adjacent vertebrae[2] • More common in male patients	• Plain radiographs (standing AP and lateral) with grading of spondylolisthesis according to Meyerding (see **Fig. 4**)[34] • Repeat radiographs recommended to monitor for progression of slippage every 3–6 mo until skeletal maturity[17] • MRI recommended if neurologic abnormalities on PE[43]	• Conservative management for slippage of the vertebral body, 50% or less[2,4] ○ PT (avoid spinal extension) ○ Anti-inflammatory drugs (NSAIDs) ○ Orthosis • Surgical referral for neurologic signs or slippage of the vertebral body beyond 50% of its width[2]

| Scheuermann disease (SD) | • Pain typically chronic, regional, activity related, and dull, aching in nature[33] | • Kyphotic posture
• Upper back pain | • Osteochondrosis of the vertebral endplate
• Caused by repetitive microtrauma and fatigue failure of immature vertebral bodies[2,34]
• Common between the ages of 12 and 17 y of age[4,23]
• More often in male patients[4,36]
• Type I (classic): Thoracic spine[36]
• Type II: Thoracic and lumbar spine[36] | • Plain radiographs (AP and lateral) may show[2,4,43]
• Rigid kyphosis (>40°)
• Irregular vertebral endplates
• Schmorl nodes
• Protrusion of disc material into the spongiosum of the vertebral body
• Narrowed disc spaces
• Anterior wedging of the vertebral bodies
• Radiographic criteria for SD met with 3 or more consecutive vertebrae wedged >5°[35] (see **Fig. 5**) | • PT: Spinal extension exercises, postural principles, and hamstring stretching.[4]
• Rest, ice, compression, elevation (RICE) protocol
• NSAIDs[4]
• Exercise is contraindicated if pain present[4,43]
• Bracing considered
  ○ TLSO for apex closer to the thoracolumbar junction in curves between 50° and 75°[2,4,43]
  ○ Milwaukee brace (Cervical TLSO) for higher thoracic apices and before skeletal maturity[24]
• Brace treatment for a minimum of 18 mo is necessary to effect vertebral wedging and control kyphosis[43]
• Surgical referral
  ○ Refractory pain
  ○ Changing neurologic status or function
  ○ Cosmetic: Patients with deformities >75°[2,4] |

(continued on next page)

Table 3
(continued)

Condition	Common Presentation	Physical Examination (PE) Findings	Cause	Evaluation	Management-Prognosis
Postural round back	• Flexible, forward posture of spine with rounded shoulders • Upper back pain • Activity-related pain • Pain with prolonged sitting[4]	• Tenderness to palpation of the cervical and upper thoracic spine, paraspinal and trapezius musculature, including associated soft tissues • Forward bend test: Smooth hump	• Muscular strain • Postural imbalance	• Plain radiographs (AP and lateral) will be negative for bony pathologic condition	• PT: Postural stabilization, cervical retraction exercises, pectoralis stretching, and periscapular strengthening[25–27] • Home exercise program compliance is paramount or reoccurrence can be anticipated[4]
Radiculopathy	• Midline back pain midline; more diffuse and less radicular compared with adults[4,28] • Neurologic symptoms (eg, numbness and weakness) worsening upon flexion of the trunk, cough, or sneeze[33,38]	• May have focal neurologic deficits • Positive straight leg raise • Positive slump test	• Congenital, traumatic, degenerative, and neoplastic causes[2,4] • Acute radiculopathy from disc herniation and related pain is less common in the pediatric and adolescent populations[37]	• MRI recommended	• Relative rest • NSAIDs • PT: Pain management, strength, function • Surgical consult, with consideration of discectomy[29,37]
Slipped vertebral ring apophysis	• Acute onset of pain associated with lifting, straining, or spine flexion[2,38] • Sudden-onset low-back pain, similar to disc herniation presentation[4]	• Similar to disc herniation presentation[4,30] • Pain radiation from low back to anterior thigh with leg extension • Intact muscle strength and reflexes • Positive straight leg raise	• Disc material displaced into vertebral canal • Unique to children occurring between the ring apophysis and vertebral body before age-appropriate fusion[2,28]	• Plain radiographs can be negative[2,38] • Lumbar CT scan preferred to identify apophyseal fracture as MRI may show just an extradural mass	• Conservative treatment: PT[30] • Epidural steroids may be considered[4] • Surgical referral for fragment excision if failed conservative care

Ankylosing spondylitis (AS)	• Morning stiffness[4] • Chronic SI joint and back pain[4] • Pain that improves with activity and not rest[4] • Hip pain • May have history of uveitis[31]	• Tenderness to palpation over SI • Stiffness • Reduced spine range of motion • Schober test[31]	• Chronic, inflammatory rheumatic disorder of the axial skeleton	• Plain radiographs • MRI pelvis with contrast considered for sacroiliitis • Laboratory evaluation including HLA-B27, CRP	• PT: Spinal mobility (promote extension), prevent lower extremity flexion contractures, lessen stiffness and pain, promote deep breathing and aerobic exercise[4] • Aquatic therapy[4,32] • Prone laying[4,32] • Referral to rheumatologist
Iliac apophysitis	• Belt-line pain along the superior iliac crests and muscular insertions • Most commonly affected: Anterior Superior Iliac Spine (ASIS), Anterior Inferior Iliac Spine (AIIS), iliac crest	• Dull, achy pain in the front side of the groin or hip • Worsening pain with activity • Swelling • Tender to palpation over the superior iliac crests and muscular insertions • Can be mistaken for a muscle strain	• Occurs in adolescents with open Risser lines on radiograph[4]	• Radiographic images • MRI	• Relative rest and RICE protocol • Activity limitations • NSAIDs[4,20]

Abbreviations: AIIS, Anterior Inferior Iliac Spine; ASIS, Anterior Superior Iliac Spine.

canal stenosis with secondary neurologic symptoms.[2,4] **Fig. 5** provides a chart for the grading of spondylolisthesis.[34]

SD, or osteochondrosis of the vertebral endplate, is considered the pediatric equivalent of the adult compression fracture. Radiographic criteria for SD is met when 3 or more consecutive vertebrae are wedged greater than 5° (**Fig. 6**).[35] Type I (classic) involves the thoracic spine; type II involves the thoracic and lumbar spine.[36] When untreated, back pain and functional disability into adulthood are more common as are cardiorespiratory conditions for kyphosis over 100°.[2,4] There is a higher incidence of SD in monozygotic twins.[36] Postural round back, distinguished from SD by its flexibility and reduced degree of pain, is a forward postural appearance of the spine involving rounded shoulders.[2,4]

Radiculopathy in the pediatric patient can be multifactorial to include congenital, traumatic, degenerative, and neoplastic causes.[2,4] Acute radiculopathy from disc herniation and related pain is less common in the pediatric and adolescent populations compared with adults.[37] The younger patient often presents with milder neurologic symptoms (eg, numbness and weakness), worsening upon flexion of the trunk, cough, or sneeze.[33,38] Greater nerve root tension, consistent with the spinal column growing faster than surrounding soft tissues, facilitates a positive straight leg test more so in this younger population.[33] MRI is the imaging of choice, and findings may be incidental

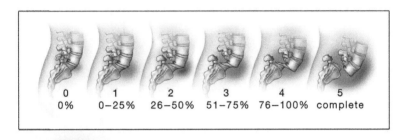

0	1	2	3	4	5
0%	0–25%	26–50%	51–75%	76–100%	complete

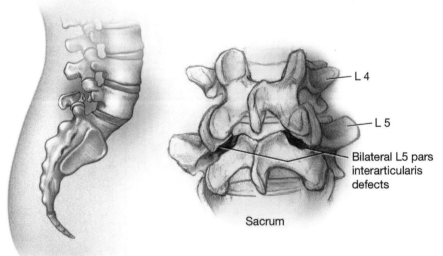

Fig. 5. Spondylolisthesis with bilateral L5 pars interarticularis defects. (c) Copyright Mayo Clinic

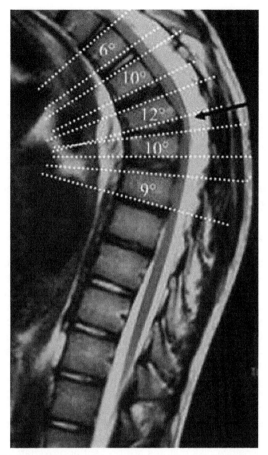

Fig. 6. Sagittal MRI demonstrating Scheuermann kyphosis. (Contributed from the Public Domain. Copyright © 2022, StatPearls Publishing LLC.)

in the pediatric population needing careful clinical correlation before any definitive diagnosis or treatment rendered.[4,33] Herniation that impacts the spinal cord resulting in neurogenic changes (loss of bowel/bladder control, saddle anesthesia) warrants emergent neurosurgical intervention.[38]

Slipped vertebral ring apophysis is unique to children, occurring between the ring apophysis and vertebral body before age-appropriate fusion.[2,38] Fusion of the ring apophysis typically occurs between the ages of 18 and 25 years.[2,4] Disc herniation in children often occurs with fracture of the adjacent vertebral end plate.[33] Up to 38% of pediatric patients presenting with symptoms of lumbar disc herniation have apophyseal ring fractures.[39]

AS is a chronic, inflammatory rheumatic disorder of the axial skeleton. A seronegative spondyloarthropathy, AS has an incidence of approximately 3 per 100,000 persons in the United States.[40] Most commonly, AS affects the sacroiliac (SI) joint as well as the spine with stiffness and pain often greatest in the morning and evenings.[4] Chronic back pain or stiffness, alternating buttock pain, pain that improves with activity and not rest, hip pain, elevated CRP, and tenderness to palpation over SI joints are all consistent with sacroiliitis.[31] Sacroiliitis can be silent with no pain upon SI joint compression testing, requiring an MRI to detect if necessary.[41] Caudal to cranial anky-losis proceeds from SI involvement to the formation of the classic "bamboo spine."[42] Stiffness is a more common complaint in children than back pain.[41] Pediatric patients are also more likely to develop enthesitis at the tendinous insertions; up to 27% re-ported having uveitis.[43] Adolescent boys commonly present with back pain; 90% are white with a positive HLA-B27.[43]

Lumbar strain of the paraspinal musculature is less common in children and adoles-cents compared with skeletally mature individuals because of the open iliac apoph-ysis.[4] The average chronologic age for closure of the iliac apophysis is 14 years in girls and 16 years in boys.[2] Iliac apophysitis is thus a more common presentation than lumbar strain in children and adolescents with radiographs having open Risser lines.[4] Sports that involve running and sprinting may be a catalyst. Lumbar interspi-nous process bursitis or kissing spines may be seen in individuals participating in lum-bar hyperextension activities, such as dance and gymnastics.[4]

RARE CONDITIONS NOT TO BE OVERLOOKED

Less than 10% of the conditions causing back pain in children are concerning for ma-jor functional loss and/or life-threatening sequelae.[1] Red flags (see **Fig. 2**) require added scrutiny for these conditions.[5] **Table 4** lists common presentations, disease category and characteristics, laboratory and pathology, imaging, management, and prognoses often associated with red flag conditions. Conditions included are discitis and vertebral osteomyelitis,[44] osteoid osteoma,[45–49] osteoblastoma,[50,51] aneurysmal bone cyst,[52–54] Langerhans cell histiocytosis (LCH),[55–60] leukemia,[61,62] fibrous dysplasia,[63,64] intramedullary spinal cord tumors,[65–67] ependymoma,[68–70] osteosar-coma,[71,72] and Ewing sarcoma.[73] Provided in later discussion are limited selected comments, thought helpful only as a supplement to **Table 4**. Discussion that is more detailed is beyond the scope of this article.

Discitis and vertebral osteomyelitis are likely a combined infectious process.[2,4,74] Infection may begin in the vascular vertebral end plates and then spread into the disc substance.[2,4] Positive disk cultures are present approximately 60% of the time and may not be necessary on a routine basis.[2] Radicular symptoms may indicate epidural involvement. Trauma with release of phospholipase A2 from disk tissue and viral infection may give rise to the more aseptic varieties.[2] Long-term back pain sequelae is present in some.[75]

Osteoid osteoma is a benign bone tumor making up about 10% of benign bone tu-mors in general. Combined with osteoblastomas, they are the most common benign spinal tumors found in children.[76] Because they are much smaller than osteoblasto-mas, neurologic deficits are rare.[2,69] Surgical excision of the central nidus can be cura-tive.[2] Accurate intraoperative localization of the nidus with CT scanning is critical for successful excision; tetracycline labeling and bone scintigraphy can be helpful also.[2]

Aneurysmal bone cysts, like osteoblastomas, are often larger (>2 cm) in size. They can be primary lesions or secondary to other lesions, such as osteosarcomas or met-astatic disease.[2] Adjunctive therapy, when appropriate and used (cementation, cryo-therapy, embolization), can help lower recurrence rates.[2]

LCH is a rare disorder that can damage tissue or cause lesions to form in one or more places in the body.[2] It occurs as part of a spectrum of conditions involving eosinophilic granulomas, including Hand-Schuller-Christian disease (HSCD) and Letterer-Siwe disease (LSD).[77] Of patients with LCH, estimates for eosinophilic gran-ulomas are solitary in 80%, multiple in 6%, with 9% having HSCD and 1.2% having LSD.[77] HSCD in classic form involves multiple eosinophilic granulomas of bone,

Table 4
Rare conditions not to be overlooked

Conditions	Common Presentations	Disease Category and Characteristics	Laboratory-Pathologic Condition	Imaging	Management-Prognosis
Discitis-vertebral osteomyelitis	• Child under age 7 most common • Stops walking, abdominal pain, constipation fever, lethargy, forward bend • Gradual onset • Pain upon palpation[2,4]	Infectious: • *Staphylococcus aureus* • Atypical organism • Brucellosis/TB Risk factors: • Immunodeficiency • History of drug abuse • Developing country[2,4,74]	• CRP, ESR, complete blood count, differential, blood cultures • White blood cell count (WBC) unremarkable • Disc biopsy if early antibiotic is ineffective • Atypical organism[2]	• AP and lateral spine • Narrowed disc space, involving vertebral bodies above and below[2] **(Fig. 7)** • MRI diagnostic[1,2,4]	• Intravenous antibiotics • Infectious disease consult • Surgery for abscess • Full functional recovery • Return to all activities[2,4,44] • Long-term back pain can be sequelae[75]
Osteoid osteoma	• Night pain over several months[2,47] • Dull ache at spinal segment • Relief with NSAIDs • Decreased spinal motion at tumor site[2,47] • Neurologic deficits rare[2] • Reactive scoliosis[2,47]	• Benign bone tumor • Male predominance[2,3] • Ages: 5 and 25 y[2,45,46] • Most often metaphyseal or diaphyseal regions • Femur, tibia, less commonly, spine[2] • Usually <2 cm in size[2] • Central nidus: Pain generator[2]	• Central nidus[2,49] • Osteoid, osteoblasts, and fibrovascular tissue • Nonmyelinated axons • Posterior spinal elements, lamina, pedicle involved[2]	• Plain radiographs • CT scan preferred **(Fig. 8)** for lesion characterization[2] • Technetium-99m demonstrates uptake in the region of the nidus: Valuable when radiographs indeterminate[2,45,48]	• Surgical excision of the painful nidus[2,49] • CT-guided percutaneous radiofrequency ablation[45] • Relief of pain immediate when nidus fully eliminated[2]

(continued on next page)

Table 4
(continued)

Conditions	Common Presentations	Disease Category and Characteristics	Laboratory-Pathologic Condition	Imaging	Management-Prognosis
Osteoblastoma	Symptoms over a few months: • Regional, painful • Dull, aching nature[2] • Pain less amenable to salicylates[50] • Tenderness over tumor site with palpable mass[50] • Radicular or myelopathic features[2,50] • Scoliosis possible: Painful and progressive[50]	• Benign bone tumor • Male-to-female ratio of 2:1[50,51] • Ages: 10 and 20 y of age (peak incidence, 20 y)[2] • 40% spinal occurrence[50,51] • >2 cm in size[2] • Common sites long bones: Metaphyseal and diaphyseal regions, femur, and tibia[2]	• Histologically, like osteoid osteoma[2] • Fibrovascular tissue with osteoid, osteoblasts, posterior spinal elements[50,51] • Aggressive osteoblastoma may be mistaken for a low-grade osteosarcoma[2,50]	• Plain radiographs show radiodensity (Fig. 9)[50] • Vertebral collapse possible[50,51] • CT scan for boundary localization and identification[2] • MRI scans helpful for involvement of soft tissue or radicular-spinal impingement[2] • Bone scan most sensitive imaging • Modality available[50]	• Surgical excision or local curettage[2,50] • Spinal or radicular involvement: neurosurgical decompression[50,51] • 95% cure rate following initial treatment[2,50] • Reoccurrence rate up to 20% with local curettage[2,50]
Aneurysmal bone cyst	Presents over weeks to months[2] • Regional pain[52] • Tenderness to palpation • Limited range of motion[53,54] • Neurologic deficits: Bowel and bladder control[2]	• Benign solitary tumor found in long bones, metaphyseal regions[2] • 30% of cases occur in spine: Most often posterior elements[52,54] • May involve spinal cord and other neurologic elements[2,52] • Genetic correlation[2]	• Vascular: Large amount of blood exuding at the time of surgery[2] • Solitary lesion, expansive[54]	• Radiolucent[2] • Plain radiographs often show a classic "blow-out" lesion (Fig. 10), outlined by a shell of new periosteal bone formation[2,54] • CT scanning helpful in localizing the spinal lesion and extent of vertebral involvement[52,54] • MRI helps localize any spinal involvement or soft tissue expansion[2]	• Preoperative embolization given vascularity[2,54] • Radiation therapy: Inoperable cysts or embolization failure[2,54] • Recurrence rates high: 10%–50%[2,54]

	Symptoms/Signs	Incidence/Pathology	Pathology	Radiographs	Treatment
Langerhans Cell Histiocytosis (LCH)	• Pain localized over the affected region • No associated neurologic deficits[2,78] Other symptoms: • Localized swelling • Low-grade fever • Elevated ESR • Torticollis (C-spine involvement)[58,78]	• Formerly histiocytosis X • Incidence in children up to 4 per million[2,78] • 2:1 male-to-female ratio[2,78] • Age: Any • Spinal lesions identified in up to 15% with back pain • Skull and femur most commonly affected with multiple lesions[2,78] • No hereditary pattern[2,57,78]	• Proliferative, reactive lesion[2] • Defect in immunologic regulation[2] • Distinct pan like histiocyte Langerhans cells[78] (**Fig. 11**) • Birbeck granules; Pathognomonic[8] • Cells can remain solitary as a local eosinophilic granuloma of bone or proliferate and spread throughout the body as a part of Hand-Schuller-Christian disease or Letterer-Siwe disease[2,56,78]	Radiographs: • Early phases may show a "moth-eaten" appearance with periosteal elevation[2] • Lytic lesions in the vertebral body and posterior elements[2,59,78] • CT delineates extent of bone lesions[2,60] • MRI for medullary or soft tissue[2,78] • Skeletal survey superior to scintigraphy for multiple lesions[2]	• Spontaneous resolution often with more solitary lesions[2,78] • Relief with bedrest and spinal bracing[2] • Indomethacin: Favorable results for healing of lesions in the appendicular skeleton[60] • Debridement and surgical spinal stabilization: Multifocal lesions or neurologic compromise[2,78] • Surgical biopsy for more atypical lesions: Rule out malignancy[2]
Leukemia	Symptoms and signs[2,61] • Fever • Bone pain • Limp • Refusal to walk • Fatigue or lethargy • Pallor • Bruising • Petechiae • Bone-joint pain in 25% with acute leukemia	• Most common malignancy of childhood[2,61] • 30% of cases of childhood cancer[61] • Most common malignancy producing back pain[2,61]	• Decreased platelet count[2] • Elevated ESR • Elevated peripheral WBC count • Anemia[61,62] • Peripheral smear can confirm the diagnosis in the presence of normal blood counts[2]	Radiograph: • Leukemic lines (lucent metaphyseal bands) in up to 50% with acute lymphoblastic leukemia[2] (**Fig. 12**) • Lines most often in distal femur, tibia (around knee), proximal humerus, distal radius, and ulna[2]	• Definitive diagnosis: Bone marrow aspiration[61,62] • Acute lymphoblastic leukemia in children has an excellent prognosis with T-cell disease now having a similar prognosis to B-cell disease[61]

(continued on next page)

Table 4
(continued)

Conditions	Common Presentations	Disease Category and Characteristics	Laboratory-Pathologic Condition	Imaging	Management-Prognosis
	• Less common are complications involving osteopenia and vertebrae[62] • Hepatosplenomegaly; central nervous system (CNS) disease occurs[61,62]				
Fibrous dysplasia	McCune-Albright syndrome (MAS): • Polyostotic bone involvement[2,63] • Precocious puberty • Café-au-lait spots[63] • Craniofacial involvement: 50% with polyostotic involvement[2]	• Benign • Nonfamilial tumor/lesion[2] • Affects any bone • Spine less common[2,64] • Polyostotic form tends to involve spine: Posterior elements, associated with scoliosis[2] Three different categories of fibrous dysplasia: • Monostotic (single bone involvement) • Polyostotic (multiple bone involvement) • Polyostotic with endocrine involvement[63,64]	• Lesion characterized by expanding intramedullary fibro-osseous tissue in 1 or more bones[2,63] • Immature bone trabeculae and collagen form a fibrocellular matrix[2,64]	• Radiographic density of lesions depends on amount of osseous tissue produced; amount of cortex replaced[2,63] • Lucent if minimal cortex replaced; ground glass with expansion and more cortex replaced[2,64] • CT helpful in defining lesion • Bone scan can be helpful determining extent of lesion[2]	• Nonoperative approach without pain, deformity, or fracture[2,64] • Bisphosphonates for pain and improving quality of life[2] • MAS consult with Endocrinology[63]
Intramedullary spinal cord tumors	• Most common symptoms: Back pain with sensory	• Exceedingly rare in children	• Occur from cervicomedullary junction to the filum terminale[2,66]	• MRI scanning with and without gadolinium: Imaging of choice[2] • Plain radiographs:	• Surgical resection[67] • Adjunctive radiation of benefit

(continued)	• and/or motor dysfunction[2,66] • Abnormal gait • Incontinence (in previously toilet-trained child) • Scoliosis[2]	• 100–200 cases annually in the United States[2,66] • Male predominance[2,65] • Mean age: 11 y[2,65]	• Common: Long segment (more than 2 vertebral levels) involvement[65] • Astrocytoma > ependymomas[65]	• Absent pedicles[2] (Fig. 13) • Widening of the intervertebral foramen[2,66]	• ± Chemotherapy[66]
Ependymoma	• Severe low-back pain[2] • Varying degrees of paraparesis • Bladder and bowel incontinence[68] • Rare in childhood and adolescent spinal cord[2,68]	• Third most common CNS tumor in childhood[2,68] • Intracranial with predilection for the posterior fossa[68]	• Intracranial seeding of tumor to the spinal canal[68,69] • Most common: Distal spinal canal[2,69]	• MRI preferred with repeat imaging given high rate of recurrence[2,68]	• Gross total surgical resection followed by postoperative radiotherapy[70] • High reoccurrence[2] • Requires long-term follow-up[68]
Osteosarcoma	• Musculoskeletal pain: Local, subacute[2,71] • Loss of range of motion • Palpable tender mass[2] • Incidence almost equal in boys and girls[2] • Peak incidence: second decade of life; rare < 5 y[71] • Requires consideration in all children[2,71]	• Most common malignant bone tumor in children and adolescents[2,71] • Aggressive malignant tumor • Most common at distal femur or proximal humerus[2,72] • Rarely affects spine; usually thoracic or lumbar levels[2,71]	• High-grade malignant osteoblasts directly form tumor osteoid or bone[2,71] • Cartilaginous and fibrous and elements may coexist[2] • Component tumor in familial cancer syndromes[2,71]	• Radiographs feature destructive and osteoblastic changes[2] • Codman triangle; sunburst patterns[2] • Bone scan or MRI: May see skip metastases (isolated foci of tumor in the same or adjacent bone)[2,72]	• Chemotherapy[2,71] • Limb salvage • Current survival rate has increased to >65%[71] • MRI scanning and CT imaging required for staging[2] • Skip metastases, go along with poorer prognosis[2]
Ewing sarcoma	• Palpable, tender mass[2] • Not systemically ill at presentation[2,71]	• Aggressive bone and soft tissue cancer: Micrometastatic disease at diagnosis[2,80]	PNETs (primitive neuroectodermal tumors)	• Radiographs: Onion peel-type periosteal new bone formation (not disease-specific)[71,73]	• Radiation therapy with chemotherapy:

(continued on next page)

Table 4
(continued)

Conditions	Common Presentations	Disease Category and Characteristics	Laboratory-Pathologic Condition	Imaging	Management-Prognosis
	• Symptoms emerge late in disease[2] • Relentless back pain: 58% with neurologic deficits[2,80] • Signs of disc herniation with lumbar spinal involvement[2] • Sacral roots involvement: Urinary and rectal complaints[2,71]	• In 20%, presenting lesion in the innominate bone[2,] • Sacrum is most common spinal site[80] • Most commonly diagnosed in the second decade of life[80]	• Common cytogenetic translocation[2] • Chromosomes 11 and 22[2,80] • Ewing sarcoma and PNET tumors create systemic diseases[2,71]	• MRI: To distinguish from other malignant bone tumors[2] • Soft tissue mass adjacent to the area of bone destruction: Indicative of cortical perforation and adjacent soft tissue spread[2,80]	• Control local disease[2] • Initial chemotherapy may decrease the size of the tumor mass making local resection an option possibly avoiding any need for postoperative radiation[79,80] • 5-y survival rates near 70%[2,71] • Central lesions (pelvis) go along with worse outcomes[2]

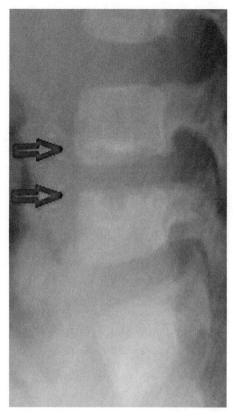

Fig. 7. Diskitis lumbar L3, L4. Infected L3, L4 disc and vertebral end plates above (*arrow*) and below (*arrow*). (*Courtesy of* Kevin P. Murphy MD, Northland Pediatric Rehabilitation Medicine LLC.)

diabetes insipidus (pituitary gland involvement), and exophthalmos (retro-orbital granulomas).[78] Significant morbidity and pathologic fractures of the spine can occur with HSCD; 70% of patients have a diagnosis before the age of 5 years.[2,78] LSD is the rare, acute disseminated form of histiocytosis with severe visceral involvement, appearing often in the first year of life.[2,78] Pulmonary parenchyma may have a granular appearance on chest radiographs with survival now possible in some using chemotherapy, steroids, and high-dose antibiotics.[2,78]

Ewing sarcoma is an aggressive malignant tumor needing consideration in all children with localized musculoskeletal pain especially in the pelvis, sacrum, and lower extremities.[2] It is a systemic condition and needs to be treated as such.[2] Initial chemotherapy may decrease the size of the tumor mass, making local resection an option, possibly avoiding any need for postoperative radiation.[79,80] In the long bones, the disease is diaphyseal in location with pathologic fractures uncommon but portending a poorer prognosis.[2]

Neuroblastoma is the most common primary cancer to metastasize to the skeleton, most commonly the spine and thoracic region.[81] Additional tumors that metastasize to the spine include Wilm tumor (associated with hemihypertrophy) and rhabdomyosarcoma.[81] Vertebral involvement can be extensive, including absent pedicles creating

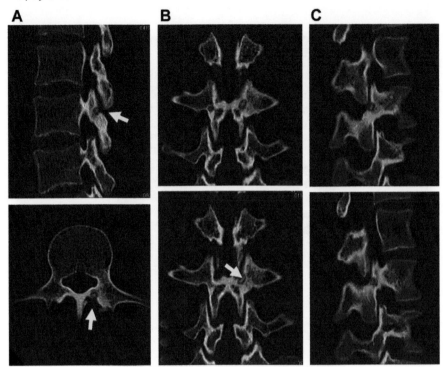

Fig. 8. Osteoid osteoma, posterior elements. Distributed under the terms of the Creative Commons NCBI Bookshelf. A service of the National Library of Medicine, National Institutes of Health. Osteoid Osteoma in posterior elements (*arrows*).

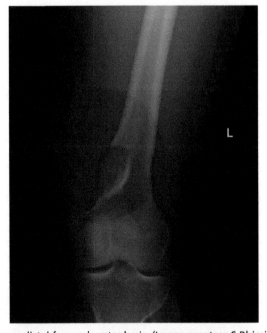

Fig. 9. Osteoblastoma distal femoral metaphysis. (Image courtesy S Bhimji MD. Contributed from Creative Commons. Copyright © 2022, StatPearls Publishing LLC.)

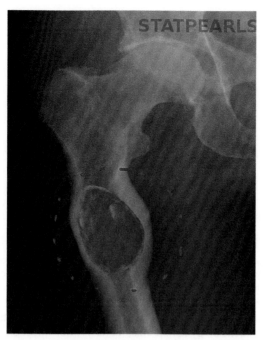

Fig. 10. Aneurysmal bone cyst proximal femoral metaphysis. Large aneurysmal bone cyst, well encapsulated in proximal femoral metaphysis (*arrow*). (Image courtesy S Bhimji MD. Contributed from Creative Commons. Copyright © 2022, StatPearls Publishing LLC.)

the appearance of a "winking owl" (**Fig. 13**).[81] Individuals with neurofibromatosis, especially type 1, have had tumors go on to degenerate into soft tissue sarcomas, adding to the vigilant surveillance required of these patients across the lifespan.[82]

Chordomas are among the rarest of malignant tumors in children, more common in the adult population.[81] The tumor arises from the primitive notochord mainly involving the sacrum and lower lumbar spine with inherent destructive behavior. Sacral chordomas may be palpable on digital examination, requiring a wide surgical resection as the surgical goal.[81]

Referred and other associated pain always needs serious consideration in the differential diagnoses of the child with a painful back.[4,83] Such conditions include pelvic

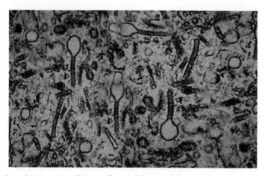

Fig. 11. Histiocytosis microscopy. (Contributed by S Bhimji MD. Contributed from Creative Commons. Copyright © 2022, StatPearls Publishing LLC.)

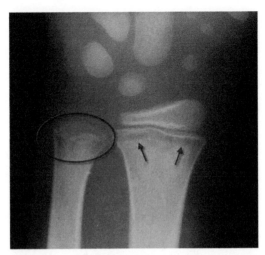

Fig. 12. Lucent metaphyseal bands in leukemia (*arrows* and *oval*). (Source: Gamuts in Radiology. Bone changes in hematologic disease. Caffey's Pediatric Diagnostic Imaging, 11th Ed. 2008. Courtesy, M. Kricun MD.)

inflammatory disease, pelvic osteomyelitis, menstrual discomforts, ovarian cysts, pregnancy, nephrolithiasis, pyelonephritis, urinary tract infection, hydronephrosis, renal osteodystrophy, pancreatitis, cholecystitis, vasculitis, constipation/ileus, megacolon, inflammatory bowel disease, pneumonia (thoracic), endocarditis, hiatal hernia/

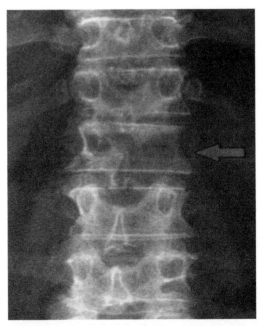

Fig. 13. Winking owl sign with metastatic neuroblastoma to the L1 pedicle. Absent L1 pedicle involved with metastatic neuroblastoma (*arrow*). (*Courtesy of* Todd Clausnitzer CMI.)

reflux, sickle cell crisis, psychogenic and conversion disorder, not to exclude others.[4,83] Further discussion of these conditions is beyond the scope of this article.

Back pain in the child with physical disability can result from all pain generators identified in the able-bodied child. In addition, the child with physical disability has features and diagnoses more common and distinct from their able-bodied peers.[2,4] Included are a host of neurologic and bone-related conditions, such as spinal cord syrinx, tethered cord, diastematomyelia, congenital vertebrae, spinal stenosis, along with other congenital and/or acquired pathologic conditions.[2,4] Some back pain generators are more condition specific, such as individuals with ambulatory spastic cerebral palsy having a higher prevalence of spondylolysis in up to 20%.[84] People with achondroplasia have an increased prevalence of spinal stenosis, whereas those with spina bifida need to be monitored more carefully for tethered cord and spinal cord syrinx.[2,4] For wheelchair users, back pain can often be more mechanical in nature and remedied with modifications to a custom seating system, tilt in space-powered wheelchair, or postural truncal orthosis.[2,4] Whatever the cause, the child with physical disability and back pain needs to be assessed with the differential diagnoses of all children while not excluding those more specific to their individual condition.[2,4]

SUMMARY

Back pain is common, estimated in up to 30% of children, and increasing with age; 80% is benign, mechanical type, improving within 2 weeks of conservative care. An in-depth evaluation often including MRI, laboratory, and specialty care consultations is required if symptoms do not improve or worsen. Spondylolysis and spondylolisthesis comprise almost 10% of pediatric back pain, often caused by lumbar hyperextension activities and treated most commonly with conservative care. Osteoid osteomas and osteoblastomas, together, constitute the most common benign spinal tumors in childhood. Aggressive and malignant tumors of the spine are rare, but when present, require tertiary care referral and a comprehensive oncology team for optimal life-sustaining outcomes.

CLINICS CARE POINTS

- When treating a child with suspected benign mechanical back pain, include rest, activity modifications, nonsteroidal anti-inflammatory drugs, and physical therapy with a focus on core strengthening, flexibility, and low-impact aerobics. Follow-up in 2 weeks is a medical necessity to assure resolution of symptoms and compliance with an ongoing home exercise program.

- Children with back pain and red flags including age 5 years and younger, systemic symptoms, night pain, incontinence of new onset, peripheral joint disease, morning stiffness, neurologic signs/symptoms, and persistent symptoms despite 4 weeks of conservative care, warrant comprehensive medical team assessment for the likelihood of aggressive pathologic condition.

- When treating a child with back pain and decreased quality of life, such as increased school days missed, decreased participation in sports and self-cares, excessive body mass index, and sedentary lifestyle, consider psychological and nutritional assessments. Cognitive behavioral therapy can be helpful, improving outcomes when combined with physical therapy.

- Children with back pain in the setting of physical disability require assessment with associated conditions in mind as well as common generators of pain found within the able-bodied pediatric population. The astute provider is aware of the possibility of a condition-specific pathologic condition and reaches out for specialty consultation where needed.

DISCLOSURE

The authors have nothing to disclose.

REFERENCES

1. Diab M, Staheli LT. Practice of paediatric orthopaedics. 3rd edition. Philadelphia, PA: Kluwer; 2015. p. 1–312. Wolters.
2. Herring JA. Tachdjian's pediatric Orthopaedics: from the Texas scottish rite hospital for children. Amsterdam, Netherlands: Elsevier Health Sciences; 2020.
3. Fabricant PD, Heath MR, Schachne JM, et al. The Epidemiology of Back Pain in American Children and Adolescents. Spine 2020;45(16):1135–42.
4. Murphy KP, Sobus KML, Moberg-Wolff E, et al. In: Musculoskeletal conditions. 6th edition. New York,New York: Springer Publishing Company; 2021. p. 371–409.
5. Achar S, Yamanaka J. Back Pain in Children and Adolescents. Am Fam Physician 2020;102(1):19–28.
6. Lamb M, Brenner JS. Back Pain in Children and Adolescents. Pediatr Rev 2020; 41(11):557–69.
7. Houghton KM. Review for the generalist: evaluation of low back pain in children and adolescents. Pediatr Rheumatol Online J 2010;8:28.
8. MacDonald J, Stuart E, Rodenberg R. Musculoskeletal Low Back Pain in School-aged Children: A Review. JAMA Pediatr. 2017;171(3):280–7.
9. Jackson C, McLaughlin K, Teti B. Back pain in children: a holistic approach to diagnosis and management. J Pediatr Health Care Sep-Oct 2011;25(5):284–93.
10. Frosch M, Mauritz MD, Bielack S, et al. Etiology, Risk Factors, and Diagnosis of Back Pain in Children and Adolescents: Evidence- and Consensus-Based Inter-disciplinary Recommendations. Children 2022;9(2). https://doi.org/10.3390/children9020192.
11. Guddal MH, Stensland SO, Smastuen MC, et al. Physical Activity Level and Sport Participation in Relation to Musculoskeletal Pain in a Population-Based Study of Adolescents: The Young-HUNT Study. Orthop J Sports Med 2017;5(1). https://doi.org/10.1177/2325967116685543. 2325967116685543.
12. Calvo-Munoz I, Kovacs FM, Roque M, et al. Risk Factors for Low Back Pain in Childhood and Adolescence: A Systematic Review. Clin J Pain 2018;34(5):468–84.
13. Macias BR, Murthy G, Chambers H, et al. Asymmetric loads and pain associated with backpack carrying by children. J Pediatr Orthop Jul-Aug 2008;28(5):512–7.
14. Booth TN, Iyer RS, Falcone RA Jr, et al. ACR Appropriateness Criteria(®) Back Pain-Child. J Am Coll Radiol 2017;14(5s): S13–s24.
15. Murphy KP. Chapter 105: Benign mechanical back pain of childhood. In: *Rehabilitation medicine Quick reference – pediatrics*. New York, NY: Springer Publishing Company; 2010.
16. Ruegsegger GN, Booth FW. Health Benefits of Exercise. Cold Spring Harb Perspect Med 2018;8(7). https://doi.org/10.1101/cshperspect.a029694.
17. Berger RG, Doyle SM. Spondylolysis 2019 update. Curr Opin Pediatr 2019; 31(1):61–8.
18. Miller R, Beck NA, Sampson NR, et al. Imaging modalities for low back pain in children: a review of spondyloysis and undiagnosed mechanical back pain. J Pediatr Orthop Apr-May 2013;33(3):282–8.
19. Beck NA, Miller R, Baldwin K, et al. Do oblique views add value in the diagnosis of spondylolysis in adolescents? J Bone Joint Surg Am 2013;95(10):e65.

20. Gum JL, Crawford CH 3rd, Collis PC, et al. Characteristics Associated With Active Defects in Juvenile Spondylolysis. Am J Orthop (Belle Mead NJ) 2015;44(10):E379–83.

21. Rush JK, Astur N, Scott S, et al. Use of magnetic resonance imaging in the evaluation of spondylolysis. J Pediatr Orthop Apr-May 2015;35(3):271–5.

22. Alqarni AM, Schneiders AG, Cook CE, et al. Clinical tests to diagnose lumbar spondylolysis and spondylolisthesis: A systematic review. Phys Ther Sport 2015;16(3):268–75. https://doi.org/10.1016/j.ptsp.2014.12.005.

23. Robin G.C., The etiology of Scheuermann's disease, In: Bridwell K.H., *The textbook of spinal surgery*, 1997, Lippincott-Raven, Philadelphia, 1169.

24. Etemadifar MR, Jamalaldini MH, Layeghi R. Successful brace treatment of Scheuermann's kyphosis with different angles. J Craniovertebr Junction Spine Apr-Jun 2017;8(2):136–43.

25. Lee JH, Cynn HS, Yoon TL, et al. The effect of scapular posterior tilt exercise, pectoralis minor stretching, and shoulder brace on scapular alignment and muscles activity in subjects with round-shoulder posture. J Electromyogr Kinesiol 2015;25(1):107–14.

26. Ruivo RM, Carita AI, Pezarat-Correia P. The effects of training and detraining after an 8 month resistance and stretching training program on forward head and protracted shoulder postures in adolescents: Randomised controlled study. Man Ther 2016;21:76–82.

27. Ruivo RM, Pezarat-Correia P, Carita AI. Effects of a Resistance and Stretching Training Program on Forward Head and Protracted Shoulder Posture in Adolescents. J Manipulative Physiol Ther 2017;40(1):1–10.

28. Jackson DW, Rettig A, Wiltse LL. Epidural cortisone injections in the young athletic adult. Am J Sports Med Jul-Aug 1980;8(4):239–43.

29. Çelik S, Göksu K, Çelik SE, et al. Benign neurological recovery with low recurrence and low peridural fibrosis rate in pediatric disc herniations after lumbar microdiscectomy. Pediatr Neurosurg 2011;47(6):417–22.

30. Farrokhi MR, Masoudi MS. Slipped vertebral epiphysis (report of 2 cases). J Res Med Sci 2009;14(1):63–6.

31. Weiss PF, Colbert RA. Juvenile Spondyloarthritis: A Distinct Form of Juvenile Arthritis. Pediatr Clin North Am 2018;65(4):675–90.

32. Powell AP, English J. Exercise for Athletes With Inflammatory Arthritis. Curr Sports Med Rep 2018;17(9):302–7.

33. Calloni SF, Huisman TA, Poretti A, et al. Back pain and scoliosis in children: When to image, what to consider. Neuroradiol J 2017;30(5):393–404.

34. Meyerding HW. Spondylolistheses. *Surg Gynecol Obstet.* 1932;54:371–7.

35. Scheuermann HW. Kyphosis dorsalis juvenilis. Ugeskr Laeger 1920;82:385.

36. Mansfield J.T., Bennett M. Scheuermann Disease. [Updated 2022 Aug 21]. In: StatPearls [Internet]. Treasure Island (FL): StatPearls Publishing; 2022. Available from: https://www.ncbi.nlm.nih.gov/books/NBK499966/.

37. Patel DR, Kinsella E. Evaluation and management of lower back pain in young athletes. Transl Pediatr 2017;6(3):225–35.

38. Sarwark JF, LaBella CR. Pediatric Orthopaedics and sports injuries: a quick reference guide. Elk Grove Village, IL: American Academy of Pediatrics; 2021.

39. Singhal A, Mitra A, Cochrane D, et al. Ring apophysis fracture in pediatric lumbar disc herniation: a common entity. Pediatr Neurosurg 2013;49(1):16–20.

40. Wright KA, Crowson CS, Michet CJ, et al. Time trends in incidence, clinical features, and cardiovascular disease in ankylosing spondylitis over three decades: a population-based study. Arthritis Care Res 2015;67(6):836–41.

41. Klein-Gitelman M. Spondyloarthritis in children. Available at: https://www.uptodate.com/contents/spondyloarthritis-in-children. Accessed Sept 25, 2022.

42. Brent L. Ankylosing Spondylitis and Undifferentiated Spondyloarthropathy. Available at: https://emedicine.medscape.com/article/332945-overview#showall. Accessed Sept 25, 2022.

43. Rossi R, Alexander M, Eckert K, et al. Pediatric rehabilitation. In: Cuccurullo S.J. New York, NY: Springer Publishing Company; 2020. p. 729–820.

44. Kang HM, Choi EH, Lee HJ, et al. The Etiology, Clinical Presentation and Long-term Outcome of Spondylodiscitis in Children. Pediatr Infect Dis J 2016;35(4): e102–6.

45. Çakar M, Esenyel CZ, Seyran M, et al. Osteoid osteoma treated with radiofrequency ablation. Adv Orthop 2015;2015:807274.

46. Jordan RW, Koç T, Chapman AW, et al. Osteoid osteoma of the foot and ankle–A systematic review. Foot Ankle Surg 2015;21(4):228–34.

47. Raskas DS, Graziano GP, Herzenberg JE, et al. Osteoid osteoma and osteoblastoma of the spine. J Spinal Disord 1992;5(2):204–11.

48. Roach JW, Klatt JW, Faulkner ND. Involvement of the spine in patients with multiple hereditary exostoses. J Bone Joint Surg Am 2009;91(8):1942–8.

49. Smolle MA, Gilg MM, Machacek F, et al. Osteoid osteoma of the foot : Presentation, treatment and outcome of a multicentre cohort. Wien Klin Wochenschr 2022; 134(11–12):434–41.

50. Galgano MA, Goulart CR, Iwenofu H, et al. Osteoblastomas of the spine: a comprehensive review. Neurosurg Focus 2016;41(2):E4.

51. Zhao JG, Wang J, Huang WJ, et al. Interventions for treating simple bone cysts in the long bones of children. Cochrane Database Syst Rev 2017;2(2): Cd010847.

52. Grigoriou E, Dormans JP, Arkader A. Primary Aneurysmal Bone Cyst of the Spine in Children: Updated Outcomes of a Modern Surgical Technique. Int J Spine Surg 2020;14(4):615–22.

53. Jaffe HL. Aneurysmal bone cyst. Bull Hosp Joint Dis 1950;11(1):3–13.

54. Zileli M, Isik HS, Ogut FE, et al. Aneurysmal bone cysts of the spine. Eur Spine J 2013;22(3):593–601.

55. Nezelof C, Basset F, Rousseau MF. Histiocytosis X histogenetic arguments for a Langerhans cell origin. Biomedicine. Sep 1973;18(5):365–71.

56. Lichtenstein L. Histiocytosis X; integration of eosinophilic granuloma of bone, Letterer-Siwe disease, and Schüller-Christian disease as related manifestations of a single nosologic entity. AMA Arch Pathol 1953;56(1):84–102.

57. Sethi A, Agarwal K, Sethi S, et al. Allograft in the treatment of benign cystic lesions of bone. Arch Orthop Trauma Surg 1993;112(4):167–70.

58. Akhaddar A, Boucetta M. Eosinophilic granuloma of the cervical spine manifesting as torticollis in a child. Pan Afr Med J 2014;19:36.

59. Velez-Yanguas MC, Warrier RP. Langerhans' cell histiocytosis. Orthop Clin North Am 1996;27(3):615–23.

60. Han I, Suh ES, Lee SH, et al. Management of eosinophilic granuloma occurring in the appendicular skeleton in children. Clin Orthop Surg 2009;1(2):63–7.

61. Kaplan JA. Leukemia in Children. Pediatr Rev 2019;40(7):319–31.

62. Lenk L, Alsadeq A, Schewe DM. Involvement of the central nervous system in acute lymphoblastic leukemia: opinions on molecular mechanisms and clinical implications based on recent data. Cancer Metastasis Rev 2020; 39(1):173–87.

63. Boyce A.M., Florenzano P., de Castro L.F., et al., Fibrous Dysplasia / McCune-Albright Syndrome. 2015 Feb 26 [Updated 2019 Jun 27]. In: Adam M.P., Everman D.B., Mirzaa G.M., et al., editors. GeneReviews® [Internet]. Seattle (WA): University of Washington, Seattle; 1993-2023. Available from: https://www.ncbi.nlm.nih.gov/books/NBK274564/. Accessed September 25, 2022.

64. Boyce AM. Fibrous Dysplasia. Available at: https://www.ncbi.nlm.nih.gov/books/NBK326740/ [Updated 2019 Mar 27]. Endotext [Internet]. Accessed Sept 25, 2022.

65. Sahu RK, Das KK, Bhaisora KS, et al. Pediatric intramedullary spinal cord lesions: Pathological spectrum and outcome of surgery. J Pediatr Neurosci Jul-Sep 2015; 10(3):214–21.

66. Ogunlade J, Wiginton JGt, Elia C, et al. Primary Spinal Astrocytomas: A Literature Review. Cureus 2019;11(7):e5247.

67. Azad TD, Pendharkar AV, Pan J, et al. Surgical outcomes of pediatric spinal cord astrocytomas: systematic review and meta-analysis. J Neurosurg Pediatr 2018; 22(4):404–10.

68. Lundar T, Due-Tønnessen BJ, Scheie D, et al. Pediatric spinal ependymomas: an unpredictable and puzzling disease. Long-term follow-up of a single consecutive institutional series of ten patients. Childs Nerv Syst 2014;30(12):2083–8.

69. Zaky W., Ater J. and Khatua S., Brain tumors in childhood, In: Kliegman R., Stanton B., St Geme J., et al., Nelson *textbook of pediatrics*, 21st edition, 2020, Elsevier, Amsterdam, Netherlands.

70. Safaee M, Oh MC, Kim JM, et al. Histologic grade and extent of resection are associated with survival in pediatric spinal cord ependymomas. Childs Nerv Syst 2013;29(11):2057–64.

71. Misaghi A, Goldin A, Awad M, et al. Osteosarcoma: a comprehensive review. Sicot j 2018;4:12.

72. Seeger LL, Gold RH, Chandnani VP. Diagnostic imaging of osteosarcoma. Clin Orthop Relat Res 1991;270:254–63.

73. Grier HE. THE EWING FAMILY OF TUMORS: Ewing's Sarcoma and Primitive Neuroectodermal Tumors. Pediatr Clin 1997/08/01/1997;44(4):991–1004.

74. Mavrogenis AF, Megaloikonomos PD, Igoumenou VG, et al. Spondylodiscitis revisited. l Open Rev 2017;2(11):447–61.

75. Jansen BR, Hart W, Schreuder O. Discitis in childhood. 12-35-year follow-up of 35 patients. Acta Orthop Scand 1993;64(1):33–6.

76. Delamarter RB, Sachs BL, Thompson GH, et al. Primary neoplasms of the thoracic and lumbar spine. An analysis of 29 consecutive cases. Clin Orthop Relat Res 1990;256:87–100.

77. Gitelis S, McDonald DJ. In: Common benign bone tumors and usual treatment, In: Simon M.A.S.D.S., *Surgery for bone and soft tissue tumors*. Philadelphia: Lippincott-Raven; 1998. p. 181–205.

78. Allen CE, Merad M, McClain KL. Langerhans-Cell Histiocytosis. N Engl J Med 2018;379(9):856–68.

79. Shamberger RC, Laquaglia MP, Krailo MD, et al. Ewing sarcoma of the rib: results of an intergroup study with analysis of outcome by timing of resection. J Thorac Cardiovasc Surg 2000;119(6):1154–61.

80. Zöllner SK, Amatruda JF, Bauer S, et al. Ewing Sarcoma-Diagnosis, Treatment, Clinical Challenges and Future Perspectives. J Clin Med 2021;14(8):10.

81. Ciftdemir M, Kaya M, Selcuk E, et al. Tumors of the spine. World J Orthop 2016; 7(2):109–16.

82. Hwang SO, Lee SH, Lee HB. Epithelioid sarcoma associated with neurofibromatosis type I. Arch Craniofac Surg 2020;21(1):41–4.

83. Anthony K. and Schanberg L., Chapter 193: Musculoskeletal pain syndromes, In: Kliegman R., Stanton B., St Geme J., et al., Nelson *textbook of pediatric*ˢ, 21st edition, 2020, Elsevier, Amsterdam, Netherlands.

84. Murphy KP. Cerebral palsy lifetime care - four musculoskeletal conditions. Dev Med Child Neurol 2009;51(Suppl 4):30–7.

Chronic Pain in Children
Interdisciplinary Management

Andrew B. Collins, MD[a,b,c,d],*

KEYWORDS

- Pediatric chronic pain • Biopsychosocial model of pain • Interdisciplinary care
- Pain psychology • Intensive interdisciplinary pain treatment

KEY POINTS

- Chronic pain in children is influenced by biological factors, such as ongoing inflammation or genetics; psychological factors, such as anxiety or catastrophizing; and social factors, such as peer relationships and family dynamics.
- Interdisciplinary care including medication management, physical and occupational therapy, and psychological treatment is the optimal treatment approach for chronic pain in children.
- Evidence is lacking for each individual aspect of interdisciplinary care for chronic pain in children, with the largest volume of research on cognitive-behavioral therapy and other psychological treatments.
- For children with high levels of pain-associated disability, intensive interdisciplinary pain treatment can improve pain intensity, function, and other associated symptoms.

INTRODUCTION
Definitions

The International Association for the Study of Pain (IASP) defines pain as an "unpleasant sensory and emotional experience associated with, or resembling that associated with, actual or potential tissue damage."[1] Although acute pain serves as an alert for damage or dysfunction, chronic pain lasts beyond this original purpose or arises without recognizable initial purpose.[2] Chronic pain is persistent or recurrent, lasting beyond typical times for healing; it is often defined as 3 to 6 months.[3,4]

[a] Department of Pediatrics, University of Cincinnati College of Medicine; [b] Department of Neurology and Rehabilitation Medicine, University of Cincinnati College of Medicine; [c] Division of Pediatric Rehabilitation Medicine, Cincinnati Children's Hospital Medical Center, 3333 Burnet Avenue MLC 4009, Cincinnati, OH 45229, USA; [d] Division of Pediatric Pain Medicine, Cincinnati Children's Hospital Medical Center, 3333 Burnet Avenue MLC 2001, Cincinnati, OH 45229, USA
* Division of Pediatric Rehabilitation Medicine, Cincinnati Children's Hospital Medical Center, 3333 Burnet Avenue MLC 4009, Cincinnati, OH 45229.
E-mail address: andrew.collins@cchmc.org
Twitter: @abcollinsmd (A.B.C.)

Pediatr Clin N Am 70 (2023) 575–588
https://doi.org/10.1016/j.pcl.2023.01.010

Epidemiology

Approximately 11% to 38% of children have chronic pain during childhood, including headache, abdominal pain, musculoskeletal pain, and widespread pain.[5,6] Prevalence is higher in women, older children/adolescents, and those with socioeconomic risk factors, such as lower income, use of public insurance, and parental educational attainment.[6] However, these estimates are complicated by inconsistent definitions and small samples; a more recent study, based on national data in the United States, showed a prevalence of chronic pain in children of about 6%.[6] As many as 5% of children have significant pain-associated functional disability.[7] Such disability can include school dysfunction, peer and social dysfunction, sleep problems, and parental burden.[8] Children with significant pain-associated disability have frequent absences from school and can struggle with academic performance.[8] They miss social events, have fewer friends, and difficulty recognizing social cues from peers.[8] Parents of such children also have significant distress and increased burden of care.[8]

Pain Mechanisms and Biopsychosocial Model

Although the exact mechanisms for the development of chronic pain are not known, multiple models have been proposed.

- The *gate control theory* describes signals propagating from peripheral fibers to ascending spinal tracts to the brainstem and brain; signals can be diminished or amplified along this course, and the brain serves a passive role in perception.[9]
- The *central sensitization model* proposes that peripheral stimulation produces hypersensitivity in the central nervous system due to changes in receptors, channels, and signaling pathways; such changes produce allodynia, hyperalgesia, and reduced pain thresholds.[10]
- The *neuromatrix model* describes a complex network of signals between peripheral nerves, the brainstem, brain, and hypothalamic-pituitary axis.[11] In this model, peripheral signaling is incorporated with cognitive and affective aspects of pain, including memories, fear, emotional responses, and associations with suffering or reward. In the neuromatrix model, the network of signals can be influenced by many factors, including genetics and past experiences.[11]

The neuromatrix model aligns with the biopsychosocial model of chronic pain and pain-associated disability. This model emphasizes that biological, psychological, and social factors can influence pain perception, pain experience, and functional ability, as illustrated in **Fig. 1**.[12] The biopsychosocial model is supported by the complex relationship between pain and anxiety, catastrophizing, peer relationships, and parental factors.[13–15]

Diagnostic Nomenclature

Terms such as primary pain syndromes, functional pain disorders, medically unexplained pain, or amplified pain syndromes have been used to describe chronic pain that is not directly associated with an underlying known painful medical diagnosis, inflammatory condition, or anatomic or structural abnormality.[16] These terms can be confusing for children, families, and providers, potentially emphasizes the psychological and social contributions to pain over the biological and physical contributions.[16]

More recently, the World Health Organization and IASP created a classification system for chronic pain, differentiating chronic primary pain syndromes, and chronic secondary pain syndromes.[4,17] Chronic primary pain syndromes describe persistent or recurrent pain that is associated with significant emotional distress or functional

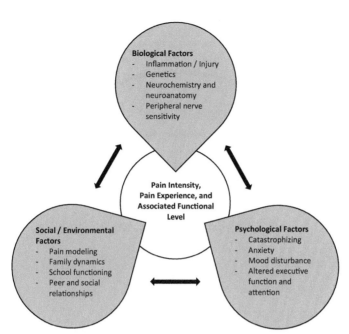

Fig. 1. Chronic pain in children is best understood through a biopsychosocial model, emphasizing the diverse factors that can contribute to ongoing pain and pain-associated disability.

disability and that is not a result of another primary diagnosis or painful condition.[4,17] Examples of chronic primary pain syndromes include fibromyalgia, irritable bowel syndrome, and complex regional pain syndrome.[4,17] Chronic secondary pain syndromes evolve from a symptom of an associated diagnosis to a distinct problem that may persist beyond treatment of the associated diagnosis; examples include chronic postsurgical pain and chronic cancer-related pain.[17]

DISCUSSION
Treatment Philosophy

Treatment of chronic pain in children emphasizes interdisciplinary rehabilitation, including psychology, physical or occupational therapy, and other services (such as acupuncture, massage, nutrition, or school services) in addition to biomedical interventions, as illustrated in **Fig. 2**.[12,18] Biomedical interventions, such as medications and procedures, have limited evidence for ongoing benefit and have potential for significant side effects including increased health-care utilization.[19–21] Instead, interdisciplinary rehabilitation focuses on adaptive functioning with an expectation that function will improve before pain intensity.[22]

An ideal treatment model for chronic pain in children includes an interdisciplinary team offering a range of treatment options and integrates clinical practice with research and education.[23] The first opportunity to emphasize this model of treatment is initial feedback with a child and family. Feedback should include validation of symptoms, diagnosis with explanation, education, and emphasis of interdisciplinary care.[24]

Although an interdisciplinary team is the ideal treatment model for pediatric pain, most patients are initially seen in primary care settings, and it can be challenging for primary care physicians to discuss chronic pain or determine a treatment plan.[25,26]

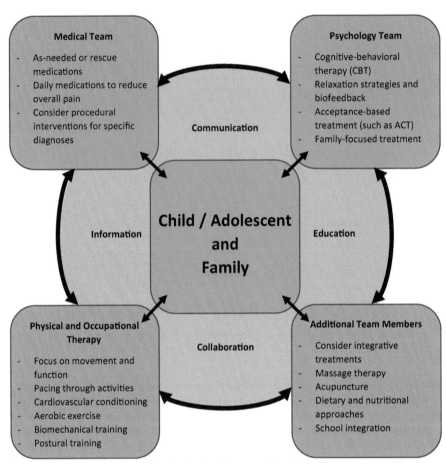

Fig. 2. Interdisciplinary treatment is the best treatment model for chronic pain in children. In this treatment model, team members work together with each other, the child, and the child's family to improve the child's pain and function.

The Pediatric Pain Screening Tool has been developed to triage services that would be most helpful for individual children.[27] This tool has 9 patient-reported items, 8 yes/no questions, and 1 rating from "not at all" to "a whole lot." These items are divided into a psychosocial subscale, which includes items such as "I worry about my pain a lot" and "I do not have as much fun as I used to," and a physical subscale, which includes items such as "My pain is in more than one body part" and "It is difficult for me to be at school all day." A child's score on each subscale and for the overall tool can guide referrals to physical therapy, psychology services, or a multidisciplinary pain clinic.[27]

Pharmacologic Treatment

Evidence for pharmacologic management of pain in children is limited, with few studies of relatively low quality, extrapolation of adult data, and concerns for side effects.[19,21] Cochrane reviews on use of antidepressants, antiepileptics, acetaminophen, nonsteroidal anti-inflammatory drugs (NSAIDs), and opioids had few or no articles that could be included for review.[28–32] However, children are often prescribed multiple medications and report high use of over-the-counter medications, such as acetaminophen and ibuprofen.[33,34] Medications for chronic pain in children can be divided into daily medications that decrease pain intensity overall and as-needed medications for worst episodes of pain. Commonly used medications are summarized in **Table 1**, including side effects and summary of evidence.[19,35–37]

Daily medications can include antiepileptics, such as gabapentin or pregabalin; tricyclic antidepressants (TCAs), such as amitriptyline; and serotonin-norepinephrine reuptake inhibitors (SNRIs), such as duloxetine.[19] Although all evidence is of low quality, these medications have been shown effective in some conditions and evidence is borrowed from adult literature for other conditions.[28,29,38–43]

As-needed medications including relatively safe and commonly used over-the-counter options, such as acetaminophen and ibuprofen.[30,32,44] Prescription options include other NSAIDs and muscle relaxing medications.[19,32,45] Opioid medications are not considered first-line treatment of chronic pain; opioids may be an option for severe acute pain as part of an interdisciplinary plan.[31,46,47]

Procedural Treatment

Interventional procedures may be recommended for certain diagnoses, such as epidural injections for radiculopathy or trigger point injections in myofascial pain. Evidence for procedures is borrowed from adult literature.[20] Interventional procedures should be part of interdisciplinary care, rather than a choice between procedures and other care.

Physical and Occupational Therapy

Physical and occupational strategies that have been proposed for the treatment of chronic pain in children include cardiovascular conditioning, aerobic exercise, functional training, postural training, and biomechanics education.[48,49] Therapists roles in pediatric chronic pain are most researched in the setting of interdisciplinary programs.[50–52]

An important role for physical and occupational therapies is teaching pacing to encourage function.[53,54] Pacing is most helpful when focused on consistency and proactive decisions around amount of activity, rather than symptom-based strategies for stopping.[55,56] One proposed strategy for mindful use of pacing is STAR (stop, think, act or ask, resume).[57]

- Stop: The child should stop or modify an activity during a planned pacing break.
- Think: This is an opportunity for the child to actively identify physical, mental, and emotional feelings that keep them from participating in an activity. Children with chronic pain can struggle to identify and name feelings other than pain, so this can be challenging.
- Act or Ask: The child should use a skill or strategy to address the feelings in the previous step or ask a designated person for help to identify a strategy. Strategies could include hydration, stretching, breathing, or another coping skill.
- Resume: After utilizing a skill or strategy, the child then resumes their activity as they were doing earlier or with appropriate adjustments.

Psychological Treatment

Psychological interventions have more supportive evidence than any other individual modality for chronic pain in children, although the overall quality of evidence is still

Table 1
Commonly used medications for chronic pain in children

Class	Example Medications	Indications	Side Effects	Evidence Per Cochrane Review
As-Needed Medications				
Acetaminophen	Acetaminophen	Acute pain, adjunctive treatment	Hepatic injury	No eligible studies to include
NSAIDs	Ibuprofen, naproxen	Acute pain, inflammatory conditions, abortive headache treatment	GI effects, kidney injury, bleeding disorders, hypertension	Small number of studies, insufficient data for analysis
Muscle relaxants	Methocarbamol, cyclobenzaprine, tizanidine, baclofen	Myofascial pain, spasmodic pain	Sedation, nausea, dizziness, serotonin syndrome for cyclobenzaprine	No review performed
Opioids	Morphine, oxycodone, hydromorphone	Acute pain, postsurgical pain	Sedation, nausea, dependence, addiction	No eligible studies to include
Daily Medications				
Antiepileptics	Gabapentin, pregabalin, oxcarbazepine	Neuropathic pain, widespread pain, primary pain disorders	Somnolence, altered mood, weight gain	Small number of studies, insufficient data for analysis
Antidepressants	Amitriptyline and other TCAs	Neuropathic pain, headache prophylaxis, abdominal pain, widespread pain, primary pain disorders	Somnolence, altered mood, dry mouth, prolonged QT interval (QTc), risk of serotonin syndrome	Small number of studies, insufficient data for analysis
	Duloxetine and other SNRIs	Neuropathic pain, widespread pain, primary pain disorders	Altered mood, nausea, risk of serotonin syndrome	

low.[58–60] Cognitive behavioral therapy (CBT), relaxation strategies, and biofeedback have the most evidence.[61]

CBT is a skill-based treatment that includes relaxation training, distraction techniques, and activity pacing, with little evidence on which aspect of CBT is more effective.[59] CBT typically starts with pain education and establishing a rationale for psychological intervention. Pain education alone is an effective intervention in adults but has not been studied in children.[59,62] In addition to pain education, CBT addresses altering maladaptive behavioral responses, challenging negative cognitions, and developing pain coping skills.

Other psychological interventions effective for some populations include problem-solving training, acceptance-based strategies, mindfulness, and positive psychology.[63,64] Acceptance and commitment therapy (ACT) is the name of one acceptance-based psychological therapy shown to improve pain, function, and engagement in activities of value in children with chronic pain.[63] Acceptance-based therapies overlap with aspects of traditional CBT, including the use of similar behavioral techniques. However, although CBT emphasizes the use of behaviors to reduce symptoms, ACT and other acceptance-based therapies emphasize accepting symptoms while continuing to engage in activities.

Because families of children with chronic pain have poorer family functioning and a child's function relates to parental distress and behaviors, parent-focused psychology is also important.[65,66] In addition to cognitive-behavioral and acceptance focused treatments, family-focused and parent-focused problem-solving skills training is effective at reducing distress and improving function.[67,68]

Pain-focused psychology is difficult to access due to lack of specifically trained psychologists and a lack of confidence in providing pain-focused treatment among therapists who do not have this specific training.[69] Some proposed methods to improve access include single day workshops, group treatment, and virtual delivery of treatment, although results have been mixed.[61,70–72] One freely available digital treatment program that can be effective for children and their parents is WebMAP mobile.[73] Another proposed option is integrating pain-focused CBT into a primary care environment to improve earlier access.[74]

Integrative Medicine

Integrative medicine is frequently used by children with pain through specialized diets, herbal supplements, manual therapies, and acupuncture; such approaches are often a part of pediatric pain clinics in the United States.[75,76] Acupuncture, the most common integrative option offered in interdisciplinary clinics in the United States, is suggested to be safe and potentially effective in children.[75,77]

Outpatient Interdisciplinary Management

Outpatient pediatric pain clinics are typically interdisciplinary, with physicians, nurses, physical therapists, and psychologists incorporating medication management, CBT, relaxation training, and pacing-focused treatments.[23] Although such clinics require significant resources, they are shown to be cost effective for both hospitals and insurance companies.[78] Although outpatient interdisciplinary treatment is effective, it can be difficult for families to access services and to adhere to recommendations.[23,79]

Intensive Interdisciplinary Pain Treatment

Some children continue to have severe pain-associated functional impairments despite appropriate outpatient treatment. Those children may benefit from either rehabilitation through intensive interdisciplinary pain treatment (IIPT) or an inpatient or day hospital program that incorporates at least 3 treatment disciplines.[52,80] Overall, IIPT programs have shown significant improvement in functional disability with smaller improvements in pain intensity.[52] These improvements occur regardless of pain intensity or pain distribution at the onset of program and can persist for multiple years following the end of intensive treatment.[81,82] IIPT can also improve depression, anxiety, sleep, school performance, and parental factors.[52,83,84] Due to the importance of parental factors, there has been increased focus on incorporating parent-focused treatment into IIPT to improve parents' mental health, behaviors, and problem-solving skills.[85–87]

IIPT programs can be costly due to the intensity of resources required. A program in the United States demonstrated cost effectiveness within 1 year with savings from decreased specialty and emergency care, decreased hospitalizations, and decreased missed work for parents.[88] Another IIPT program in Germany showed no change in cost but showed a change in expenditures with increased goal-directed treatment such as psychology and decreased hospitalization.[89] Longer term, this program showed decrease in health-care utilization and subjective financial burden.[82]

In addition to IIPT, which is resource-intensive and requires a large team, lower intensity outpatient programs have been introduced to address chronic pain in children.[90,91] Such lower intensity options may provide a lower cost alternative for some children or help to bridge the gap between traditional outpatient management and IIPT.

SUMMARY

Chronic pain, or pain that persists or recurs for 3 to 6 months, is relatively common in children and can be associated with significant functional impairments. Although mechanisms for the development of chronic pain are not fully understood, the biopsychosocial model can help to identify contributing factors. In addition to biomedical factors such as ongoing inflammation or genetic predisposition to pain, children with chronic pain often have higher levels of catastrophizing, anxiety, and mood disturbance. Children with chronic pain also can have family dysfunction, parental distress, and poor peer relationships.

Interdisciplinary treatment is the best treatment approach for children with chronic pain, including medical, psychological, and physical or occupational therapy treatments. Medical treatment can include daily medications, as-needed medications, and potentially procedural interventions. Physical and occupational therapy should focus on function, movement, and pacing. Psychological treatment centers on pain education and CBT, with potential for acceptance-and-mindfulness-based treatments.

Although evidence is lacking for individual aspects of treatment, interdisciplinary care is considered the best treatment approach for children with chronic pain. Interdisciplinary care can include medication management with daily and as-needed medications, physical and occupational therapies focusing on function and movement, and psychological treatment with cognitive-behavioral therapy and acceptance-focused treatment. In children with severe pain and disability that does not improve outpatient, IIPT can improve pain intensity and function.

CLINICS CARE POINTS

- Chronic pain in children is best treated through an interdisciplinary approach with medication management, psychology, and physical or occupational therapy. The Pediatric Pain Screening Tool can help to efficiently identify children who are at higher risk and would benefit from such treatments.

- Systematic review of multiple medication classes showed insufficient evidence for treating chronic pain in children. However, there is some support for daily use of specific antiepileptics or antidepressants and as-needed use of acetaminophen or nonsteroidal anti-inflammatory medications.
- Psychological strategies have the best evidence for treating chronic pain in children, specifically CBT. Treatment should also include parents to address family factors.
- Children with chronic pain and severe pain-associated disability may benefit from specialized care through an IIPT program.

DECLARATION OF INTERESTS

The authors declare no competing interests.

REFERENCES

1. Terminology | International Association for the Study of Pain. International Association for the Study of Pain (IASP). Available at: https://www.iasp-pain.org/resources/terminology/. Accessed September 3, 2022.
2. Grichnik KP, Ferrante FM. The difference between acute and chronic pain. Mt Sinai J Med N Y 1991;58(3):217–20.
3. Merskey H. Classification of chronic pain: Descriptions of chronic pain syndromes and definitions of pain terms. Pain 1986;(Suppl 3):226.
4. Nicholas M, Vlaeyen JWS, Rief W, et al. The IASP classification of chronic pain for ICD-11: chronic primary pain. Pain 2019;160(1):28–37.
5. King S, Chambers CT, Huguet A, et al. The epidemiology of chronic pain in children and adolescents revisited: a systematic review. Pain 2011;152(12):2729–38.
6. Tumin D, Drees D, Miller R, et al. Health care utilization and costs associated with pediatric chronic pain. J Pain 2018;19(9):973–82.
7. Huguet A, Miró J. The severity of chronic pediatric pain: an epidemiological study. J Pain 2008;9(3):226–36.
8. Palermo TM. Impact of recurrent and chronic pain on child and family daily functioning: a critical review of the literature. J Dev Behav Pediatr 2000;21(1):58–69.
9. Melzack R, Wall PD. Pain mechanisms: a new theory. Science 1965;150(3699):971–9.
10. Fitzgerald M. The neurobiology of chronic pain in children. In: McClain BC, Suresh S, editors. Handbook of pediatric chronic pain: current science and integrative practice. Springer; 2011. p. 15–25. https://doi.org/10.1007/978-1-4419-0350-1_2.
11. Melzack R. From the gate to the neuromatrix. Pain 1999;Suppl 6:S121–6.
12. Gatchel RJ, Peng YB, Peters ML, et al. The biopsychosocial approach to chronic pain: scientific advances and future directions. Psychol Bull 2007;133(4):581–624.
13. Tran ST, Jastrowski Mano KE, Hainsworth KR, et al. Distinct influences of anxiety and pain catastrophizing on functional outcomes in children and adolescents with chronic pain. J Pediatr Psychol 2015;40(8):744–55.
14. Vetter TR, McGwin G, Bridgewater CL, et al. Validation and clinical application of a biopsychosocial model of pain intensity and functional disability in patients with a pediatric chronic pain condition referred to a subspecialty clinic. Pain Res Treat 2013;2013:143292.

15. Forgeron PA, King S, Stinson JN, et al. Social functioning and peer relationships in children and adolescents with chronic pain: a systematic review. Pain Res Manag 2010;15(1):27–41.

16. Schechter NL. Functional pain: time for a new name. JAMA Pediatr 2014;168(8):693–4.

17. Treede RD, Rief W, Barke A, et al. Chronic pain as a symptom or a disease: the IASP classification of chronic pain for the international classification of diseases (ICD-11). Pain 2019;160(1):19–27.

18. Namerow LB, Kutner EC, Wakefield EC, et al. Pain amplification syndrome: a biopsychosocial approach. Semin Pediatr Neurol 2016;23(3):224–30.

19. Mathew E, Kim E, Goldschneider KR. Pharmacological treatment of chronic non-cancer pain in pediatric patients. Pediatr Drugs 2014;16(6):457–71.

20. Shah RD, Cappiello D, Suresh S. Interventional procedures for chronic pain in children and adolescents: a review of the current evidence. Pain Pract Off J World Inst Pain 2016;16(3):359–69.

21. Boulkedid R, Abdou AY, Desselas E, et al. The research gap in chronic paediatric pain: a systematic review of randomised controlled trials. Eur J Pain Lond Engl 2018;22(2):261–71.

22. Lynch-Jordan AM, Sil S, Peugh J, et al. Differential changes in functional disability and pain intensity over the course of psychological treatment for children with chronic pain. Pain 2014;155(10):1955–61.

23. Miró J, McGrath PJ, Finley GA, et al. Pediatric chronic pain programs: current and ideal practice. PAIN Rep 2017;2(5):e613.

24. Schechter NL, Coakley R, Nurko S. The golden half hour in chronic pediatric pain—feedback as the first intervention. JAMA Pediatr 2021;175(1):7–8.

25. De Inocencio J. Epidemiology of musculoskeletal pain in primary care. Arch Dis Child 2004;89(5):431–4.

26. Jandial S, Myers A, Wise E, et al. Doctors likely to encounter children with musculoskeletal complaints have low confidence in their clinical skills. J Pediatr 2009;154(2):267–71.

27. Simons LE, Smith A, Ibagon C, et al. Pediatric Pain Screening Tool (PPST): Rapid identification of risk in youth with pain complaints. Pain 2015;156(8):1511–8.

28. Cooper TE, Heathcote LC, Clinch J, et al. Antidepressants for chronic non-cancer pain in children and adolescents. Cochrane Database Syst Rev 2017;8. https://doi.org/10.1002/14651858.CD012535.pub2.

29. Cooper TE, Wiffen PJ, Heathcote LC, et al. Antiepileptic drugs for chronic non-cancer pain in children and adolescents. Cochrane Database Syst Rev 2017;8. https://doi.org/10.1002/14651858.CD012536.pub2.

30. Cooper TE, Fisher E, Anderson B, et al. Paracetamol (acetaminophen) for chronic non-cancer pain in children and adolescents. Cochrane Database Syst Rev 2017;8. https://doi.org/10.1002/14651858.CD012539.pub2.

31. Cooper TE, Fisher E, Gray AL, et al. Opioids for chronic non-cancer pain in children and adolescents. Cochrane Database Syst Rev 2017;7. https://doi.org/10.1002/14651858.CD012538.pub2.

32. Eccleston C, Cooper TE, Fisher E, et al. Non-steroidal anti-inflammatory drugs (NSAIDs) for chronic non-cancer pain in children and adolescents. Cochrane Database Syst Rev 2017;8. https://doi.org/10.1002/14651858.CD012537.pub2.

33. Stinson J, Harris L, Garofalo E, et al. Understanding the use of over-the-counter pain treatments in adolescents with chronic pain. Can J Pain Rev Can Douleur 2017;1(1):84–93.

34. Gmuca S, Xiao R, Weiss PF, et al. Opioid prescribing and polypharmacy in children with chronic musculoskeletal pain. Pain Med Malden Mass 2019;20(3): 495–503.

35. Pereira A, Gitlin MJ, Gross RA, et al. Suicidality associated with antiepileptic drugs: implications for the treatment of neuropathic pain and fibromyalgia. Pain 2013;154(3):345–9.

36. Hengartner MP, Plöderl M. Suicidality and other severe psychiatric events with duloxetine: Re-analysis of safety data from a placebo-controlled trial for juvenile fibromyalgia. Int J Risk Saf Med 2021;32(3):209–18.

37. Patra KP, Sankararaman S, Jackson R, et al. Significance of screening electrocardiogram before the initiation of amitriptyline therapy in children with functional abdominal pain. Clin Pediatr (Phila) 2012;51(9):848–51.

38. Rusy LM, Troshynski TJ, Weisman SJ. Gabapentin in phantom limb pain management in children and young adults: report of seven cases. J Pain Symptom Manage 2001;21(1):78–82.

39. Butkovic D, Toljan S, Mihovilovic-Novak B. Experience with gabapentin for neuropathic pain in adolescents: report of five cases. Paediatr Anaesth 2006;16(3): 325–9.

40. Arnold LM, Schikler KN, Bateman L, et al. Safety and efficacy of pregabalin in adolescents with fibromyalgia: a randomized, double-blind, placebo-controlled trial and a 6-month open-label extension study. Pediatr Rheumatol Online J 2016; 14(1):46.

41. de Leeuw TG, der Zanden T van, Ravera S, et al. diagnosis and treatment of chronic neuropathic and mixed pain in children and adolescents: results of a survey study amongst practitioners. Child Basel Switz 2020;7(11):E208.

42. Teitelbaum JE, Arora R. Long-term efficacy of low-dose tricyclic antidepressants for children with functional gastrointestinal disorders. J Pediatr Gastroenterol Nutr 2011;53(3):260–4.

43. Upadhyaya HP, Arnold LM, Alaka K, et al. Efficacy and safety of duloxetine versus placebo in adolescents with juvenile fibromyalgia: results from a randomized controlled trial. Pediatr Rheumatol Online J 2019;17(1):27.

44. Pierce CA, Voss B. Efficacy and safety of ibuprofen and acetaminophen in children and adults: a meta-analysis and qualitative review. Ann Pharmacother 2010;44(3):489–506.

45. Chou R, Peterson K, Helfand M. Comparative efficacy and safety of skeletal muscle relaxants for spasticity and musculoskeletal conditions: a systematic review. J Pain Symptom Manage 2004;28(2):140–75.

46. Wren AA, Ross AC, D'Souza G, et al. Multidisciplinary Pain Management for Pediatric Patients with Acute and Chronic Pain: A Foundational Treatment Approach When Prescribing Opioids. Children 2019;6(2):33.

47. Schechter NL. Pediatric Pain Management and Opioids: The Baby and the Bathwater. JAMA Pediatr 2014;168(11):987–8.

48. Eccleston Z, Eccleston C. Interdisciplinary management of adolescent chronic pain: developing the role of physiotherapy. Physiotherapy 2004;90(2):77–81.

49. Landry BW, Fischer PR, Driscoll SW, et al. Managing chronic pain in children and adolescents: a clinical review. Pharm Manag PM R 2015;7(11 Suppl):S295–315.

50. Sherry DD, Wallace CA, Kelley C, et al. Short- and long-term outcomes of children with complex regional pain syndrome type I treated with exercise therapy. Clin J Pain 1999;15(3):218–23.

51. Klepper SE. Effects of an eight-week physical conditioning program on disease signs and symptoms in children with chronic arthritis. Arthritis Care Res 1999; 12(1):52–60.

52. Hechler T, Kanstrup M, Holley AL, et al. Systematic review on intensive interdisciplinary pain treatment of children with chronic pain. Pediatrics 2015;136(1): 115–27.

53. McCracken LM, Samuel VM. The role of avoidance, pacing, and other activity patterns in chronic pain. Pain 2007;130(1–2):119–25.

54. Revivo G, Amstutz DK, Gagnon CM, et al. Interdisciplinary pain management improves pain and function in pediatric patients with chronic pain associated with joint hypermobility syndrome. PM&R 2019;11(2):150–7.

55. Antcliff D, Keeley P, Campbell M, et al. Activity pacing: moving beyond taking breaks and slowing down. Qual Life Res Int J Qual Life Asp Treat Care Rehabil 2018;27(7):1933–5.

56. Cane D, Nielson WR, Mazmanian D. Patterns of pain-related activity: replicability, treatment-related changes, and relationship to functioning. Pain 2018;159(12): 2522–9.

57. Kempert H. Teaching and applying activity pacing in pediatric chronic pain rehabilitation using practitioner feedback and pace breaks. Pediatr Pain Lett 2021; 23(2):12.

58. Birnie KA, Ouellette C, Do Amaral T, et al. Mapping the evidence and gaps of interventions for pediatric chronic pain to inform policy, research, and practice: a systematic review and quality assessment of systematic reviews. Can J Pain Rev Can Douleur 2020;4(1):129–48.

59. Coakley R, Wihak T. Evidence-based psychological interventions for the management of pediatric chronic pain: new directions in research and clinical practice. Children 2017;4(2):9.

60. Fisher E, Law E, Dudeney J, et al. Psychological therapies for the management of chronic and recurrent pain in children and adolescents. Cochrane Database Syst Rev 2018;9. https://doi.org/10.1002/14651858.CD003968.pub5.

61. Palermo TM, Eccleston C, Lewandowski AS, et al. Randomized controlled trials of psychological therapies for management of chronic pain in children and adolescents: An updated meta-analytic review. Pain 2010;148(3):387–97.

62. Lee H, McAuley JH, Hübscher M, et al. Does changing pain-related knowledge reduce pain and improve function through changes in catastrophizing? Pain 2016;157(4):922–30.

63. Gauntlett-Gilbert J, Connell H, Clinch J, et al. Acceptance and values-based treatment of adolescents with chronic pain: outcomes and their relationship to acceptance. J Pediatr Psychol 2013;38(1):72–81.

64. Cousins LA, Tomlinson RM, Cohen LL, McMurtry CM. The power of optimism: applying a positive psychology framework to pediatric pain. Pediatric Pain Letter 2016;18(1):5.

65. Lewandowski AS, Palermo TM, Stinson J, et al. Systematic review of family functioning in families of children and adolescents with chronic pain. J Pain 2010; 11(11):1027–38.

66. Chow ET, Otis JD, Simons LE. The longitudinal impact of parent distress and behavior on functional outcomes among youth with chronic pain. J Pain 2016; 17(6):729–38.

67. Law EF, Fisher E, Fales J, et al. Systematic review and meta-analysis of parent and family-based interventions for children and adolescents with chronic medical conditions. J Pediatr Psychol 2014;39(8):866–86.

68. Palermo TM, Law EF, Essner B, et al. Adaptation of problem-solving skills training (PSST) for parent caregivers of youth with chronic pain. Clin Pract Pediatr Psychol 2014;2(3):212–23.
69. Darnall BD, Scheman J, Davin S, et al. Pain psychology: a global needs assessment and national call to action. Pain Med 2016;17(2):250–63.
70. Coakley R, Wihak T, Kossowsky J, et al. The comfort ability pain management workshop: a preliminary, nonrandomized investigation of a brief, cognitive, biobehavioral, and parent training intervention for pediatric chronic pain. J Pediatr Psychol 2018;43(3):252–65.
71. Fisher E, Law E, Dudeney J, et al. Psychological therapies (remotely delivered) for the management of chronic and recurrent pain in children and adolescents. Cochrane Database Syst Rev 2019;4. https://doi.org/10.1002/14651858. CD011118.pub3.
72. Huestis SE, Kao G, Dunn A, et al. Multi-family pediatric pain group therapy: capturing acceptance and cultivating change. Children 2017;4(12):106.
73. Palermo TM, de la Vega R, Murray C, et al. A digital health psychological intervention (WebMAP Mobile) for children and adolescents with chronic pain: results of a hybrid effectiveness-implementation stepped-wedge cluster randomized trial. Pain 2020;161(12):2763–74.
74. Salamon KS, Cullinan CC. The integrated prevention model of pain—Chronic pain prevention in the primary care setting. Clin Pract Pediatr Psychol 2019; 7(2):183–91.
75. Bodner K, D'Amico S, Luo M, et al. A cross-sectional review of the prevalence of integrative medicine in pediatric pain clinics across the United States. Complement Ther Med 2018;38:79–84.
76. Groenewald CB, Beals-Erickson SE, Ralston-Wilson J, et al. Complementary and alternative medicine use by children with pain in the United States. Acad Pediatr 2017;17(7):785–93.
77. Yang C, Hao Z, Zhang LL, et al. Efficacy and safety of acupuncture in children: an overview of systematic reviews. Pediatr Res 2015;78(2):112–9.
78. Mahrer NE, Gold JI, Luu M, et al. A cost-analysis of an interdisciplinary pediatric chronic pain clinic. J Pain 2018;19(2):158–65.
79. Simons LE, Logan DE, Chastain L, et al. Engagement in multidisciplinary interventions for pediatric chronic pain: parental expectations, barriers, and child outcomes. Clin J Pain 2010;26(4):291–9.
80. Stahlschmidt L, Zernikow B, Wager J. Specialized rehabilitation programs for children and adolescents with severe disabling chronic pain: indications, treatment and outcomes. Child Basel Switz 2016;3(4):E33.
81. Williams SE, Homan KJ, Crowley SL, et al. The impact of spatial distribution of pain on long-term trajectories for chronic pain outcomes after intensive interdisciplinary pain treatment. Clin J Pain 2020;36(3):181–8.
82. Zernikow B, Ruhe AK, Stahlschmidt L, et al. Clinical and Economic long-term treatment outcome of children and adolescents with disabling chronic pain. Pain Med 2018;19(1):16–28.
83. Krietsch KN, Beebe DW, King C, et al. Sleep among youth with severely disabling chronic pain: before, during, and after inpatient intensive interdisciplinary pain treatment. Children 2021;8(1):42.
84. Harbeck-Weber C, Sim L, Morrow AS, et al. What about parents? A systematic review of paediatric intensive interdisciplinary pain treatment on parent outcomes. Eur J Pain 2022;26(7):1424–36.

85. Law EF, Fales JL, Beals-Erickson SE, et al. A single-arm feasibility trial of problem-solving skills training for parents of children with idiopathic chronic pain conditions receiving intensive pain rehabilitation. J Pediatr Psychol 2017; 42(4):422–33.

86. Kemani MK, Kanstrup M, Jordan A, et al. Evaluation of an intensive interdisciplinary pain treatment based on acceptance and commitment therapy for adolescents with chronic pain and their parents: a nonrandomized clinical trial. J Pediatr Psychol 2018;43(9):981–94.

87. Benjamin JZ, Harbeck-Weber C, Ale C, et al. Becoming flexible: Increase in parent psychological flexibility uniquely predicts better well-being following participation in a pediatric interdisciplinary pain rehabilitation program. J Context Behav Sci 2020;15:181–8.

88. Evans JR, Benore E, Banez GA. The cost-effectiveness of intensive interdisciplinary pediatric chronic pain rehabilitation. J Pediatr Psychol 2016;41(8):849–56.

89. Ruhe AK, Frosch M, Wager J, et al. Health Care utilization and cost in children and adolescents with chronic pain: analysis of health care claims data 1 year before and after intensive interdisciplinary pain treatment. Clin J Pain 2017; 33(9):767–76.

90. Black WR, DiCesare CA, Thomas S, et al. Preliminary evidence for the fibromyalgia integrative training program (FIT Teens) improving strength and movement biomechanics in juvenile fibromyalgia : secondary analysis and results from a pilot randomized clinical trial. Clin J Pain 2021;37(1):51–60.

91. Dekker C, Goossens M, Winkens B, et al. Functional disability in adolescents with chronic pain: comparing an interdisciplinary exposure program to usual care. Children 2020;7(12):288.

Pediatric Functional Neurologic Disorders

Angela Garcia, MD

KEYWORDS

- Functional neurologic disorder • Functional neurologic symptom disorder
- Functional movement disorder • Functional seizure • Pediatric • Children
- Rehabilitation

KEY POINTS

- Functional neurologic disorders are common in the pediatric population, taking the forms of functional seizures, functional movement disorders, and functional vision disorders.
- Functional movement disorders are now a "rule in" diagnosis, with specific physical examination signs that are characteristic of the diagnosis.
- Timely diagnosis and treatment by a multidisciplinary team can lead to improvement and resolution of functional neurologic disorder symptoms in the pediatric population.

INTRODUCTION

Functional neurologic disorder (FND) is a common and disabling medical condition where patients experience neurologic symptoms with clinical findings that are inconsistent with a neurologic diagnosis.[1] Common manifestations of FND include functional movement disorder (FMD), functional seizure disorder (FSD), and functional vision disorders (FVDs).

HISTORY

Historically, physicians have proposed many potential etiologies to explain the symptoms of an FND. Raynor and colleagues[2] reviewed these etiologies, which included supernatural causes (eg, a god sending a spirit to "punish," causing the symptoms in Mesopotamia and Ancient Greece or a devil causing the symptoms in the Middle Ages), to being related to uterine dysfunction or "Hysteria." Physicians in the sixteenth to eighteenth centuries hypothesized that FND symptoms were related to a mental disorder, melancholy, or hypochondria.[2] In the late nineteenth century, the connection to the uterus was discouraged (but the term continued to be used until the 1960s), and

Department of Physical Medicine and Rehabilitation, University of Pittsburgh, UPMC Children's Hospital of Pittsburgh, 4401 Penn Avenue, Suite 1200, Pittsburgh, PA 15201, USA
E-mail address: garciaam@upmc.edu
Twitter: @pghconcussionmd (A.G.)

Pediatr Clin N Am 70 (2023) 589–601
https://doi.org/10.1016/j.pcl.2023.01.006
0031-3955/23/© 2023 Elsevier Inc. All rights reserved.

pediatric.theclinics.com

FND was thought to be a neurologic or mental disorder.[2] At the beginning of the twentieth century, with the split between psychiatry and neurology, other clinicians, including Sigmund Freud and Josef Breuer, attempted to use the psychoanalytic theory and categorize the symptoms as either "conversion symptoms," which included somatic symptoms; or "dissociative" symptoms-symptoms with altered level of consciousness. Later, in the 1960s, the term "hysteria" was retired, and divided into other diagnoses, including somatoform disorders, conversion disorder, and body dissociative disorders. The more recent editions of the Diagnostic and Statistical Manual of Mental Disorders (DSM) have de-emphasized theory and etiology and have altered the definition of an FND to only include the presence of neurologic symptoms not consistent with a known neurologic diagnosis and eliminated the need to have had a traumatic experience or stressful event.[2,3]

EPIDEMIOLOGY

Although the exact incidence is unknown, a 2021 JAMA Neurology study[4] looking at the prevalence and costs of FNDs from 2008 to 2017 found that approximately 1% of Pediatric Emergency Department visits with neurologic symptoms were related to an FND (3800 out of 328,609 patients). It is estimated that in 2016, total hospitalization costs for children diagnosed with an FND were 35.7 million dollars.[4] This has likely increased during the coronavirus disease-2019 pandemic, as Hull and colleagues[5] found that the incidence of FND increased in their pediatric population by 90% when comparing the incidence in March to October 2020 with the same period in 2019.[5]

Recent studies have explored the characteristics of pediatric patients with FND.[6,7] In these studies, the patients diagnosed with FND were mostly female, around the ages of 13 to 14 years old, had a normal or "functional" neurologic examination, and an identifiable stressor at the time of diagnosis.[6,7] In Pal and colleagues,[6] 38% of the patients had a co-current psychiatric diagnosis, 58% had a co-current physical illness, and 20% of their patients had a history of verbal, sexual or physical abuse. In Watson and colleagues,[7] 33% had a co-current psychiatric diagnosis, 35% had a co-current neurologic diagnosis, and 65% of the patients had pain as a co-presenting complaint.

PATHOPHYSIOLOGY

Although the exact pathophysiology of FND is unknown, recent research has gained insight into potential mechanisms. One theory is that it is a dysfunction of brain circuitry affecting specific constructs including emotional processing (including salience), attention, agency (our sense of free will that governs voluntary movement), interoception (the way the body senses and processes bodily signals on an unconscious and conscious level), and predictive processing/interference (the way we generate beliefs about the causes and effects of events occurring within and outside the body).[8] A recent study[8] showed that patients with FMDs had impairment in the executive control of attention compared with healthy controls and patients with organic neurologic disorders, whereas another study showed that patients with FMD had impaired inhibitory controls compared with healthy subjects.[9]

Recently, the use of functional neuroimaging (FMRI) has identified structural alterations in the neural circuitry associated with FND, as highlighted in reviews by Perez and colleagues[10] and Baizabal-Carvallo and colleagues.[11]

In addition to functional MRI studies, diffusion tensor imaging shows which pathways may be involved in FND.[12] A recent study by Diez and colleagues[13] found that patients with FND had reduced fractional anisotropy (which is a measure of white matter integrity) in the areas associated with our limbic system (stria terminalis/fornix, medial forebrain bundle, extreme capsule, uncinate fasciculus, cingulum bundle, corpus callosum, and striatal-postcentral gyrus projections). These networks are involved in emotional regulation and awareness, fear extinction, viscerosomatic processing (interoception, multimodal integration), and salience (homeostatic balance).

DIAGNOSIS
Diagnostic Criteria

Traditionally, FND was a "diagnosis of exclusion" but is now a "rule in" diagnosis.[12] To be diagnosed with an FND, per the DSM-5, the following four criteria must be met:[3]

1. Criteria A: One or more symptoms of altered voluntary motor or sensory function.
2. Criteria B: Clinical findings provide evidence of incompatibility between the symptom and recognized neurologic or medical conditions. To show this, you must have physical examination (PE) findings that support the incompatibility.
3. Criteria C: The symptom or deficit is not better explained by another medical or mental (health) disorder.
4. Criteria D: The symptom or deficit causes clinically significant distress or impairment in social, occupational, or other important areas of functioning or warrants medical evaluation.

Motor Symptoms

Motor symptoms can be classified into negative symptoms, where you have loss of function (eg, weakness, reduced movement), or positive symptoms, where you have excessive movement (tremor, jerks, dystonia). The movements can last or be in short episodes, which permits the diagnosis of pseudoseizure to be under this category.

Physical Examination

The PE is an important component for the diagnosis of FND. In general, the examiner evaluates for inconsistencies in what is being reported compared with what is observed during the evaluation.[14,15] Signs of increased effort such as expressive behavior[16] or grimacing, huffing, and puffing[17] before a motor movement, and changes with distraction, are consistent with FND.[14,15] Aybek and Perez[15] published an excellent review of the examination findings that help "rule in" FND, as summarized in **Table 1**. PE findings that correlate with specific FND subtypes are discussed below.

Neurodiagnostic Studies

To support Criterion C of the DSM-5 criteria for diagnosis of an FND, a medical workup, including imaging and other studies, may be necessary to rule out other neurologic conditions or comorbidities. Studies that may be consider include CT-head, MRI studies, electromyography (EMG), electroencephalogram (EEG), and lumbar punctures (LPs). In a study of patients with FND by Watson and colleagues,[7] head CTs were normal, MRIs and LPs were unremarkable, and EEG findings did not correlate with the PE. A recent study by Pal and colleagues[6] found that head CTs were normal, and there were some abnormalities seen on MRI and in the LP in patients diagnosed with FND that strongly correlated with focal abnormalities found during the neurologist's PE. Thomsen and colleagues[18] performed a systematic review of potential biomarkers and found very few that have been validated in the diagnosis of FND.

Table 1
Physical examination signs suggestive of a functional movement disorder

Sign		Description	
Convergence spasm—oculomotor test		The patient stares at your finger that is 10 cm away at lateral end range for 5 s, then move your finger toward midline. If you see the presence of disconjugate gaze and miosis, it is a positive sign for a functional neurologic disorder.[15,62]	
Monoplegic leg drag		During gait, the "affected" leg is dragged like a piece of wood, without circumduction.[15,16,25]	
Falls toward support		When the patient loses their balance, they fall toward a source of support[15,16,25]	
Noneconomic posture		Look for postures while walking that require increased effort and balance, for example, excessive knee flexion[15,16,25]	
Discordance of arm/leg weakness		When assessing isolated motor strength, the movement cannot be performed, but the muscle is used during another maneuver[15,63]	
Co-contracture		When testing a muscle, no movement at a joint is noted due to co-contracture of the agonist and antagonist muscles.[15,16]	
Hoover sign		Ask the patient to flex the hip on the strong side, while evaluating the hip extensors on the "weak" side for involuntary movement (if lying, put hand under heel; if sitting, place hand under thigh). Then test the hip extensor on the "weak" side. If involuntary movement is stronger than voluntary, then positive for a functional neurologic disorder.[15,16]	
Abductor sign		While sitting, ask the patient to abduct the legs against resistance. Observe or feel for involuntary abduction of the weak leg- if it occurs, it is a sign of FND[15,64]	
Functional Romberg		Large amount of imbalance during Romberg task without falling, usually gets better with distraction (drawing number in the back, cognitive task)[15,16]	
Functional tremors	Distractibility	The tremor pauses or changes amplitude/ frequency during a different motor and/ or mental task	Presence of two out of three signs is highly specific and sensitive for a functional tremor[15,24]
	Increase amplitude with weight	The tremor increases in amplitude when a 50 g weight is wrapped around the wrists (or holding a larger weight).	
	Entrainment	Have the patient imitate a tapping motion with one hand and watch the tremor affecting the other hand change in frequency	

(continued on next page)

Table 1 (continued)	
Sign	**Description**
Whack a mole sign	Tremors spreads to other limbs if the affected limb is restrained

COMMON SUBTYPES
Functional Seizure Disorder

FSD, otherwise known as pseudoseizures, or psychogenic non-epileptic seizures are a common presentation of FND. They are paroxysmal and self-limiting, and consist of "alterations in physical or cognitive functioning, behaviors, sensations (paresthesias) or awareness."[19] These may be accompanied by jerking movements, eye rolling or excessive blinking, and grunting. One study of patients with seizure-like activity admitted to a tertiary care children's hospital found that approximately 25% of all admissions to their Epilepsy Monitoring Unit were secondary to an FSD.[20]

Research is ongoing to help identify behaviors that help distinguish an FSD from an epileptic seizure. Izadyer and colleagues[21] evaluated the following behaviors in a population of patients with FSD: (1) abrupt, brief, and rapid blinking or shaking of the head as if regaining sensorium or "coming out" of the ictal event; (2) looking around the room with a scanning and uncertain look; and (3) posing a question of "what happened?" or a similar question to the others present in the room. They found that they were highly specific but not necessarily sensitive, as only 20.1% of the patients on chart review had one of these findings.[21] Compared with patients with an epileptic seizure, patients with an FSD had a longer ictal state, but a shorter time to follow commands after the event. They were more likely to have an altered voice when responding and perform the initial command incorrectly.[21] The gold standard to diagnosis FSD is to capture the event using Video EEG.[19]

Functional Movement Disorder

FMDs are characterized by abnormal, involuntary, hypo-or hyperkinetic movements that are inconsistent with a known neurologic disorder.[12,19] Movements can be tremors, tics, myoclonus, dystonia (blepharospasm, focal limb dystonia), weakness, or gait abnormalities.[22] PE findings are inconsistent and variable. For example, movements will increase with attention and decrease with distraction. FMDs are more likely to be chronic and disabling when compared with movements related to functional seizures.[19] There are several validated clinical examination findings (see **Table 1**) that can "rule in" the diagnosis.[16] Specific subtypes of FMD include the following:

- *Functional tremor disorder:* These tremors tend to start abruptly. They will affect the arms, legs, head, and whole body. During the PE, the tremor can increase in severity and complexity during direct observation but will attenuate during tasks that distract the patient. Common examination findings consistent with a functional tremor include entrainment, attenuation with distraction, increase of the tremor with the limb weighted down, and the "whack-a-mole" sign.[15,23,24]
- *Functional gait disorder:* One study found that approximately 40% of patients diagnosed with an FMD in a movement disorder clinic had a gait component.[25] Nonnekes and colleagues[25] suggested classifying the gait disturbance into one of seven categories (ataxic gait, spastic gait, weak gait, antalgic gait,

parkinsonism gait, hemiparetic gait, and dystonic gait), and then looking for PE findings that are inconsistent with that gait pattern.

- *Functional dystonia:* Functional dystonia was one of the earliest movements identified as an FMD, and historically, many organic dystonias were initially misclassified as an FMD. Limbs with a fixed posture at rest are highly suggestive of a functional dystonia, as most organic dystonias worsen with movement. Postures, including unilateral jaw or lip deviation, laterocollis with ipsilateral shoulder elevation and contralateral shoulder depression, fixed ankle plantarflexion with inversion, and fixed finger and wrist flexion with sparing of the first and second fingers are highly common in functional dystonias.[26]
- *Functional tic disorder:* These tic movements are identical to movements made by patients with Tourette's syndrome, which complicates the diagnosis of a functional tic disorder. Ways to distinguish a functional tic from a tic related to Tourette's include: an inability to "suppress" the tics, interference with motor movements, lack of premotion, and atypical response to tic medications.[26–29]
- *Social media tic disorder:* This is a newer FMD phenomenon. With the advent of social media, videos of various neurologic symptoms and behaviors are now widely available. Hull and colleagues[27] described a cohort of patients who developed a functional tic disorder after watching a specific patient with tics on TikTok. These tics consisted of neck movements (flexion/extension/shoulder elevation and concurrent "whoo" sound), punching/slapping of the face, punching the contralateral hand, clapping, clicking, whistling, "jazz hands," "hang-loose sign," throwing objects and blowing kisses. They would have a "Tic attack" which was an "episode of insuppressible involuntary movements and vocalizations of increased frequency and severity, with a clear beginning and end."[26,27]

Functional Vision Disorders

FVDs are characterized by a "decrease in vision acuity or visual field without an anatomic or physiologic basis."[30] It can present as central or peripheral vision loss, affecting one or both eyes; or, as diplopia, distortions, gaze palsy, ptosis, or accommodation spasm.[31] The incidence can range from 0.5% to 5% in ophthalmology practices,[31] A recent study by Daniel found the incidence in a pediatric clinic to be 3.5% (95% confidence interval of 2.9% to 4.4%).[32]

Diagnosing an FVD begins with close observation. Patients may exaggerate their movements or bump into objects more often than expected for their degree of vision loss if from an organic condition. The "sunglasses sign," where the patient comes into the office wearing sunglasses but does not have an underlying reason for photophobia, is a common finding in FVDs.[30] PE maneuvers that can help distinguish an FVD from a non-FVD for both monocular and binocular FVD are specified in **Table 2**.[30]

MANAGEMENT
Communicating the Diagnosis

As FNDs cause significant distress to the patient and family, appropriate communication of the diagnosis, including what symptoms are consistent with an FND, and setting the expectation for recovery, is essential in helping patients and families accept the diagnosis and prepare for treatment.[33,34] Pierce and Albert[35] recommend the following while communicating the diagnosis.

- Name the diagnosis
- Legitimatize concerns

Table 2
Specialized tests for functional vision disorders

Fogging test	The ophthalmologist will use a stronger lens to "fog" the patient's good eye and use a weaker lens on the affected eye. The stronger lens is increased gradually to the point where the visual acuity seen is what is in the "weaker eye"[30,65]
Prism test	Prism is placed in front of the good eye, and patient is asked if they see one or two objects. If they report two, that is suspicious for a functional vision disorder[30,66]
Red-green color test	The patient is given glasses with one red lens and one green lens, and read a chart with red and green letters. The letters can only be seen with their respective lens, and if they can read them, that is suspicious for a functional vision disorder.[30,67]
Pupil response	Using a light to check the pupillary light reflex.
Optokinetic test	An optokinetic drum (or any black and white object) is rotated slowly in front of the patient, which leads to a smooth pursuit, and quick saccade as patient refocus. If fast and slow nystagmus reflexes are seen, it suggests that the vision is 20/200.[30,68]
Saccadic test for visual field loss	The examiner can frame this as a test of eye movements rather than vision. The patient starts by looking at a small target in their visual field, which is then moved outside the alleged visual field in random. If the patient has saccadic movement to the target, it shows the visual field is intact.[30,65]

- Explain the mechanism (analogies help, ie, the hardware is intact, but the software is malfunctioning)
- Show the examination. Point out any "rule-in" signs.
- Lastly, the physician should make a treatment plan with the patient and emphasize that the condition can improve.

Stone and colleagues[36] produced a series of videos[37,38] that can help clinicians explain the diagnosis of FND, which are available to view online. Online sources (www.neurosymptoms.org [39], Functional Neurologic Disorder | National Institute of Neurologic Disorders and Stroke [nih.gov]),[40] can also assist with explaining the disorder and various treatments.

Once the diagnosis has been communicated, it is important to create an action plan for when functional symptoms occur, to minimize the use of the emergency room and prevent iatrogenic harm (especially in the situation of receiving treatment of FS). Depending on the subtype of FND, the patient may benefit from different treatment modalities.

Interdisciplinary Care

Treatment of FND often involves multiple specialists, including physiatry, neurology, psychiatry, psychology, and rehabilitation therapies. Interdisciplinary care can occur in the inpatient setting or as part of a multidisciplinary outpatient clinic. Interventions in these settings can have medical, psychological, rehabilitative, and educational components.[41] Interdisciplinary care has been effective in treating FSD[42] and FMDs[43,44] In Pediatrics, the pediatric physiatrist is uniquely positioned to act as a team coordinator to manage patients with FNDs in the inpatient and outpatient setting with our expertise in function and experience leading multidisciplinary teams.

Psychotherapy

Psychotherapy appears to be beneficial for all patients with an FND.[12,33,41,45] Psychotherapy can consist of Psychoeducation, Cognitive Behavioral Therapy, Behavioral Approaches, Biofeedback, Eye Movement and Desensitization Reprocessing (EMDR), and Hypnosis.[41]

- *Psychoeducation* explaining the diagnosis of FND and the underlying psychological components is usually the first part of an FND treatment program. It is difficult to say that it is beneficial independently, but it has been associated with positive outcomes in case studies and as part of clinical pathways for FND.[41]
- *Cognitive behavioral therapy (CBT)* has the most evidence to support its use in FND. It addresses the underlying psychological and behavioral mechanisms of the disorder. CBT can help the patient's identify and recognize their warning signs and triggers, and provide ways for the patient to regain control of their body.[19] Retraining and control therapy (ReACT) has been shown in a randomized control trial to be effective for functional seizures,[46] and a study by Robinson and colleagues[47] found that CBT facilitated a reduction in movement symptoms in children with FMD with 78% achieving full remission.[41]
- *Behavioral approaches* have been used to *treat* FND. These approaches focus on decreasing reinforcement of the child's functional symptoms and increasing reinforcement for other more desirable behaviors. The use of a reward system for achieving daily goals is an example of a behavioral approach.[48]
- *Biofeedback* is a procedure to enable the voluntary modulation of physiologic responses through the provision of explicit (visual or auditory) feedback of covert physiologic signal.[49] Although biofeedback has been used in the treatment of FNDs, its effectiveness is largely unstudied.[41] Only one study has looked at using biofeedback with CBT as part of a treatment program in CBT, but they were unable to definitively determine how effective Biofeedback was, as it was part of the comprehensive program.[50]
- *Eye movement and desensitization reprocessing (EMDR) therapy* is an 8-phase treatment protocol that utilizes eye movements, taps, and tone during the desensitization and reprocessing phases.[51] A case series by Demiri and Sagaltici in 2021 found that EMDR therapy was helpful for two patients with functional seizures and suggestive that it may be helpful in other FND's.[41,51]
- *Hypnosis* is another therapy that is being evaluated as potentially beneficial for patients with FND. A recent case report by Coogle and colleagues[52] used the "Magic Glove Technique," which is a form of hypnosis, to help a child with pain and lower limb weakness in their recovery. Hypnosis was originally used in the historical treatment of FND by Charcot,[2] and may have more utilization in the future.

Intensive Inpatient Rehabilitation Programs

An inpatient rehabilitation program (IPR) should be considered when the patient has a significant loss of function such as the inability to perform their age-appropriate self-care activities or ambulate independently secondary to FND. To determine eligibility for an IPR for FND, children should be assessed by a physiatrist, physical therapist, and occupational therapist to assess their current level of function in the domains of activities of daily living and mobility, along with a psychologist. If their current level of function is below their baseline, then they are eligible to participate in an IPR program. During the IPR program, the child must show ongoing improvements in function as evidence that the program is effective. In the IPR programs described by Bolger and colleagues[53] and Butz and colleagues,[43] children participated in a multidisciplinary treatment program consisting of physical therapy (PT), occupational therapy (OT), recreational therapy (RT), a school liaison, and psychology. Butz and colleagues[43] program used a "goal mountain," which listed the skills required to achieve their goals in a hierarchical manner, which was communicated to the patient and family. The patient needed to master each "step" before advancing to the next higher goal during their therapy sessions, until they were ready for discharge.[43] In both studies, patients in IPR showed improvements in the motor domains of the pediatric version of the Functional Independence Measure (WEEFIM) indicating more functional independence.[43,53]

Physical Therapy

PT has been shown to be a first-line intervention as part of a comprehensive program for patients with FND.[41,45,54] It is most commonly used with the following symptoms: motor symptoms, physical deconditioning, pain, and orthostasis.[41,55] PT works by encouraging normal movement patterns to improve a patient's physical functioning.[55] This can occur as part of an IPR[43,48,53,56,57] or an outpatient PT program. .[41,54,58]

More recently, the term "psychologically informed PT" has been used to describe a focus on wellness in PT.[44] The goal is to improve an individual's resilience and their ability to respond to changes in their body. Gray and colleagues[59] published an excellent review of psychologically based PT. In psychological-based PT, the physical therapist utilizes active listening, and acknowledgment of the child's experience while providing reassurance to improve interpersonal relationships and create a "safe space" for PT. The PT actively shifts the focus of attention from the symptoms experienced by the patient to the task at hand, bringing attention to and reinforcing the appropriate movement patterns during the activity, and emphasize the mind-body strategies being taught by psychology to control any symptoms experienced by the child during the PT session.[59] In three cohorts of children with mixed FND symptoms (motor, seizure-like, sensory, cognitive, and pain) using this approach as part of a multidisciplinary rehabilitation program, there were improvements in 54/57 (95%), 51/60 (85%), and 22/25 (88%) of children.[41,44]

PROGNOSIS

Long-term outcomes of FNDs are not well described in the literature. A systemic review by Gelauff and colleagues in 2014[60] of 24 studies looking at patients with functional movement symptoms showed that 39% of patients had the same or worsening symptoms at follow-up, with high levels of disability. A recent chart review by Raper and colleagues[61] showed that out of 114 children who were diagnosed with FND (of which, 18% had functional seizure, 18% had sensory loss and 16% had motor symptoms), 23% continued to have symptoms at age 21.[35,61] Positive prognostic factors include short duration of symptoms, early diagnosis, and high satisfaction with care.[30,60,45]

SUMMARY

FNDs are common in the pediatric population. Timely diagnosis and use of a multidisciplinary team including pediatric physiatrists, neurologists, psychiatrists, psychologists, and physical therapists can lead to improvement in a patient's symptoms.

CLINICS CARE POINTS

- Functional neurologic disorders are common in the pediatric population, but the exact incidence is unknown.
- Functional neurologic disorders can present as movement disorders, seizure-like activity, and vision disorders.
- Inconsistencies in the physical examination can rule in a diagnosis of a functional neurologic disorder.
- Communication of the diagnosis of functional neurologic disorder can impact the patient's response to treatment of the functional neurologic disorder.
- Psychological therapies and physical therapies are effective for treating functional neurologic disorders.
- Pediatric physiatrists are uniquely positioned to lead an interdisciplinary team for the management of functional neurologic disorders.

DISCLOSURE

The author has nothing to disclose.

REFERENCES

1. Functional Neurologic Disorder. 09-04-2022. Available at: https://rarediseases.org/rare-diseases/fnd/.
2. Raynor G, Baslet G. A historical review of functional neurological disorder and comparison to contemporary models. Epilepsy Behav Rep 2021;16:100489.
3. Association AP. Diagnostic and statistical manual of mental disorders. 5th edition. Washington, DC: American Psychiatric Publishing; 2013.
4. Stephen CD, Fung V, Lungu CI, et al. Assessment of Emergency Department and Inpatient Use and Costs in Adult and Pediatric Functional Neurological Disorders. JAMA Neurol 2021;78(1):88–101.
5. Hull M, Parnes M, Jankovic J. Increased Incidence of Functional (Psychogenic) Movement Disorders in Children and Adults Amid the COVID-19 Pandemic: A Cross-sectional Study. Neurol Clin Pract 2021;11(5):e686–90.
6. Pal R. Pediatric Functional Neurological Disorder:Demographic and Clinical Factors Impacting Care. J Child Neurol 2022. https://doi.org/10.1177/08830738221113899.
7. Watson C, Sivaswamy L, Agarwal R, et al. Functional Neurologic Symptom Disorder in Children: Clinical Features, Diagnostic Investigations, and Outcomes at a Tertiary Care Children's Hospital. J Child Neurol 2019;34(6):325–31.
8. Huys AML, Bhatia KP, Edwards MJ, et al. The Flip Side of Distractibility-Executive Dysfunction in Functional Movement Disorders. Front Neurol 2020;11:969.
9. van Wouwe NC, Mohanty D, Lingaiah A, et al. Impaired Action Control in Patients With Functional Movement Disorders. J Neuropsychiatry Clin Neurosci. Winter 2020;32(1):73–8.
10. Perez DL, Nicholson TR, Asadi-Pooya AA, et al. Neuroimaging in Functional Neurological Disorder: State of the Field and Research Agenda. Neuroimage Clin 2021;30:102623.
11. Baizabal-Carvallo JF, Hallett M, Jankovic J. Pathogenesis and pathophysiology of functional (psychogenic) movement disorders. Neurobiol Dis 2019;127:32–44.

12. Kola S, LaFaver K. Updates in Functional Movement Disorders: from Pathophysiology to Treatment Advances. Curr Neurol Neurosci Rep 2022;22(5):305–11.
13. Diez I. Reduced limbic microstructural integrity in functional neurological disorder. Psychology Medicine 2021;51(3):485–93.
14. Baizabal-Carvallo JF, Jankovic J. Functional (psychogenic) stereotypies. J Neurol 2017;264(7):1482–7.
15. Aybek S, Perez DL. Diagnosis and management of functional neurological disorder. BMJ 2022;376:o64.
16. Daum C, Gheorghita F, Spatola M, et al. Interobserver agreement and validity of bedside 'positive signs' for functional weakness, sensory and gait disorders in conversion disorder: a pilot study. J Neurol Neurosurg Psychiatry 2015;86(4):425–30.
17. Laub HN, Dwivedi AK, Revilla FJ, et al. Diagnostic performance of the "Huffing and Puffing" sign in psychogenic (functional) movement disorders. Mov Disord Clin Pract 2015;2(1):29–32.
18. Thomsen BLC, Teodoro T, Edwards MJ. Biomarkers in functional movement disorders: a systematic review. J Neurol Neurosurg Psychiatry 2020;91(12):1261–9.
19. Kola S, LaFaver K. Functional movement disorder and functional seizures: What have we learned from different subtypes of functional neurological disorders? Epilepsy Behav Rep 2022;18:100510.
20. Doss JL, Plioplys S. Pediatric Psychogenic Nonepileptic Seizures: A Concise Review. Child Adolesc Psychiatr Clin N Am 2018;27(1):53–61.
21. Izadyar S, Shah V, James B. Comparison of postictal semiology and behavior in psychogenic nonepileptic and epileptic seizures. Epilepsy Behav 2018;88:123–9.
22. Espay AJ, Lang AE. Phenotype-specific diagnosis of functional (psychogenic) movement disorders. Curr Neurol Neurosci Rep 2015;15(6):32.
23. Schwingenschuh P, Espay AJ. Functional tremor. J Neurol Sci 2022;435:120208.
24. van der Stouwe AM, Elting JW, van der Hoeven JH, et al. How typical are 'typical' tremor characteristics? Sensitivity and specificity of five tremor phenomena. Parkinsonism Relat Disord 2016;30:23–8.
25. Nonnekes J, Ruzicka E, Serranova T, et al. Functional gait disorders: A sign-based approach. Neurology 2020;94(24):1093–9.
26. Larsh T, Wilson J, Mackenzie KM, et al. Diagnosis and Initial Treatment of Functional Movement Disorders in Children. Semin Pediatr Neurol 2022;41:100953.
27. Hull M, Parnes M. Tics and TikTok: Functional Tics Spread Through Social Media. Mov Disord Clin Pract 2021;8(8):1248–52.
28. Baizabal-Carvallo JF, Jankovic J. The clinical features of psychogenic movement disorders resembling tics. J Neurol Neurosurg Psychiatry 2014;85(5):573–5.
29. Baizabal-Carvallo JF, Fekete R. Recognizing uncommon presentations of psychogenic (functional) movement disorders. Tremor Other Hyperkinet Mov (N Y) 2015;5:279.
30. Raviskanthan S, Wendt S, Ugoh PM, et al. Functional vision disorders in adults: a paradigm and nomenclature shift for ophthalmology. Surv Ophthalmol 2022;67(1):8–18.
31. Phansalkar R, Lockman AJ, Bansal S, et al. Management of Functional Vision Disorders. Curr Neurol Neurosci Rep 2022;22(4):265–73.
32. Daniel MC, Coughtrey A, Heyman I, et al. Medically unexplained visual loss in children and young people: an observational single site study of incidence and outcomes. Eye 2017;31(7):1068–73.

33. Weiss KE, Steinman KJ, Kodish I, et al. Functional Neurological Symptom Disorder in Children and Adolescents within Medical Settings. J Clin Psychol Med Settings 2021;28(1):90–101.
34. Yam A, Rickards T, Pawlowski CA, et al. Interdisciplinary rehabilitation approach for functional neurological symptom (conversion) disorder: A case study. Rehabil Psychol 2016;61(1):102–11.
35. Pierce ME, Albert DVF. Delivering the Diagnosis: A Practical Approach to a Patient With a Functional Neurological Disorder. Semin Pediatr Neurol 2022;41: 100948. https://doi.org/10.1016/j.spen.2021.100948.
36. Stone J, Hoeritzauer I. How Do I Explain the Diagnosis of Functional Movement Disorder to a Patient? Mov Disord Clin Pract 2019;6(5):419.
37. Stone J. How Do I Explain the Diagnosis of Functional Movement Disorder to a Patient?. Available at: https://www.youtube.com/watch?v=w4lqr4Mo32M. Accessed 12.07.2022.
38. Stone J. How Do I Explain the Diagnosis of Functional Movement Disorder to a Patient?. Available at: https://movementdisorders.onlinelibrary.wiley.com/page/journal/23301619/homepage/mdc312785-sup-v001.htm. Accessed 12.07.2022.
39. FND guide JS. Available at: www.neurosymptoms.org. Accessed 09.23.22.
40. Stroke NIoNDa. Updated 8-22-2021. Available at: https://www.ninds.nih.gov/functional-neurologic-disorder. Accessed 09.23.2022.
41. Elliott L, Carberry C. Treatment of Pediatric Functional Neurological Symptom Disorder: A Review of the State of the Literature. Semin Pediatr Neurol 2022;41: 100952.
42. Terry D, Enciso L, Trott K, et al. Outcomes in Children and Adolescents With Psychogenic Nonepileptic Events Using a Multidisciplinary Clinic Approach. J Child Neurol 2020;35(13):918–23.
43. Butz C, Iske C, Truba N, et al. Treatment of Functional Gait Abnormality in a Rehabilitation Setting: Emphasizing the Physical Interventions for Treating the Whole Child. Innov Clin Neurosci 2019;16(7–08):18–21.
44. Kasia K, Nicola G, Stephen S, et al. Psychologically informed physiotherapy as part of a multidisciplinary rehabilitation program for children and adolescents with functional neurological disorder: Physical and mental health outcomes. J Paediatr Child Health 2021;57(1):73–9.
45. Espay AJ, Aybek S, Carson A, et al. Current Concepts in Diagnosis and Treatment of Functional Neurological Disorders. JAMA Neurol 2018;75(9):1132–41.
46. Fobian AD, Long DM, Szaflarski JP. Retraining and control therapy for pediatric psychogenic non-epileptic seizures. Ann Clin Transl Neurol 2020;7(8):1410–9.
47. Robinson S, Bhatoa RS, Owen T, et al. Functional neurological movements in children: Management with a psychological approach. Eur J Paediatr Neurol 2020; 28:101–9.
48. Gooch JL, Wolcott R, Speed J. Behavioral management of conversion disorder in children. Arch Phys Med Rehabil 1997;78(3):264–8.
49. Nagai Y. Autonomic biofeedback therapy in epilepsy. Epilepsy Res 2019; 153:76–8.
50. Sawchuk T, Buchhalter J, Senft B. Psychogenic nonepileptic seizures in children-Prospective validation of a clinical care pathway & risk factors for treatment outcome. Epilepsy Behav 2020;105:106971.
51. Demirci OO, Sagaltici E. Eye movement desensitization and reprocessing treatment in functional neurological symptom disorder with psychogenic nonepileptic seizures: A study of two cases. Clin Child Psychol Psychiatry 2021;26(4): 1196–207.

52. Coogle J, Coogle B, Quezada J. Hypnosis in the Treatment of Pediatric Functional Neurological Disorder: The Magic Glove Technique. Pediatr Neurol 2021; 125:20–5.
53. Bolger A, Collins A, Michels M, et al. Characteristics and Outcomes of Children With Conversion Disorder Admitted to a Single Inpatient Rehabilitation Unit, A Retrospective Study. Pharm Manag PM R 2018;10(9):910–6.
54. Maggio JB, Ospina JP, Callahan J, et al. Outpatient Physical Therapy for Functional Neurological Disorder: A Preliminary Feasibility and Naturalistic Outcome Study in a U.S. Cohort. *J Neuropsychiatry Clin Neurosci*. Winter 2020;32(1):85–9.
55. Kim YN, Gray N, Jones A, et al. The Role of Physiotherapy in the Management of Functional Neurological Disorder in Children and Adolescents. Semin Pediatr Neurol 2022;41:100947.
56. Kanarek SL, Stevenson JE, Wakefield H, et al. Inpatient rehabilitation approach for a young woman with conversion hemiparesis and sensory deficits. *PM R*. Jan 2013;5(1):66–9.
57. Chudleigh C, Kozlowska K, Kothur K, et al. Managing non-epileptic seizures and psychogenic dystonia in an adolescent girl with preterm brain injury. Harv Rev Psychiatry 2013;21(3):163–74.
58. Nielsen G, Buszewicz M, Stevenson F, et al. Randomised feasibility study of physiotherapy for patients with functional motor symptoms. J Neurol Neurosurg Psychiatry 2017;88(6):484–90.
59. Gray N, Savage B, Scher S, et al. Psychologically Informed Physical Therapy for Children and Adolescents With Functional Neurological Symptoms: The Wellness Approach. *J Neuropsychiatry Clin Neurosci*. Fall 2020;32(4):389–95.
60. Gelauff J, Stone J, Edwards M, et al. The prognosis of functional (psychogenic) motor symptoms: a systematic review. J Neurol Neurosurg Psychiatry 2014;85(2): 220–6.
61. Raper J, Currigan V, Fothergill S, et al. Long-term outcomes of functional neurological disorder in children. Arch Dis Child 2019;104(12):1155–60.
62. Fekete R, Baizabal-Carvallo JF, Ha AD, et al. Convergence spasm in conversion disorders: prevalence in psychogenic and other movement disorders compared with controls. J Neurol Neurosurg Psychiatry 2012;83(2):202–4.
63. Chabrol H, Peresson G, Clanet M. Lack of specificity of the traditional criteria for conversion disorders. Eur Psychiatry 1995;10(6):317–9.
64. Sonoo M. Abductor sign: a reliable new sign to detect unilateral non-organic paresis of the lower limb. J Neurol Neurosurg Psychiatry 2004;75(1):121–5.
65. Chen CS, Lee AW, Karagiannis A, et al. Practical clinical approaches to functional visual loss. J Clin Neurosci 2007;14(1):1–7.
66. Mojon DS, Flueckiger P. A new optotype chart for detection of nonorganic visual loss. Ophthalmology 2002;109(4):810–5.
67. Bruce BB, Newman NJ. Functional visual loss. Neurol Clin 2010;28(3):789–802.
68. Beatty S. Non-organic visual loss. Postgrad Med J 1999;75(882):201–7.

Physical Activity and Sports Participation among Children and Adolescents with Disabilities

Mary E. Dubon, MD[a,b,c,*], Stephanie Tow, MD[d,e,1],
Amy E. Rabatin, MD[f,g,h]

KEYWORDS

- Disability • Sport • Children • Physical activity

KEY POINTS

- Physical activity is important for everyone.
- In general, children with disabilities should participate in the same amount of physical activity as their peers.
- Children with disabilities generally participate in less physical activity than recommended.
- Health care providers can be key players in helping to improve physical activity participation in children with disabilities.

INTRODUCTION

Physical activity has known physical, social, and mental health benefits, yet there are known disparities in access to physical activity for children and adolescents with disabilities. It is of paramount importance for all health care providers who care for

[a] Division of Pediatric Rehabilitation Medicine, Department of Physical Medicine and Rehabilitation, Spaulding Rehabilitation Hospital/Harvard Medical School, Boston, MA, USA; [b] Department of Physical Medicine and Rehabilitation, Kelley Adaptive Sports Research Institute, Spaulding Rehabilitation Hospital, Harvard Medical School, Boston, MA, USA; [c] Department of Orthopedics & Sports Medicine, Boston Children's Hospital, 300 Longwood Avenue, Boston, MA 02115, USA; [d] US Paralympics Swimming; [e] University of Colorado, Anschutz Medical Campus, Children's Hospital Colorado, Aurora, USA; [f] Division of Pediatric Rehabilitation Medicine, Department of Physical Medicine and Rehabilitation, 200 1st Street Southwest, Rochester, MN 55905, USA; [g] Department of Pediatric, Mayo Clinic, 200 1st Street Southwest, Rochester, MN 55905, USA; [h] Department of Adolescent Medicine, Mayo Clinic, 200 1st Street Southwest, Rochester, MN 55905, USA

[1] Present address: 2342 N Xenia Street, Denver, CO 80238.
* Corresponding author. Department of Sports Medicine, Boston Children's Hospital, 300 Longwood Avenue, Boston, MA 02115.
E-mail address: Mary.dubon@childrens.harvard.edu

Pediatr Clin N Am 70 (2023) 603–614
https://doi.org/10.1016/j.pcl.2023.01.009
0031-3955/23/© 2023 Elsevier Inc. All rights reserved.

pediatric.theclinics.com

children and adolescents with disabilities to promote physical activity for the health and well-being of the population they serve.[1] In this article, we review the basics of physical activity and sports for children with disabilities and ways to help overcome barriers to participation.

Definitions

When discussing physical activity and sports participation with individuals with disabilities, it is important to understand some basic definitions and organizations. Para sports refers to sports that are in "parallel" to sports in the general population. It is an umbrella term for sports for individuals with disabilities and generally refers to Paralympic-style sports.[2] The Paralympics is the elite sporting competition that is in parallel to the Olympics.[3] There are a number of eligible impairments, including blindness/low vision and numerous physical disabilities. There are also some Paralympic-style sports where athletes with intellectual disabilities can qualify.[4]

Some Paralympic-style sports are adaptive sports, meaning that they are adapted from sports in the general population. An example of this is wheelchair basketball, which is adapted from mainstream basketball to accommodate athletes with disabilities. Other Paralympic-style Para sports, such as goalball, are not adaptive sports as there is no comparable sport in the general population.[2]

As mentioned, although there are some Paralympic-style sports where athletes with intellectual disabilities can qualify, Special Olympics is the largest organization for sports programs and competitions for athletes with intellectual disabilities and includes novice to elite programming and events. Special Olympics sports programs start at age 8, but the Young Athlete Program serves athletes ages 2 through 7.[5,6] The International Committee of Sports for the Deaf (ICSD) is the committee that organizes the Deaflympics and World Deaf Championships for elite deaf athletes.[7,8]

Although the above are organized sporting organizations with mostly elite-level programs and competitions, there are many other community programs that provide sports opportunities for athletes with disabilities. It is also important to note that athletes with disabilities may participate in sporting programs specific to athletes with disabilities, as those mentioned above, and/or participate in programs that are inclusive of athletes with and without disabilities (eg, Unified Sports, a program through Special Olympics in which athletes with intellectual disabilities participate alongside athletes without intellectual disabilities),[6,9] and/or participate in mainstream sports programs that are not specifically for athletes with disabilities (eg, a child with a lower limb amputation may participate on his/her local community baseball team). Health care providers should work together with their patients and their families on promoting physical activity and sports participation that best meets the needs of their patients.

History of Adaptive Sports

Opportunities for sports and physical activity for athletes with disabilities have evolved immensely over the past two centuries (**Table 1**).[10–16] The population of people with disabilities increased in the late 1700s as advances in medicine drastically improved the survival rates and recovery from medical conditions that previously had high complication and mortality rates. Attention to a growing population of people with disabilities again increased in the 1900s as veterans from World Wars I and II returned with disabilities but otherwise in good health. Gradually, as society's medical understanding of conditions causing disability and civil rights in this population improved, attention shifted toward other needs, such as physical activity, sports, and recreation.[10]

Founded in 1888, the Sports Club for the Deaf is one of the first organizations developed for athletes benefiting from sports adaptations. The first International Silent Games

Table 1	
History of adaptive sports[1,10–15]	
Year	**Historical Event**
1888	Sports Club for the Deaf founded
1924	First International Silent Games for deaf athletes
1948	Stoke Mandeville Games organized by Sir Ludwig Guttmann
1956	National Wheelchair Athletic Association (later became Adaptive Sports USA) founded
1967	National Amputee Skiers Association (later became Disabled Sports USA) founded
1968	First International Special Olympics event hosted in Chicago, Illinois
1978	Cerebral Palsy International Sports and Recreation Association founded
2020	Adaptive Sports USA and Disabled Sports USA merge to become Move United

for deaf athletes occurred in 1924 in Paris, France, and has since evolved into the Deaflympics—the oldest known adaptive sporting event. In 1948, Sir Ludwig Guttmann, a German-British neurologist who opened a spinal cord injury center at Stoke Mandeville Hospital in Great Britain during World War II, organized the Stoke Mandeville Games in England, an Olympic-style wheelchair archery competition.[10] Held on the Opening Ceremony day of the London 1948 Olympic Games, the Stoke Mandeville Games is often credited to be the origin of the Paralympic Movement.[11] Over time, the Stoke Mandeville Games grew to be an international movement and eventually into the Paralympic Games, inclusive of athletes with physical, visual, and intellectual impairments.[12,13]

Thereafter, the mid-1900s saw a significant increase in organizations, events, and opportunities focused on adaptive sports, recreation, and physical activity. In the United States, organizations such as Adaptive Sports USA (founded as the National Wheelchair Athletic Association in 1956) and Disabled Sports USA (founded as the National Amputee Skiers Association in 1967) increased organized sporting opportunities nationwide for people with disabilities in the United States.[10,14] Organized sporting opportunities for people with intellectual disabilities were developed and by 1968, the first International Special Olympics event was hosted in Chicago, Illinois.[10] In 1978, the Cerebral Palsy International Sports and Recreation Association (CPISRA) was founded to serve as the sporting organization for athletes with cerebral palsy (CP).[10,15] In 2020, Adaptive Sports USA and Disabled Sports USA merged to become Move United, a national organization dedicated to community-based adaptive sports programming.[16] Today, many organizations at the local, regional, national, and international levels exist to support the needs of adaptive sports, recreation, and physical activity opportunities, thus increasing opportunities for physical activity and participation in organized sports and recreation by children and adolescent athletes with disabilities.

DISCUSSION
Participation Trends

Participation in physical activity supports many aspects of development for children, including physical literacy, mobility, physical and mental health, and socialization.[17,18] In general, however, children are not participating in enough physical activity. An estimated 25% of children in the general population are participating in appropriate levels of physical activity.[19] For children with disabilities this rate is comparable or even lower.[1,18] General physical activity participation in children with CP is a fraction of that of peers and less than 30% of the recommended guidelines.[18] Children with disabilities are less likely to participate in sports if their level of participation in physical activity is low. In addition, sports participation is lower in children with functional and mobility impairments when compared with their peers with sensory, cognitive, or intellectual impairments.[20] Unfortunately, the low rate of physical activity participation in children with disabilities continues as they become adults with even a wider gap when compared with their peers without disabilities.[17] Physical literacy, enabling ability, confidence, and interest in physical activity, is also correlated with preference for physical activity as a child and into adulthood.[21] This can be positively influenced as well. Children with motor delays who receive programming to maximize potential and are encouraged to participate in free play and recess develop fundamental movement skills that may foster interest in physical activity, thus supporting long-term physical literacy.[1,21] In addition, in families where physical activity is a priority or who participate in physical activities themselves, promotion of and participation in physical activity increases for children with disabilities.[1]

Physical Activity Guidelines and Recommendations

The Department of Health and Human Services Physical Activity Guidelines for Americans, 2nd edition, was released in 2018. This guideline provides recommendations for physical activity for children and adolescents with and without disabilities, noting that, whenever possible, children and adolescents with disabilities should meet the same guidelines recommended for their age.[22] The American Academy of Pediatrics follows the same recommendations.[19] See **Table 2** for general recommendations.[19,22,23]

Physical activity recommendations for children with disabilities should consider their overall health status including exercise limitations due to medical conditions such as cardiac or pulmonary restrictions, individual activity preferences, safety precautions, and availability and feasibility of appropriate programs and equipment.[1,17,23] Programs should also include recommendations for balance, flexibility, and agility, as appropriate.[1] Referral to experts including pediatric rehabilitation medicine physicians, sports medicine physicians, and/or recreational, physical, and occupational therapists is also appropriate.

A "physical activity prescription" may also serve as a motivation and reminder supporting the physical activity guidelines.[1,23] A prescription may include goals for participation including amount and frequency, referrals to programs or resources, functional activity that may require adaptation, preparticipation planning, and evidence regarding risks and benefits.[1] For children, self-propelling a wheelchair for mobility, participating in wheelchair basketball or riding an adaptive bike might be recommended. For a child with more significant mobility limitations, a program for standing, mobilizing in a gait trainer, or playing on the floor with siblings or friends may provide an opportunity for increased heart rate and socialization.[17] Exercise programs may require adjustments based on specific disability-specific and patient-specific precautions and considerations.[17]

The goal is to promote participation and inclusion for all children in appropriate activities and empower them with a "can do" message. Again, referral to providers specializing in these type of adjustments and adaptations can be helpful.

Facilitators and Barriers

Personal factors and environmental factors can be either barriers or facilitators to physical activity participation in children and adolescents with disabilities. Knowledge of health benefits of physical activity, having self-confidence in athletic capabilities, social networks supportive of physical activity, and access to adaptive physical

Table 2		
Physical activity recommendations for children and adolescents with and without disabilities[19,22,23]		
Age	**Physical Activity Amount and Type**	**Examples**
Infants and young children	"Tummy time" and other interactive play, spread throughout each day	Tummy time, standing during activities, reaching activities
Preschool-aged children (3 to 5 years old)	Physical activity daily • Guidance includes target of 3 h daily of activity combining all intensities: light, moderate, and vigorous	Riding a bicycle or tricycle, playing throwing games and tag
Children and adolescents (6 to 17 years old)	Moderate-to-vigorous intensity physical activity at least 1 h daily—should be fun, varied and age-appropriate • *Aerobic exercises* that raise heart rate—at least 3 days per week • *Muscle-strengthening exercises* through strengthening/resistance exercises of muscles—at least 3 days per week • *Bone-strengthening exercises* through weight-bearing exercises—at least 3 days per week	• Aerobic exercises— swimming, running, jumping • Muscle-strengthening exercises—push-ups, tug-of-war, resistance bands, weights • Bone-strengthening exercises—running, jumping

activity resources are known facilitators for physical activity.[1,18] Medical/physical condition limitations, absence of social networks supportive of physical activity, and lack of access to adaptive physical activity resources are known barriers for physical activity.[1,18] Health care providers can be facilitators by being part of the positive social network encouraging children with disabilities to participate in physical activity and can help patients overcome barriers by working together on strategies for participation.[1] Health care providers can positively influence participation by asking physical activity vital sign questions, which is noted to increase participation in adults.[1,21] Health care providers are encouraged to "take the pledge" to discuss physical activity with their patients with disabilities through the Foundation for Physical Medicine and Rehabilitation Rx for Exercise website.[1,24] This website also includes additional information about prescribing exercise for individuals with disabilities, including a link to an instructional video on how to talk to pediatric patients with disabilities about physical activity.[25–27]

Benefits and risks

The benefits of physical activity are broad and universal. Just as for children and adolescents without disabilities, the benefits of physical activity for children and adolescents with disabilities include optimizing physical function, minimizing deconditioning, improving muscle and bone strength, increasing aerobic capacity, maintaining a healthy weight and body composition, supporting mental health and cognitive skills, and enhancing overall well-being.[1,17,18,23] When participating in physical activity, functional independence, quality of life, and social and community integration may be positively impacted throughout their lives.[18] As an example, exercise in children with autism has been correlated with reduced stereotypic movements, reduced maladaptive behaviors, and improved participation in school. Forming friendships, expressing creativity and self-identity are positive outcomes noted with sports participation.[1]

High rates of sedentary behavior are more common in children with disabilities putting them at higher risk of obesity and associated health conditions.[17] Inactivity can lead to earlier age-related cardiovascular, metabolic, and musculoskeletal changes, including reduced cardiovascular fitness, impaired fasting glucose, elevated blood lipids, and osteoporosis.[1,17,23] Higher rates of chronic medical conditions including coronary artery disease, diabetes, joint pain, and hypertension are seen in adults with CP than in age-matched peers without CP.[17] Psychosocial impact of reduced physical activity includes, for example, decreased self-esteem, decreased social acceptance, and possibly greater dependence on others for daily living.[1] Regular physical activity for children with disabilities has been shown to help in controlling or slowing the progression of chronic diseases.[1,17]

Consideration of risks for injury or illness is imperative before and during participation in physical activity and sports to ensure safe participation. Children with neuromuscular conditions may have abnormalities of thermoregulation secondary to impaired vasomotor control, decreased muscle mass, and impaired central temperature-regulating mechanisms putting them at risk for heat illness or hyperthermia. Children with spinal cord injuries at the T6 level or above are at risk of autonomic dysreflexia, and excessive sympathetic nervous system output, in the setting of noxious stimuli below the level of injury. It may also be self-inflicted as a method of "boosting," though this is a dangerous practice and is banned by sporting organizations.[1,28,29] Medications and side effects must also be taken into consideration. Musculoskeletal injuries and overuse injuries may occur in children with impaired motor coordination, apraxia, decreased endurance, limited mechanical efficiency, and osteopenia. Attention should also be paid to training, nutrition and hydration, clothing, and equipment type, including helmets as appropriate, and fit to promote safe participation.[1,29] Helmets are typically used in sports in which athletes may move at a rapid speed and therefore have an increased risk of head injury if they were to lose control and impact their head on a surface. Examples of such sports include wheelchair racing, cycling, adaptive skiing, sled hockey, and wheelchair motocross. Referral to experts including pediatric rehabilitation medicine physicians, sports medicine physicians, and/or recreational, physical, and occupational therapists may be beneficial in providing specialized guidance related to safe sports participation.

RECOMMENDATIONS
Approach to Physical Activity Participation during Patient Clinical Encounters

Once a comprehensive medical history and physical exam is performed and a patient is determined to be appropriate to actively participate in physical activity, it is important to discuss physical activity participation with patients and their families. Such discussions may require multiple clinical visits depending on the complexity of a patient and family's situation. A multidisciplinary approach including pediatric rehabilitation medicine or sports medicine physicians; physical, occupational, and/or recreational therapists; and school nurses, physical education teachers, and coaches also may be helpful and needed in some situations.[1,21] The Centers for Disease Control and

Prevention recommends that providers start by understanding the physical activity guidelines and to then ask their patients about physical activity participation, goals, and barriers. If a patient is already involved in physical activity, providers should consider if there is capacity to increase physical activity levels or need to modify routines. If the patient is not already involved in physical activity, recommendations and resources should be provided.[30]

Adapted from the International Classification of Functioning, Disability, and Health (ICF) of the World Health Organization (WHO), Rosenbaum and colleagues created the "5 F-words" as a framework to think about a well-rounded approach to the care of children with disabilities.[31,32] Carbone and colleagues, in a 2021 American Academy of Pediatrics Clinical Report on the topic of physical activity promotion for children and adolescents with disabilities, summarized a way to incorporate Rosenbaum's framework into discussions surrounding physical activity (**Table 3**).[1,31]

Risks such as sport-related injury or illness should also be discussed, taking into consideration the patient's unique medical history.[29] Patients and families should be educated about the signs and symptoms of such issues and potential strategies for injury or illness prevention.[1,29] Follow-up appointments to continually evaluate patients' physical activity status and if any modifications should be made are also recommended.[1]

Resources

Table 4 summarizes adaptive sports, recreation, and physical activity resources that providers may find useful to share with patients.[33–44] This list is not all-inclusive and there may be additional opportunities that are available more locally for patients. We recommend finding resources locally by searching online for local adaptive physical activity programs, connecting with your local departments of parks and recreation, or local physical medicine and rehabilitation departments that may have providers who are aware of additional resources.

Case presentation

- *Title*: A Child Who Loves to Dance
- *Case presentation*: We present a case of a 12-year-old girl with spastic quadriplegic CP who loves to dance. She would like to participate in an adaptive dance class, but the closest adaptive dance class to her is 2 h driving distance from her house. She lives in a rural setting where there are limited public transportation options, but this is her main means of transportation as she uses a power wheelchair, and her family does not have an accessible vehicle.
- *Clinical question*: As her health care provider, how can you best help decrease barriers to physical activity for your patient?
  - Access:
    - You can connect this patient to accessible resources for physical activity involvement. During the coronavirus disease-2019 pandemic, there was an increase in virtual adaptive sports opportunities that have improved access to adaptive physical activity programming for individuals who may have more limited local opportunities.[45]
    - You or a social worker can also help your patient and her family explore other local opportunities, such as local dance programs that may incorporate adaptations into their general programs. You can provide a letter supporting her physical activity and providing safety guidance with relevant medical precautions.

Table 3
"5 F-words" for physical activity discussions[1,31]

"F-word"	Recommendation
Fitness	• *Assess for facilitators or barriers* on the part of the child that affects physical activity participation and connect the child/family with local resources that would align with the child's goals and needs.
Function	• *Assess the patient's and family's physical literacy*, including understanding of and motivation regarding physical activity. • *Assess physical gross motor and fine motor skills* and if necessary, refer to appropriate therapists and specialists as indicated.
Friendships	• *Counsel patients and families on the social benefits of organized physical activity and sports* (eg, social bonds with other athletes that can create ongoing friendships even outside of sports/physical activity time).
Family factors	• *Assess family factors that may contribute to physical activity participation*—either as facilitators or as barriers. • Work with the family and patient together so the family's needs and the patient's needs are being met (eg, finding physical activity opportunities that are fun and healthy for the patient while also being feasible with the family's schedule).
Fun	• *Emphasize that physical activity should be fun!* • Encourage the patient/family to explore physical activities that may be fun for the patient and may provide a sense of joy, confidence, and accomplishment.

Table 4
Adaptive sports, recreation, and physical activity resources[33]

Resource/Organization	Website
America the Beautiful—National Parks & Federal Recreational Lands Access Pass (free, lifetime pass for US citizens or permanent residents with a permanent disability)	https://store.usgs.gov/access-pass.[33]
Challenged Athletes Foundation (offer grants for adaptive sports equipment)	https://www.challengedathletes.org/.[34]
Deaflympics	https://www.deaflympics.com/.[35]
Easter Seals	https://www.easterseals.com/.[36]
International Paralympic Committee	https://www.paralympic.org/.[37]
Miracle League	https://www.miracleleague.com/.[38]
Move United	https://moveunitedsport.org/.[39]
National Centers on Health Promotion for People with Disabilities—National Center on Health, Physical Activity, and Disability	https://www.nchpad.org/.[40]
Special Olympics	https://www.specialolympics.org/.[41]
Team US Paralympic Sports Clubs	https://www.teamusa.org/Team-USA-Athlete-Services/Paralympic-Sport-Development/Getting-Started.[42]
US Association of Blind Athletes	https://www.usaba.org/.[43]
US Deaf Sports Federation	https://usdeafsports.org/.[44]

- You or a social worker can help your patient and her family explore transportation options and can explore grant funding to cover transportation expenses for transportation to adaptive dance programs.
- You can provide a list of adaptive physical activity options available locally. Although this patient may be most interested in adaptive dance, she also may find other opportunities of interest in the local list.
  ○ Advocacy:
    - You can educate the community about the importance of inclusive and adaptive physical activity to allow access to physical activity opportunities for all. Physician allies and advocates will be critical to continue the forward momentum toward improved access to physical activity for all.[46]
  • *Discussion*: When thinking about this case and others like it, we recommend using the framework of the ICF of the WHO (**Fig. 1**).[1,32] Using this framework, it is clear to see that the environmental factors of far distance to the closest adaptive dance program and poor public transportation options are major barriers to adaptive physical activity participation in this example. Exploring the barriers through this framework allows health care providers to explore best next steps for overcoming barriers and to identify facilitators and opportunities to support participation through consideration of the 5 Fs (see **Table 3**).[1,31]

FUTURE DIRECTIONS

Although research exists regarding physical activity, sports participation, and barriers/facilitators to participation in children and adolescents with disabilities, there is still

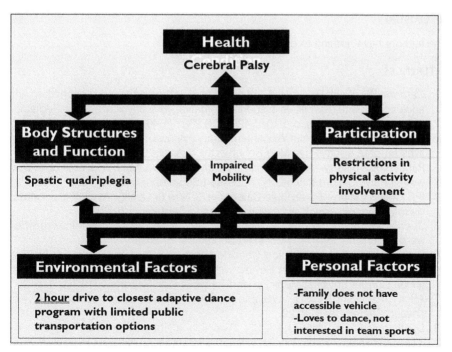

Fig. 1. Case example of a child with cerebral palsy who likes to dance—using the framework of the ICF of the WHO.[1,32]

more work to be done in this area. Future work should focus on identifying these patterns in patients with specific diagnoses/disability types. Additional work should also focus on physical activity/sport-related injury and illness patterns in pediatric athletes with disabilities, as there is little available evidence in the literature in this arena.[29]

SUMMARY

Approximately 25% of children in the United States participate in appropriate amounts of physical activity. That percentage is even lower for children with disabilities. Adaptive sports and physical activity opportunities are increasing in the United States. Health care providers are encouraged to discuss physical activity in the clinical setting and help to promote physical activity for all individuals, including children with disabilities.

CLINICS CARE POINTS

- Physical activity is important for everyone.
- In general, children with disabilities should participate in the same amount of physical activity as their peers.
- Children with disabilities generally participate in less physical activity than recommended.
- Health care providers can be key players in helping to improve physical activity participation in children with disabilities.

DISCLOSURE

The authors have nothing to disclose.

REFERENCES

1. Carbone PS, Smith PJ, Lewis C, et al. Promoting the participation of children and adolescents with disabilities in sports, recreation, and physical activity. Pediatrics 2021;148(6). https://doi.org/10.1542/PEDS.2021-054664/183444.
2. Tuakli-Wosornu Y, Derman W. Contemporary medical, scientific & social perspectives on para sport. Phys Med Rehabil Clin N Am 2018;29(2).
3. Paralympics history—evolution of the paralympic movement. Available at: https://www.paralympic.org/ipc/history. Accessed September 5, 2022.
4. IPC Classification—Paralympic Categories & How to Qualify. Available at: https://www.paralympic.org/classification. Accessed September 5, 2022.
5. Special Olympics: Sports. Available at: https://www.specialolympics.org/what-we-do/sports?locale=en. Accessed September 5, 2022.
6. Chandan P, Dubon ME. Clinical Considerations and Resources for Youth Athletes with Intellectual Disability: a Review with a Focus on Special Olympics International. Current Physical Medicine and Rehabilitation Reports 2019;7(2):116–25.
7. About the ICSD | ICSD. Available at: https://www.deaflympics.com/icsd. Accessed September 5, 2022.
8. Deaflympics—Regulations | ICSD. Available at: https://www.deaflympics.com/icsd/deaflympics-regulations. Accessed September 5, 2022.
9. Unified Sports. Available at: https://www.specialolympics.org/what-we-do/sports/unified-sports?locale=en. Accessed September 5, 2022.

10. Scholz J, Chen YT. History of Adaptive and Disabled Rights within Society, Thus Creating the Fertile Soil to Grow, Adaptive Sports. Adaptive Sports Medicine 2018;3–19. https://doi.org/10.1007/978-3-319-56568-2_1.

11. Stoke Mandeville 70: celebrating Sir Ludwig Guttmann. Available at: https://www.paralympic.org/news/stoke-mandeville-70-celebrating-sir-ludwig-guttmann. Accessed September 5, 2022.

12. About the international paralympic committee. Available at: https://www.paralympic.org/ipc/who-we-are. Accessed September 5, 2022.

13. 2015 athlete classification code. Available at: https://www.paralympic.org/classification-code. Accessed September 5, 2022.

14. WASUSA History. Available at: http://www.tswaa.com/wheelchair_sports_usa_history.htm. Accessed September 6, 2022.

15. CPISRA History—CPISRA. Available at: https://cpisra.org/cpisra-history/. Accessed September 6, 2022.

16. Disabled Sports USA and Adaptive Sports USA join forces to become Move United, the nation's leading community-based adaptive sports organization. Available at: https://moveunitedsport.org/disabled-sports-usa-and-adaptive-sports-usa-join-forces-to-become-move-united-the-nations-leading-community-based-adaptive-sports-organization-a/. Accessed Februrary 21, 2023.

17. Driscoll SW, Conlee EM, Brandenburg JE, et al. Exercise in Children with Disabilities. Current Physical Medicine and Rehabilitation Reports 2019;7(1):46–55.

18. Bloemen MAT, Backx FJG, Takken T, et al. Factors associated with physical activity in children and adolescents with a physical disability: a systematic review. Dev Med Child Neurol 2015;57(2):137–48.

19. Making Physical Activity a Way of Life: AAP Policy Explained—HealthyChildren. org. Available at: https://www.healthychildren.org/English/healthy-living/fitness/Pages/Making-Fitness-a-Way-of-Life.aspx. Accessed September 5, 2022.

20. Ross SM, Smit E, Yun J, et al. Updated national estimates of disparities in physical activity and sports participation experienced by children and adolescents with disabilities: NSCH 2016-2017. J Phys Activ Health 2020;17(4):443–55.

21. Lobelo F, Muth ND, Hanson S, et al. Physical activity assessment and counseling in pediatric clinical settings. Pediatrics 2020;145(3). https://doi.org/10.1542/PEDS.2019-3992.

22. Department of Health and Human Services. Physical Activity Guidelines for Americans 2 nd edition. Available at: https://health.gov/sites/default/files/2019-09/Physical_Activity_Guidelines_2nd_edition.pdf. Accessed September 5, 2022.

23. Murphy KP, Sobus KML, Moberg-Wolff E, et al. Musculoskeletal conditions. In: Murphy KP, McMahon MA, Houtrow AJ, editors. Pediatric rehabilitation: principles and practice. 6th ed. Springer Publishing Company; 2020. p. 371–409.

24. #doctalk : take a pledge to talk about physical activity : NCHPAD—building healthy inclusive communities. Available at: https://www.nchpad.org/pledge/doctalk. Accessed September 5, 2022.

25. How to talk about Physical Activity with your patient—YouTube. Available at: https://www.youtube.com/watch?v=S48DEvG0lpl. Accessed September 6, 2022.

26. Rx for Exercise: Pediatrics | Foundation for Physical Medicine and Rehabilitation. Available at: http://foundationforpmr.org/old/physicians/diagnostic-population/rx-for-exercise-pediatrics-new/. Accessed September 6, 2022.

27. Rx for Exercise: Physicians | Foundation for Physical Medicine and Rehabilitation. Available at: http://foundationforpmr.org/old/physicians/rx-for-exercise-physicians/. Accessed September 6, 2022.

28. The IPC tightens rules to clamp down on boosting. Available at: https://www. paralympic.org/news/ipc-tightens-rules-clamp-down-boosting.   Accessed September 6, 2022.

29. Dubon ME, Rovito C, van Zandt DK, et al. Youth Para and Adaptive Sports Medicine. Current Physical Medicine and Rehabilitation Reports 2019;7(2):104–15.

30. Increasing Physical Activity Among Adults with Disabilities | CDC. Available at: https://www.cdc.gov/ncbddd/disabilityandhealth/materials/infographic-increasing-physical-activity.html. Accessed September 5, 2022.

31. Rosenbaum P, Gorter JW. The "F-words" in childhood disability: I swear this is how we should think. Child Care Health Dev 2012;38(4):457–63.

32. Centers for Disease Control and Prevention. The ICF: An Overview Introducing The ICF. Available at: https://www.cdc.gov/nchs/data/icd/icfoverview_finalforwho10sept.pdf. Accessed November 24, 2022.

33. America the Beautiful—National Parks & Federal Recreational Lands Access Pass | USGS Store. Available at: https://store.usgs.gov/access-pass. Accessed September 5, 2022.

34. Challenged Athletes Foundation. Available at: https://www.challengedathletes. org/. Accessed September 5, 2022.

35. Welcome! | ICSD. Available at: https://www.deaflympics.com/. Accessed September 5, 2022.

36. Easterseals | Supporting Full Equity, Inclusion, and Access. Available at: https:// www.easterseals.com/. Accessed September 5, 2022.

37. International Paralympic Committee | IPC. Available at: https://www.paralympic. org/. Accessed September 5, 2022.

38. The Miracle League. Available at: https://www.miracleleague.com/. Accessed September 5, 2022.

39. Move United. Available at: https://moveunitedsport.org/. Accessed September 5, 2022.

40. NCHPAD—Building Healthy Inclusive Communities. Available at: https://www. nchpad.org/. Accessed September 5, 2022.

41. Special Olympics. Available at: https://www.specialolympics.org/. Accessed September 5, 2022.

42. Getting Started. Available at: https://www.teamusa.org/Team-USA-Athlete-Services/Paralympic-Sport-Development/Getting-Started. Accessed September 5, 2022.

43. Home—U.S. Association of Blind Athletes. Available at: https://www.usaba.org/. Accessed September 5, 2022.

44. USADSF | Welcome!. Available at: https://usdeafsports.org/. Accessed September 5, 2022.

45. Blauwet CA, Robinson D, Riley A, et al. Developing a Virtual Adaptive Sports Program in Response to the COVID-19 Pandemic. Pharm Manag PM R 2021;13(2): 211–6.

46. Legg D, Dubon M, Webborn N, et al. Advancing sport opportunities for people with disabilities: from grassroots to elite. Br J Sports Med 2022. https://doi.org/ 10.1136/BJSPORTS-2022-106227.

Disability Justice and Anti-ableism for the Pediatric Clinician

Christopher D. Lunsford, MD[a,b,*], Marion Quirici, PhD[c]

KEYWORDS

- Disability • Advocacy • Equity • Ableism • Child development • Clinical etiquette
- Accessibility • Inclusion

KEY POINTS

- Ableism and anti-disability bias continue to go underrecognized as a source of harm in patient care.
- Although certain jargon is required for the practice of medicine, the persistent use of some words and phrases, even as technical language, reveals anti-disability bias.
- Unlike medical understandings of the term "disability," disability studies scholars and advocates use the term to refer to the consequences of a society failing to meet the needs of a person with an impairment, resulting in inaccessibility, stigma, and discrimination.
- Although still used in most medical literature, person first language is not always appropriate outside of that context as many disabled people prefer identity first language.
- Even the busiest clinician can be an effective anti-ableist advocate.

INTRODUCTION
How Can Any Baby Be a Failure?

R62. 51... That's the International Classification of Diseases, Tenth Revision, Clinical Modification (ICD-10 CM) code for a diagnosis of failure to thrive (FTT), which is, essentially, a lack of appropriate weight gain. Although certain jargon is required for the practice of medicine, the persistent use of some words and phrases, even as technical language, can also reveal bias. In the early twentieth century, Meinhard von

The authors have no commercial or financial conflicts of interest or any funding sources outside of their University affiliations.
[a] Department of Orthopaedics, Duke University Health System, 3000 Erwin Road, DUMC Box 2911, Durham, NC 27705, USA; [b] Department of Pediatrics, Duke University Health System, 3000 Erwin Road, DUMC Box 2911, Durham, NC 27705, USA; [c] Disability Studies and Global Anglophone Literature, Department of English, Kennesaw State University, 440 Bartow Avenue, Kennesaw, GA 30144, USA
* Corresponding author. Department of Orthopaedics, Duke University Health System, 3000 Erwin Road, DUMC Box 2911, Durham, NC 27705.
E-mail address: cdl40@duke.edu

Pfaundler first coined the term, FTT, to describe institutionalized orphaned infants with poor weight gain that was attributed to "the lack of maternal influences."[1] Over time this theory of maternal deprivation lost favor, but the term persisted in use for difficult-to-explain weight issues in infants.[2] FTT also seems to be correlated with disability. In a cohort of subjects with cerebral palsy, a condition defined by lifelong motor disability, over half of the subjects had a history of FTT in their medical charts.[3] The concern with FTT is the strongly negative connotation embedded within. This language could easily be replaced with other terminology such as "idiopathic lack of weight gain," but to date, this language shift has not occurred. On the surface, FTT may not seem to carry a value judgment, but the term *cripple* also had medical status in the past that did not seem to carry a value judgment at the time. Although not an official diagnosis, the acronym FLK, or "Funny Looking Kid," which clinicians still sometimes use among themselves to convey suspicions of genetic conditions, would be beyond offensive to any parent.[4] Although there are many different types of issues arising from medical jargon,[5] FTT and FLK are prime examples of anti-disability related words that persist in health care longer than they should. Health care professionals may perceive this language as technical and therefore innocuous, but that does not change how those outside of medicine interpret such terms. Ultimately, these words both reveal and reinforce our implicit biases. Continued use of ableist language negatively impacts doctor-patient interactions. When it comes to understanding disability, it is health care as a whole, not individual patients, that are failing to thrive.

We petition health care providers to develop and advocate for disability consciousness by using the principles of disability justice to improve health care in medical education, residency training, and practice.[6,7] Although staying fully up to date with disability justice activism and critical disability studies scholarship is an unattainable standard for most practicing clinicians, we believe learning the basic principles of disability justice and preferred disability language is possible and necessary. This article provides a primer on disability justice, disability language, and clinical best practices to show how every pediatrician can resist ableism in their work with children and families. Using FTT as a representative example of how the language derived from the medical model of disability, based on impairment, is harmful to children with disabilities and their families, we offer alternatives to ableist language that are either disability-positive or value-neutral. By simply being more aware of the language we use, health care providers can help, rather than hinder, the development of empowered disability identities in young people. This is the first step for any person who aspires to be an effective advocate for disability inclusion and equity.

KEY TERMS FOR UNDERSTANDING DISABILITY JUSTICE AND ANTI-ABLEISM

Health care professionals and disability studies scholars use many of the same words, but not always with the same meaning, which creates confusion and distracts from efforts to acknowledge and address ableism. The word "disability" itself represents a complex concept that is affected by the context in which it is used. At either ends of a broad spectrum are the medical and social models of disability; as their names suggest each of these models place disability in a different sphere: one wholly biologic and organic and the other wholly societal and political. The medical model of disability is impairment-based, in that disability is simply understood as the impact of an impairment on a person's function. Linking the definitions of disability and impairment provides theoretic structure to study and learn about the relationship between impairments, disability, and health at the individual level. However, the focus of the medical model solely on individual biology fails to appropriately recognize societal

forces that create and sustain "disablement."[8] Further, it relies on a subjective definition of "normal" human function and ability.[9,10]

In contrast to the medical model of disability is the social model, where disability is
not defined by a perceived deficiency, but by the failure of sociopolitical institutions to
address a person's needs, resulting in participation restriction and often societal dis-
advantages, discrimination, and/or stigma.[11] This theory defines disability without
reference to the biology of any specific impairments, which is a starkly different
approach from the current medical usage of the word.

Building upon an appreciation of the medical and social models of disability, **Table 1**
reviews other key terms and definitions related to disability per various medical,
educational, legal, and scholarly institutions. Some of the definitions are also classified
as a representative of the medical model, whereas others are] labeled as "binocular
view," as described by Eric Parens to indicate an appreciation of both the medical
and the social models of disability.[12]

Many clinicians are familiar with the biopsychosocial (BPS) model of disability,
which understands disability as dynamic and the disability experience as informed
by biology, personal factors, and social, political, and other environmental factors.
Parens' binocular view of disability is essentially another interpretation of the BPS
approach to health-related conditions, first developed by Engel in 1977.[25] However,
the traditional understanding and implementation of BPS models have not usually
appreciated any aspect of disability as a social construct as described by social
model, and by extension, the binocular view. In fact, one of the more prominent
uses of BPS overtly created disability stigma. Gordon Waddell, an orthopedic surgeon, used the BPS in the context of disability, disability insurance, and chronic low
back pain, to advance the idea of nonorganic factors affecting the phenomenon of
chronic low back pain.[26] Waddell's interpretation of BPS delineated how a clinical
assessment of a patient's back pain should consider psychological (eg, hypochondria)
and social (eg, disability insurance fraud) aspects.[27] Even today, medical students are
taught the five Waddell signs to test for during a physical examination, which are used
as evidence that a patient is either in denial about somatizing their pain or "faking
it."[28] By promoting the concept of patient malingering due to financial incentives to
stay disabled, Waddell's variant of the BPS added significant stigma to the conversation around disability.[29] However, there are many other disability-neutral versions of
the BPS,[30–33] and as shown in **Table 1**, we classify both the UN and the WHO definitions of disability as the binocular view, and the WHO does self-describes its framework as a BPS approach.[16]

ADDRESSING BIAS TO ACHIEVE ANTI-ABLEIST HEALTH CARE PRACTICE

Ableism in society leads to everyday assumptions about disability, and these assumptions contribute to and perpetuate health care access inequities for patients with
disability, creating a new risk to their health. The causal relationship between bias
and poor health care outcomes has been shown in many different scenarios, thus
bias due to ableism must be considered as a source of health care disparities.[34,35]
For example, we already know that health care providers generally underestimate
the quality of life of those with disabilities, whereas those with disabilities themselves
report quality of life ratings in line with the general population.[36,37] Erroneous assumptions about quality of life suggests a strong bias against disability, and although we do
not yet know the full extent of harm done by such bias, we can work to dispel such
assumptions about disability that lead to bias. In the following sections, specific examples of ableism experienced during clinical care are shared by author, Christopher

Table 1
Disability justice and anti-ableism terminology[a]

Term	Definitions and Examples
Disability (medical model)	*Centers for Disease Control and Prevention (CDC)*: "any condition of the body or mind (impairment) that makes it more difficult for the person with the condition to do certain activities (activity limitation) and interact with the world around them (participation restrictions)."[13] *Americans with Disabilities Act (ADA)*: "a physical or mental impairment that substantially limits one or more major life activities, a person who has a history or record of such an impairment, or a person who is perceived by others as having such an impairment."[14] *Individuals with Disabilities Education Act (IDEA)*: "a child with a disability means a child evaluated in accordance with [specific policies] as having an intellectual disability, a hearing impairment (including deafness), a speech or language impairment, a visual impairment (including blindness), a serious emotional disturbance (referred to in this part as "emotional disturbance"), an orthopedic impairment, autism, traumatic brain injury, another health impairment, a specific learning disability, deaf-blindness, or multiple disabilities, and who, by reason thereof, needs special education and related services."[15]
Disability (social model)	Occurs when societal institutions have failed to address a person's basic needs resulting in activity restriction and often societal disadvantages, discrimination, and/or stigma.[11]
Disability (binocular view)	*World Health Organization (WHO)*: the results of the interaction between individuals with a health condition, such as cerebral palsy, Down syndrome, and depression, with personal and environmental factors including negative attitudes, inaccessible transportation and public buildings, and limited social support.[16] *United Nations (UN)/Convention on the Rights of Persons with Disabilities (CRPD)*: evolving concept and that disability results from the interaction between persons with impairments and attitudinal and environmental barriers that hinders their full and effective participation in society on an equal basis with others.[17]
Intersectionality	A theory developed by Kimberlé Crenshaw to describe how race, gender, class, and other aspects of identity intersect and overlap, such that an attempt to address one aspect of a person's identity discretely from the others is problematic.[18]
Disability rights movement	A social movement, similar to and in parallel with other civil rights movements, that works to ensure equal opportunities and rights for all people with disabilities. The movement has been criticized by Disability Justice activists for focusing singularly on ableism and neglecting intersectionality, such that issues of race, ethnicity, class, gender, and sexuality, are separated from other social and political issues.[19]
Disability justice	A framework and movement, developed by queer and trans-disabled activists of color, that builds solidarity across all disabled communities by capturing the voices left unheard by the Disability Rights Movement.[19,20] Per the advocacy coalition, Sins Invalid, Disability Justice has these core values: • Solidarity across different types of disability • All bodies have needs and are interdependent with others

(continued on next page)

Table 1 *(continued)*	
Term	**Definitions and Examples**
	• All persons have value outside notions of productivity • Ableism is part of intersectional oppression that also draws upon racism, sexism, and classism • Collective access and collective liberation are the goals of our movements.[19]
Ableism	The privileging of people without disabilities and a structural system of stigma, prejudice, discrimination, and oppression of people with disabilities. Per Talila Lewis, this system of valuation is "deeply rooted in eugenics, anti-Blackness, misogyny, colonialism, imperialism, and capitalism."[21]
Disability studies	An academic multi-disciplinary area of scholarship focused on disability in both individuals and society, considering not only the medical and psychological foundations of the term, but also the cultural, political, legal, historical, and interpersonal context, influences, and impact.[22,23]
Disability humility	Per Reynolds, "learning about experiences, cultures, histories, and politics of disability, recognizing that one's knowledge and understanding of disability will always be partial, and acting and judging in light of that fact." With respect to the doctor-patient relationship, this is especially important for health care professionals to cede power and respect the patient's authority over their own lived experience.[24]
Disability consciousness	An understanding that competency alone in the care of those with disabilities is insufficient for health care providers. At all levels of health care education, training, and practice, both individuals and institutions have a duty to learn from disability humility, disability scholarship, and disability justice, which compels anti-ableism and action for change.

[a] This table was prepared for the busy clinician, and as such, it contains many over-simplifications of complex topics and ongoing scholarship. The authors urge readers to explore the reference cited herein as well as these resources: The Disability Visibility Project Website: https://disabilityvisibility-project.com/. Wong, A. (ed), (2018). Resistance and Hope: Essays by Disabled People, Disability Visibility Project. Wong, A. (ed) (2020). Disability Visibility: First-Person Stories from the Twenty-First Century, Penguin. Piepzna-Samarasinha, L. L. (2018). Care Work: Dreaming Disability Justice, Arsenal Pulp Press.

Lunsford, both a proudly disabled individual and a pediatric rehabilitation medicine physician.

"Failure to Thrive" and the Fallacy of Normal

The mother of a 5-year-old patient with diplegic cerebral palsy and I had just discussed the likelihood of needing hip surgery. It was clear the thought of another surgery was triggering PTSD for the mother. She spent nearly half a year in the NICU with her child and another half year in the hospital for various other reasons since then. When faced with the surgery and resulting hospital admission related to her child's disability, she finally asked a question that she had been holding onto for years: "I know my child has cerebral palsy, but why do they also have 'failure to thrive' as a diagnosis?" As we discussed it, she admitted that she worried her son would also be failing to thrive. I tried to explain the meaning of the diagnosis, but it almost made the situation worse. She couldn't understand what purpose we, the doctors, had for labeling sick infants as failures. Ultimately, I knew I could not defend the medical institution for still using this term, the same way I would not defend how long it took to retire terms like "mental retardation" or "crippled."

FTT is one of many vague medical diagnoses that signal deviation from a norm and a negative judgment of that deviation. Critiquing *normality* is a core focus of disability studies that medical institutions can learn from. Though it is impossible to dispense entirely with statistics and norms in medical practice, we must consider where they are needed to preserve health through diagnostic or treatment value, and where they do harm by conveying implicit biases. Vital signs can be abnormal in a quantitative sense. The shape and color of a mole can be abnormal in a qualitative sense. Ableism in health care goes deeper than individual physicians, but they can still be agents of positive change by earnestly confronting conscious and unconscious anti-disability bias. One can still work to address the negative consequences of health conditions and optimize functioning without attaching the negative label to the child with disabilities. A child with disabilities is no less worthy than any other child of high-quality health care and the love and support they need to thrive; and yet, clinicians may subtly or overtly express anti-disability bias to their patients and families. As physicians, the process of examining one's biases must be ever-evolving to lessen the impact of discrimination on health. For those looking for resources on implicit bias against disability, the American Bar Association has a fantastic guide.[38]

Do we Really Need a Wheelchair?

For the child who may or may not be able to walk into adulthood, another ableist quandary arises when the child who cannot ambulate effectively to keep up with their peers and family gets too large for a commercial stroller. Whether I bring it up or they do, some parents request a 'medical stroller': essentially the next size up from what is sold in stores. However, I invest the time to educate and counsel on the alternate option of ordering a manual wheelchair for the child. A manual wheelchair allows the child the chance for some independence, but some parents share with me that they didn't think we needed this. Usually with more discussion, the parent expresses concern with the appearance of their child in a wheelchair; for some families, this would mark the first time they would go to the mall and have to adjust to the feeling of being different than other families. Getting the wheelchair makes the disability real in a way that they hadn't come to terms with prior to this decision. The wheelchair is a tool for learning independent mobility, but is treated like the 'scarlet letter' of disability. However, the stroller, especially with the slightly reclined position that most have, creates a situation where the child is always dependent on others to explore their environment. From a developmental standpoint, exploring one's environment is a crucial cognitive milestone that unlocks many other areas of cognitive growth. Explaining this to a parent can be difficult, but as a physician, it is my role to get ahead of these ableist assumptions for the health of my patient.

Parents' preference for a stroller in this example reflects their desire to seem nondisabled and avoid the stigma, bias, and discrimination associated with disability. *Normality* encapsulates a judgment on the value of human experience and identity, as it leaves no space for alternative yet value-neutral experiences and identities. For example, it is now widely recognized that having autism, or other forms of neurodiversity, should be value-neutral in medical contexts, but still, bias against these diverse experiences and identities leads to discrimination and even harmful medical practice. For children especially, being different than others and feeling excluded due to these differences leads to negative self-esteem and self-valuation. To our knowledge, there is no developmental psychology research about the impact of ableism and ableist language on children's self-image. However, it seems clear that children do not assume being different is in any way negative until society teaches them these value judgements.

Developmental Delay and "Special Needs": Disability as Diversity

In realm of pediatric medicine, the failure to develop physical and cognitive abilities age-appropriately may be labeled with the nebulous diagnosis of "Developmental Delay." In and of itself, there is nothing concerning about using the word "delay" to signify that a person's development is two standard deviations behind the mean timeline of all individuals. However, there is a concern when this diagnosis lingers indefinitely in a child's medical chart. In my role for families, children are already diagnosed with developmental delay and I'll ask parents: "Do you remember getting this diagnosis? What did they tell you about this?" I often find that families were never told how this delay fits into a "bigger picture," and they were not told how delays could actually just be their child's expected baseline even into adulthood. The lack of discussion around a possible persistent disability is a result of ableism, as some doctors do not want to be the one to make that call, or they do not have the time or confidence to have an on open-ended conversation about disability. I have been asked by the parents of middle school-aged children, "When exactly is my child going to catch up on this delay?" These parents still cling to an outside chance that their child will become what the world calls "normal." When we delay further discussions to resolve "developmental delay," we allow no space for disability to be acceptable, and ableism persists.

Health care providers often share sites like the CDC's milestone checklist with families.[39] Families are told to act early on possible missed milestones, but they are not prepared for the fact that some delays may not have a treatment or a reversible cause; some delays are not delays at all when the child is not expected to reach that milestone. Physicians are trained to screen for delays in development and treat or cure the cause of that delay, but they must also be trained how to support families and promote disability advocacy when permanent disability may be present in childhood. When developmental delay lasts until kids are school-aged, then a new code-word for disability in used: "special needs," Rather than segregated as "special," disability should be considered a feature of diversity,[40] because it leads to a diversity of lived experiences. More accurately, there is nothing "special" about the needs of kids with disabilities, as all humans have needs, but the fact that facilitating the needs of some individuals is different, and perhaps less common, than others, should not make those needs "special" at a societal level. The Disability Africa blog made the case in 2016 that so-called special needs are nothing more or less than human rights.[41] The term, special needs, stigmatizes disability, and simply saying "disabled needs" is both more clear and less belittling. The conflation of disability with illness and poor health also prevents some from seeing disability as diversity, but one can also be disabled and healthy.[42,43] Treating people with disability with respect and humility, while also hoping to minimize or prevent the negative health implications, is not only possible, but pivotal. The lack of recognition that disability is part of what makes society diverse is an obstacle to optimizing health care.

CONFRONTING ABLEIST LANGUAGE

To offer pediatricians an actionable strategy for undermining ableism in their practice, we close with examples of ableist language paired with recommended alternatives in **Tables 2–4**. Recognizing the ableism inherent in common language choices is an important first step toward resisting the ableism of our culture. As disability studies scholar Simi Linton remarks, language "reinforces the dominant culture's views of

Table 2 Ableist language to avoid	
Avoid	**Say Instead**
"Suffers from" or "is afflicted with"	Has
"Victim of"	Survivor
"Confined" to a wheelchair	Uses a wheelchair/wheelchair user
"Bed bound" or "wheelchair bound"	In a bed/wheelchair much of the time
"Handicapped stall" or "handicapped parking space"	Accessible stall/parking space
"The disabled"	Disabled people/people with disabilities
"Normal," "able-bodied," and "typically developing"[a]	Nondisabled people/people without disabilities/(for medical literature only: people with typical development)

[a] Typical or atypical would be acceptable if they were only used to describe parts of a person's medical history, but when these adjectives are attributed to the person themselves, this terminology ultimately carries the same value-negative judgment of normal and abnormal.

disability."[44] Health care providers should recognize ableist language as an obstacle to good health care delivery, comparable to racist and sexist language. Of course, language choices alone are not sufficient to address social and structural injustices. Although the tables below present the reader with straightforward dos and don'ts, we preface this material with a reminder that we are calling for a paradigm shift toward disability justice in medicine. This paradigm shift takes much more than replacing word choices, and we therefore recommend, while considering the seemingly subtle revisions outlined below, you consider the totality of the mindset these changes represent.

One of the more recognizable language choices related to disability is the rise of so-called "person first" language (PFL), presented by mainstream disability etiquette as the respectful, politically correct way to name disability. However, as Emily Ladau has remarked, "PFL intentionally separates a person from their disability. Although this supposedly acknowledges personhood, it also implies that "disability" or "disabled" are negative, derogatory words."[45] As an alternative to PFL, some disabled people prefer "identity first" language (IFL). We call attention to these efforts to destigmatize disability by noting that the person with the disability should be given the space to decide if and how the disability relates to their identity. If you are unsure if you should call your next patient an autistic man or a man with autism, you can simply ask that person if they have a preference on this. Of note, for medical journals, the use of PFL is acceptable and, in some instances, still required, but we encourage authors to push against those rules when appropriate. In some cases, identity-first language might be more "patient-centered."

Our language recommendations are the result of many influences, but also a product of original thought that shares similarity to other scholarship and advocacy through

Table 3 Disability metaphors to avoid	
Avoid	**Say Instead**
He "blindly" followed orders	Ignorantly; thoughtlessly
My request "fell on deaf ears"	Was ignored
His argument was "crippled" by her defense	Taken apart; vanquished; disproven
That test was "crazy/insane/lame"	Difficult, unfair

Table 4 Disability euphemisms to avoid	
Avoid	**Say Instead**
"Special needs"	Disabled
"Differently abled"	Disabled
"Physically challenged"; "mentally challenged"	Disabled
"Handicapable"	Disabled
"Person of diverse ability"	Disabled
"Diffability"	Disability

convergent evolution, such as the work of Kristen Bottema-Beutel and colleagues and Michigan Medicine.[46,47] However, **Table 2** was specifically adapted from Simi Linton's *Claiming Disability*, and reflects some of the most common ableist expressions.[44] The first three examples, referencing suffering, victimhood, and confinement, are all negative value judgments that assume disability is reducible to hardship and misfortune. An expression like "confined to a wheelchair" is not only negative, but also inaccurate. The wheelchair does not "confine" the user; the opposite is closer to the truth. Enabling movement from place to place, the wheelchair would be better characterized as a tool of liberation. Swapping the adjective "handicapped" for "accessible" is similarly a matter of accurate description. We recommend avoiding "the disabled" as a blanket term for the community because it erases the humanity and diversity of what is likely the most heterogenous minority group. Our final recommendation in this table, to avoid using terms like "able-bodied" or "normal" to describe those without disabilities, is perhaps the most important. We have discussed the stigmatizing and marginalizing consequences of the suggestion that having a disability makes a person "not normal." In clinical settings, "typically developing" is often used as a replacement for "normal," and many authors have used the phrase in peer-reviewed literature for at least 40 years, but we recommend using the term "nondisabled" instead. Despite best intentions, "typically developing" marginalizes disability as "atypical." Although we concede that a person's developmental history may be described as statistically "typical" or "atypical," these words should not be used as adjectives for the whole person. A term like "nondisabled," as a preferable alternative, re-centers the disabled perspective and avoids implying a hierarchy. As a comparable example, using the term "non-Hispanic" as a contrast to "Hispanic" avoids value judgements in a society where non-Hispanics are the majority. We acknowledge that it is easy to make mistakes when updating our language choices, but learning new terminology has always been part of medical training. Choosing language that centers rather than marginalizes the lived experience of a young patients with a disability promotes child health.

Table 3 outlines expressions that use disability as a metaphor. These phrases are commonplace in our language, but their cumulative effect is to equate disability to all things negative. Expressions like these are both a sign of how deeply ingrained ableism is, as well as a means for reinforcing ableism. Our alternatives, again, appeal to accuracy. When you catch yourself reaching for one of these common expressions, consider how it could hurt the development of a young person that identifies with the related disability. More often than not, there are a multiplicity of other words available to express your intended meaning, and although most disabled people will not take offense to phrases like "Do you see what I mean?" or "I won't stand for that," avoiding negative disability metaphors helps to resist ableism. Of note, despite our recommendation to avoid the use of, "crippled," as a metaphor, some members of the disabled community have purposefully reclaimed the term, crip, to call out ableism. Although we encourage readers to learn about the #CripTheVote movement and to enjoy the Netflix documentary, *Crip Camp*, the term "crip" should only be used by those who identify as physically disabled.

Finally, some disability etiquette guidelines recommend avoiding the word "disability" and replacing it with other languages, but we argue that these efforts do harm rather than good. To treat "disability" as a bad word is to accept the stigmatizing view that disability itself is bad. Children who come through our care, perhaps not yet knowing if they will have their disability for life, are sensitive to the value judgments we assign to their differences. As they are in the vulnerable process of identity formation, it is essential not to associate disability with the idea of "something wrong." Avoiding the word makes it into something unspeakable, rather than a valid difference. Consider the examples in **Table 4**.

Discussed also above, "special needs" seems unlikely to be eradicated if only due to its pervasiveness and the fact that the whole field of education is named for it. However, Disabled activists have long expressed their frustration with avoidance tactics, because the refusal to say "disabled" or "disability" reflects the belief that disability is shameful or embarrassing, and thus better left unmentioned. In 2016, disabled activist Lawrence Carter-Long led a social media campaign around the hashtag #SayTheWord. He wrote on Facebook, "If you 'see the person not the disability' you're only getting half the picture. Broaden your perspective. You might be surprised by everything you've missed. DISABLED. #SayTheWord."

For a more thorough list of terms to avoid and recommended alternatives, we direct the reader to the National Center on Disability and Journalism.[48] Disability language is constantly evolving; however, terms like "feeblemindedness" and "mental retardation" were medical diagnoses in the past, they are clearly regarded as disability slurs today.

DISABILITY-CONSCIOUS BEST PRACTICES FOR PATIENT CARE

What does disability consciousness look like in practice? The answer can take many shapes, but at the foundation of all strategies to support the health of disabled people must be an understanding of ableism and anti-disability bias. Although no list of clinical best practices for anti-ableism in health care could be exhaustive and the road to achieving disability justice is long, we recommend the following strategies as a starting point for the disability-conscious physician.

General

- Ask the patient/parent if they feel comfortable with the terms/diagnoses that you use.

For example, "In my notes, you may see that I'll say your child has cerebral palsy, intellectual disability, and seizures. Do you feel like we've talked about all those enough that it makes sense and are you comfortable with that description?"

- Ask the patient and/or ask a caregiver what is the best way to address and interact with the patient.

For example, often physicians may forget to directly address a child with an alternative or limited expressive communication skills during a visit. This is not only a missed opportunity to build rapport, but also could be received as an insult by the family. Do not assume that a patient cannot understand/communicate based on chart review.

- Be respectful of patient autonomy.

Be mindful to avoid paternalistic pats on the head or other mannerisms, nicknames, or touching that could be demeaning if the patients were not disabled. Related to mobility equipment: ask before moving a patient or their device.

- Remember to examine patients with disabilities as closely as how you would examine any other patient.

If you are unsure how to adapt your usual examination, then explain what you are hoping to do and ask the patient or their parent for advice on how to proceed. For example, if you are concerned that examining a child out of a wheelchair could be difficult or painful, ask how they feel about being transitioned to an examination table, rather than just skipping the examination.

Primary Care and Preventative Health

- Clinical research, screening tools, and practices can all have the bias of the people and systems that created them.

Many educational tests and development screens were not developed with certain populations and disability statuses in mind and therefore are not able to accurately capture or assess a person's capabilities. Refer instead to developmental specialists and/or adaptive rehabilitation experts when appropriate.

- Children with disabilities deserve the same standard of care as nondisabled children.

Often key aspects of child health maintenance are neglected for children with disabilities, such as puberty screening/counseling, sexual health education, depression screening, and educational/vocational planning. Importantly, this is a form of discrimination and must be addressed.

Inaccessible Spaces and Attitudes

- Ask patients or parents if they have had accessibility issues with your clinic.

It is also important to be prepared to address any issues that you are alerted to.

- Ask health care team members and staff if they are comfortable with the needs of patients with disability.

For example, what does the check-in team do if a patient arrives who only communicates in American Sign Language? Be prepared to help engage the team with support, resources, and time to learn as needed.

- Ensure all medical equipment is present and working for those with disability.

Does your clinic have a functional Hoyer lift for transfers? Do staff know when to offer it and how to assist in that type of transfer?

SUMMARY

Every child deserves the chance to thrive, regardless of their relationship to the milestones of typical childhood development. Physicians must address ableism and implicit biases against disability, or they will "fail to thrive" as disability advocates. Returning to the example of FTT as a medical diagnosis, it is one of many terms in medicine that convey negative connotations that go unaddressed by health care professionals. Although we recommend FTT no longer be used as a medical diagnosis, the larger point of this work is to state that simply striking offensive language from medical records or daily conversations is insufficient to address disability injustice in health care. The onus of addressing ableism in health care should not fall to people with disabilities, who have already spoken out and told us their lived experiences for many years. Disability humility compels us to listen to these voices, and disability consciousness compels us to act. Pediatric health care providers are a guiding force in the lives of individuals with disability, and that force must be trained to examine how ableism is a threat to child development, just as racism, sexism, transphobia and homophobia are threats to our youth. Children deserve anti-ableist childhoods, communities, and especially doctors.

POST-ARTICLE DISCUSSION QUESTIONS

When have you observed or experienced ableism in a health care setting?
   Were you the victim, a witness, or ableist yourself?
   What happened?
   How could disability consciousness have led to a different result?

CLINICS CARE POINTS

Disability-conscious best practices for patient care include but are not limited to:
- Ask the patient/parent if they feel comfortable with the terms/diagnoses that you use or that they might find in medical documentation.
- Ask the patient and/or ask a caregiver what is the best way to address, communication with, and interact with the patient.
- Be respectful of patient autonomy by avoiding avoid paternalistic pats on the head or other mannerisms, nicknames, or touching that could be demeaning. Related to mobility equipment: ask before touching or moving a patient or their wheelchair/mobility device.
- Examine patients with disabilities as close to how you would examine any other patient.
- Children with disabilities deserve the same standard of care as nondisabled children, but often key aspects of child health maintenance are neglected for children with disabilities, such as puberty screening/counseling, sexual health education, depression screening, and educational/vocational planning.
- Ask patients or parents if they have had accessibility issues with your clinic and be prepared to address any issues that you are alerted to.
- Ask health care team members and staff if they are comfortable with the needs of patients with disability, such as does the check-in team do if a patient arrives who only communicates with American Sign Language or does the clinic staff know how to use assist with a two-person transfer if needed.
- Ensure all adaptive medical equipment is present and working for those with a disability, such as a functional Hoyer lift for transfers.

REFERENCES

1. Estrem HH, Pados BF, Park J, et al. Feeding problems in infancy and early childhood: evolutionary concept analysis. J Adv Nurs 2017;73(1):56–70.
2. Hughes I. Confusing terminology attempts to define the undefinable. Arch Dis Child 2007;92(2):97–8.
3. Reyes AL, Cash AJ, Green SH, et al. Gastrooesophageal reflux in children with cerebral palsy. Child Care Health Dev 1993;19(2):109–18.
4. Robinow M. A syndrome's progress. Am J Dis Child 1973;126(2):150.
5. Pitt MB, Hendrickson MA. Eradicating Jargon-Oblivion-A Proposed Classification System of Medical Jargon. J Gen Intern Med 2020;35(6):1861–4.

6. Doebrich A, Quirici M, Lunsford C. COVID-19 and the need for disability conscious medical education, training, and practice. J Pediatr Rehabil Med 2020;13(3):393–404.
7. Roush SE, Sharby N. Disability reconsidered: the paradox of physical therapy. Phys Ther 2011;91(12):1715–27.
8. Reddy CR. From impairment to disability and beyond: Critical explorations in disability studies. Socio Bull 2011;60(2):287–306.
9. Söder M. Disability as a social construct: the labelling approach revisited. Eur J Spec Needs Educ 1989;4(2):117–29.
10. Jones SR. Toward inclusive theory: Disability as social construction. NASPA J 1996;33(4):347–54.
11. Thomas P, Gradwell L, Markham N. Defining impairment within the social model of disability. Manchester, England, UK: Greater Manchester Coalition of Disabled People; 1997.
12. Parens E. Choosing flourishing: toward a more" binocular" way of thinking about disability. Kennedy Inst Ethics J 2017;27(2):135–50.
13. Prevention CfDCa. Disability and Health Overview. https://www.cdc.gov/ncbddd/disabilityandhealth/disability.html. Accessed September 4, 2022.
14. Rights DoJ-DoC. Introduction to the ADA. https://www.ada.gov/ada_intro.htm. Accessed September 5, 2022.
15. Education USDo. Individuals with Disabilities Education Act. 1990. Available at: https://sites.ed.gov/idea/regs/b/a/300.8. Accessed April 20, 2023.
16. Organization WH. Disability. Available at: https://www.who.int/health-topics/disability. Accessed September 5, 2022.
17. Assembly UG. Convention on the Rights of Persons with Disabilities. 13 December 2006. Available at: www.un.org/en/development/desa/population/migration/generalassembly/docs/globalcompact/A_RES_61_106.pdf. Accessed April 20, 2023.
18. Runyan AS. What Is Intersectionality and Why Is It Important? American Association of University Professors 2018. Available at: https://www.aaup.org/article/what-intersectionality-and-why-it-important#.Yw4TYnbMKpc. Accessed September 4, 2022.
19. Invalid S. 10 Principles of Disability Justice. Available at: https://www.sinsinvalid.org/blog/10-principles-of-disability-justice. Accessed September 4, 2022.
20. Ellis K, Garland-Thomson R, Kent M, et al. Manifestos for the future of critical disability studies, vol. 1. England, UK: Routledge Oxon; 2019.
21. Lewis T. Working Definition of Ableism 2022. Available at: https://www.talilalewis.com/blog. Accessed September 4, 2022.
22. Program UoWDS. What is Disability Studies? 2022. Available at: https://disabilitystudies.washington.edu/what-is-disability-studies. Accessed September 4, 2022.
23. 101 DS. What is disability studies?. Available at: https://disstudies101.com/definitions/what-is-disability-studies/. Accessed September 4, 2022.
24. Reynolds JM. Three Things Clinicians Should Know About Disability. AMA J Ethics Dec 1 2018;20(12):E1181–7.
25. Engel GL. The need for a new medical model: a challenge for biomedicine. Science 1977;196(4286):129–36.
26. Waddell G. Volvo award in clinical sciences. A new clinical model for the treatment of low-back pain. Spine 1987;12(7):632–44.
27. Shakespeare T, Watson N, Alghaib OA. Blaming the victim, all over again: Waddell and Aylward's biopsychosocial (BPS) model of disability. Crit Soc Pol 2017;37(1):22–41.

28. Novy DM, Collins HS, Nelson DV, et al. Waddell signs: distributional properties and correlates. Archives of physical medicine and rehabilitation 1998;79(7): 820–2.

29. Kennedy A. The biopsychosocial model: A response to Shakespeare, Watson and Alghaib (2017). Crit Soc Pol 2017;37(2):310–4.

30. Havelka M, Despot Lučanin J, Lučanin D. Biopsychosocial model–the integrated approach to health and disease. Coll Antropol 2009;33(1):303–10.

31. Mescouto K, Olson RE, Hodges PW, et al. A critical review of the biopsychosocial model of low back pain care: time for a new approach? Disabil Rehabil 2020;1–15.

32. Hunt J. Holistic or harmful? Examining socio-structural factors in the bio-psychosocial model of chronic illness, 'medically unexplained symptoms' and disability. Disability & Society 2022;1–30.

33. Wade DT, Halligan PW. The biopsychosocial model of illness: a model whose time has come. London, England: SAGE Publications Sage UK; 2017. p. 995–1004.

34. FitzGerald C, Hurst S. Implicit bias in healthcare professionals: a systematic review. BMC Med Ethics 2017;18(1):1–18.

35. Chapman EN, Kaatz A, Carnes M. Physicians and implicit bias: how doctors may unwittingly perpetuate health care disparities. J Gen Intern Med 2013;28(11): 1504–10.

36. Iezzoni LI, Rao SR, Ressalam J, et al. Physicians' Perceptions Of People With Disability And Their Health Care. Health Aff (Millwood). Feb 2021;40(2):297–306.

37. Albrecht GL, Devlieger PJ. The disability paradox: high quality of life against all odds. Social science & medicine 1999;48(8):977–88.

38. Rights ACoD. Implicit Biases & People with Disabilities. Available at: https://www.americanbar.org/groups/diversity/disabilityrights/resources/implicit_bias/. Accessed 2022.

39. Prevention CfDCa. CDC's Developmental Milestones. Available at: https://www.cdc.gov/ncbddd/actearly/milestones/index.html. Accessed September 5, 2022.

40. Meeks LM, Neal-Boylan L. Disability as diversity: a guidebook for inclusion in medicine, nursing, and the health professions. Cham, Switzerland: Springer Nature; 2020.

41. Africa D. This is why we must stop searching for ways to say 'special needs' 2016. Available at: https://www.disability-africa.org/blog/2016/7/29/this-is-why-we-must-stop-searching-for-ways-to-say-special-needs. Accessed September 5, 2022.

42. Brown JM. Relational equality and disability injustice. J Moral Philos 2019;16(3): 327–57.

43. Mont D. Measuring health and disability. Lancet 2007;369(9573):1658–63.

44. Linton S. Claiming disability: knowledge and identity. New York: NyU Press; 1998.

45. Ladau E. Why Person-First Language Doesn't Always Put the Person First 2015. Available at: https://www.thinkinclusive.us/post/why-person-first-language-doesnt-always-put-the-person-first. Accessed September 5, 2022.

46. Bottema-Beutel K, Kapp SK, Lester JN, et al. Avoiding ableist language: Suggestions for autism researchers. Autism in Adulthood 2021;3(1):18–29.

47. Communication MMDo. Using Inclusive Language: A Handy Guide. Available at: https://mmheadlines.org/2022/11/using-inclusive-language-a-handy-guide/. Accessed December 2, 2022.

48. Journalism NCoDa. Disability Language Style Guide 2022. Available at: https://ncdj.org/style-guide/. Accessed December 2, 2022.

Moving?

Make sure your subscription moves with you!

To notify us of your new address, find your **Clinics Account Number** (located on your mailing label above your name), and contact customer service at:

Email: journalscustomerservice-usa@elsevier.com

800-654-2452 (subscribers in the U.S. & Canada)
314-447-8871 (subscribers outside of the U.S. & Canada)

Fax number: 314-447-8029

Elsevier Health Sciences Division
Subscription Customer Service
3251 Riverport Lane
Maryland Heights, MO 63043

*To ensure uninterrupted delivery of your subscription, please notify us at least 4 weeks in advance of move.

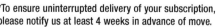

ELSEVIER

Printed and bound by CPI Group (UK) Ltd, Croydon, CR0 4YY

03/10/2024

01040468-0013